Venous Thromboembolism

Guest Editors

TERENCE K. TROW, MD
C. GREGORY ELLIOTT, MD

CLINICS IN CHEST MEDICINE

www.chestmed.theclinics.com

December 2010 • Volume 31 • Number 4

SAUNDERS an imprint of ELSEVIER, Inc.

W.B. SAUNDERS COMPANY
A Division of Elsevier Inc.

1600 John F. Kennedy Boulevard • Suite 1800 • Philadelphia, Pennsylvania 19103

http://www.theclinics.com

CLINICS IN CHEST MEDICINE Volume 31, Number 4
December 2010 ISSN 0272-5231, ISBN-13: 978-1-4377-2435-6

Editor: Sarah E. Barth
Developmental Editor: Jessica Demetriou

Clinics in Chest Medicine (ISSN 0272-5231) is published quarterly by Elsevier Inc., 360 Park Avenue South, New York, NY 10010-1710. Months of issue are March, June, September, and December. Periodicals postage paid at New York, NY and additional mailing offices. Subscription prices are $293.00 per year (domestic individuals), $475.00 per year (domestic institutions), $140.00 per year (domestic students/residents), $321.00 per year (Canadian individuals), $583.00 per year (Canadian institutions), $399.00 per year (international individuals), $583.00 per year (international institutions), and $195.00 per year (international and Canadian students/residents). International air speed delivery is included in all Clinics subscription prices. All prices are subject to change without notice. **POSTMASTER:** Send address changes to Clinics in Chest Medicine, Elsevier Health Sciences Division, Subscription Customer Service, 3251 Riverport Lane, Maryland Heights, MO 63043. **Customer Service: Telephone: 1-800-654-2452** (U.S. and Canada); **1-314-447-8871** (outside U.S. and Canada). **Fax: 1-314-447-8029. E-mail: journalscustomerservice-usa@elsevier.com** (for print support); **journalsonlinesupport-usa@elsevier.com** (for online support).

Reprints. For copies of 100 or more of articles in this publication, please contact the Commercial Reprints Department, Elsevier Inc., 360 Park Avenue South, New York, NY 10010-1710. Tel.: 212-633-3812; Fax: 212-462-1935; E-mail: reprints@elsevier.com.

Clinics in Chest Medicine is covered in *MEDLINE/PubMed (Index Medicus), Current Contents/Clinical Medicine, EMBASE/ Excerpta Medica, Science Citation Index,* and *ISI/BIOMED.*

Printed and bound by CPI Group (UK) Ltd, Croydon, CR0 4YY

Transferred to Digital Print 2011

Contributors

GUEST EDITORS

TERENCE K. TROW, MD
Director, Pulmonary Vascular Disease
Program; Assistant Professor of Medicine,
Yale University School of Medicine,
Section of Pulmonary and Critical Care,
New Haven, Connecticut

C. GREGORY ELLIOTT, MD
Chairman, Department of Medicine,
Intermountain Medical Center, Murray,
Utah; Professor of Medicine, University
of Utah School of Medicine,
Salt Lake City, Utah

AUTHORS

DANIEL ADAMS, MD
Department of Medicine, Intermountain
Medical Center, Murray, Utah

JULIA A.M. ANDERSON, MD
Consultant Hematologist, Department
of Clinical and Laboratory Hematology,
Royal Infirmary of Edinburgh, Scotland,
United Kingdom; Associate Professor (P/T),
Department of Medicine, McMaster
University, Hamilton, Ontario, Canada

WILLIAM R. AUGER, MD
Professor of Clinical Medicine, Division
of Pulmonary and Critical Care Medicine,
University of California, San Diego,
La Jolla, California

LYNETTE M. BROWN, MD, PhD
Pulmonary Division, Intermountain
Medical Center, Murray, Utah; Assistant
Professor of Medicine, University of Utah
School of Medicine, Salt Lake City, Utah

HILARY CAIN, MD
Medical Director, CCU/MICU, Acting Chief,
Pulmonary and Critical Care Section,
Veterans Affairs Connecticut Healthcare
System, Section of Pulmonary and Critical
Care Medicine, West Haven, Connecticut

**JAMES D. DOUKETIS, MD, FRCP(C),
FACP, FCCP**
Associate Professor of Medicine, Department
of Medicine, McMaster University, Hamilton,
Ontario, Canada

C. GREGORY ELLIOTT, MD
Chairman, Department of Medicine,
Intermountain Medical Center, Murray,
Utah; Professor of Medicine, University
of Utah School of Medicine,
Salt Lake City, Utah

ESTEBAN GANDARA, MD
Thrombosis Program, Department
of Medicine, Division of Hematology,
The Ottawa Hospital and The University
of Ottawa; Clinical Epidemiology Program,
Ottawa Health Research Institute, Ottawa,
Ontario, Canada

RUSSELL D. HULL, MBBS, MSc, FRCPC
Professor of Medicine, Department of
Medicine; Director, Thrombosis Research Unit,
University of Calgary, Calgary, Alberta,
Canada

CLIVE KEARON, MB, MRCPI, FRCPC, PhD
Professor of Medicine, McMaster University,
Hamilton, Ontario, Canada

NICK H. KIM, MD
Associate Clinical Professor of Medicine,
Division of Pulmonary and Critical Care
Medicine, University of California,
San Diego, La Jolla, California

STAVROS KONSTANTINIDES, MD
Department of Cardiology, Democritus
University of Thrace, University General
Hospital, Alexandroupolis, Greece

MAREIKE LANKEIT, MD
Department of Cardiology and Pulmonology,
Georg August University of Göttingen,
Germany

TODD D. LOVELACE, MD
Chairman, Department of Radiology,
Intermountain Medical Center, Murray, Utah

PAUL E. MARIK, MD, FCCM, FCCP
Chief, Division of Pulmonary and Critical Care
Medicine, EVMS Internal Medicine, Eastern
Virginia Medical School, Norfolk, Virginia

PETER S. MARSHALL, MD, MPH
Assistant Professor, Pulmonary and Critical
Care Section, Department of Internal Medicine,
Yale School of Medicine, New Haven,
Connecticut

FADI MATTA, MD
Visiting Research Scientist, Department of
Internal Medicine and Research and Advanced
Studies Program, College of Osteopathic
Medicine, Michigan State University,
MSU/COM Venous Thromboembolism
Research Unit, Pontiac, Michigan

TIMOTHY A. MORRIS, MD, FACCP
Professor of Medicine, Clinical Service Chief,
Division of Pulmonary and Critical Care
Medicine, University of California, San Diego
School of Medicine, San Diego, California

ROBERT C. PENDLETON, MD
Associate Professor, Department of Medicine;
Director, University Healthcare Thrombosis
Service, University of Utah,
Salt Lake City, Utah

GEORGE M. RODGERS, MD, PhD
Professor of Medicine and Director,
Hemostasis and Thrombosis Laboratory,
ARUP Laboratories; Department of Medicine,
University of Utah, Salt Lake City, Utah

PAUL D. STEIN, MD
Visiting Professor, Department of Internal
Medicine and Research and Advanced
Studies Program, College of Osteopathic
Medicine, Michigan State University,
MSU/COM Venous Thromboembolism
Research Unit, Pontiac, Michigan

SCOTT M. STEVENS, MD, FACP
Department of Medicine, Intermountain
Medical Center, Murray; Associate Clinical
Professor of Medicine, University of Utah,
Salt Lake City, Utah

VICTOR F. TAPSON, MD, FCCP, FRCP
Professor of Medicine and Director,
Center for Pulmonary Vascular Disease,
Division of Pulmonary and Critical Care
Medicine, Duke University Medical Center,
Durham, North Carolina

TERENCE K. TROW, MD
Director, Pulmonary Vascular Disease
Program; Assistant Professor of Medicine,
Yale University School of Medicine,
Section of Pulmonary and Critical Care,
New Haven, Connecticut

JEFFREY I. WEITZ, MD
Professor, Departments of Medicine and
Biochemistry and Biomedical Sciences,
McMaster University, HSFO/J.F. Mustard
Chair in Cardiovascular Research Canada,
Research Chair (Tier 1) in Thrombosis,
Thrombosis and Atherosclerosis Research
Institute, Hamilton, Ontario, Canada

PHILIP S. WELLS, MD, MSc
Professor, Chair and Chief, Department
of Medicine, The Ottawa Hospital and
The University of Ottawa; Canada Research
Chair in Thromboembolic Diseases, Ottawa
Health Research Institute, Ottawa,
Ontario, Canada

Contents

The proportion of hospitalized patients with pulmonary embolism (PE) is increasing. Whether this represents more admissions with PE or more diagnoses made in hospitalized patients is uncertain. The proportion of hospitalized patients with deep venous thrombosis has decreased precipitously as a result of home treatment. Asians and Native Americans have a lower incidence of PE than whites or African Americans. The incidence of PE increases exponentially with age, but no age group, including infants and children, is immune. Several medical illnesses have now been shown to be associated with a higher risk for venous thromboembolism. Epidemiologic data and new information on risk factors provide insight into making an informed clinical assessment and evaluation for antithrombotic prophylaxis.

Evidence suggests that patients with suspected pulmonary embolism are managed better with a diagnostic strategy that includes clinical pretest probability assessment, D-dimer test, and/or imaging. Several clinical prediction rules have been described in the literature during the last decade. This review focuses on the role of clinical prediction rules in the diagnostic process and their clinical application into diagnostic algorithms.

The diagnosis of venous thromboembolism (VTE) cannot be confirmed or excluded by the medical history and physical examination alone. Objective testing is required in all cases of clinically suspected VTE; for most patients, this includes imaging modalities such as compression ultrasonography, ventilation-perfusion lung scintigraphy, or computed tomography pulmonary angiography (CTPA). Conventional pulmonary arteriography remains useful when CTPA is nondiagnostic or when an intervention such as catheter embolectomy is planned. Although CTPA is important in the evaluation of suspected VTE, ultimately the clinician must balance the risks against the benefits of CTPA for individual patients. Bedside echocardiography may be most appropriate for patients with hypotension or shock and suspected pulmonary embolism.

Hypercoagulable states can be inherited or acquired. Inherited hypercoagulable states can be caused by a loss of function of natural anticoagulant pathways or a gain of function in procoagulant pathways. Acquired hypercoagulable risk factors include a prior history of thrombosis, obesity, pregnancy, cancer and its treatment, antiphospholipid antibody syndrome, heparin-induced thrombocytopenia, and myeloproliferative disorders. Inherited hypercoagulable states combine with acquired risk factors to establish the intrinsic risk of venous thromboembolism for each individual. Venous thromboembolism occurs when the risk exceeds a critical threshold. Often a triggering factor, such as surgery, pregnancy, or estrogen therapy, is required to increase the risk above this critical threshold.

Venous thromboembolism (VTE), which encompasses deep vein thrombosis and pulmonary embolism, is a leading cause of preventable morbidity and mortality following hospitalization. In the last decade, investigators have used randomized controlled trials to assess the efficacy and safety of various methods of VTE prevention for more than 20,000 medical patients. Identifying medical patients at risk for VTE and providing effective prophylaxis is now an important health care priority to reduce the burden of this morbid and sometimes fatal disease. Pharmacologic prophylaxis is the mainstay of VTE prevention. It is effective, safe, and cost effective. Multiple scientific guidelines support VTE prophylaxis in medical patients. Regulatory and accreditation agencies have mandated that hospitals use formalized systems to assess VTE risk and provide clinically appropriate prophylaxis measures to patients at risk.

For a majority of patients with venous thromboembolism (VTE), initial treatment is straightforward and necessitates the immediate initiation of a parenteral anticoagulant (eg, heparin or low molecular weight heparin), simultaneous initiation of long-term therapy (eg, vitamin K antagonist), and discontinuation of the parenteral anticoagulant after 5 days assuming that the vitamin K antagonist is therapeutic. This standardized approach is based on numerous pivotal clinical trials completed over the past 3 decades. Yet, advances in standardized VTE treatment continue to evolve and include issues related to the selection and dosing of parenteral anticoagulants (eg, relative efficacy and dosing in the obese patient, patients with renal impairment, and pregnant patients), optimal location of initial care delivery, use of dosing initiation nomograms for vitamin K antagonists with the potential of gene-based dosing, and demonstration that longterm low molecular weight heparin therapy may be optimal for some patient populations (eg, those with active cancer). Further, in parallel with the evolution of VTE treatment, there have been remarkable advances in our understanding of heparin-induced thrombocytopenia, a prothrombotic complication of parenteral anticoagulant use.

Heparin and low molecular weight heparins have limitations in their efficacy and safety for the prevention and treatment of venous thromboembolism (VTE). New synthetic antithrombotic drugs, designed with the intention of improving the therapeutic window for prophylaxis and treatment, are in various stages of development. Synthetic pentasaccharides include fondaparinux and its long-acting analogue idraparinux. Dabigatran is a direct thrombin inhibitor that has undergone clinical trials for VTE prophylaxis and treatment. Direct factor Xa inhibitors include rivaroxiban, which has shown promising results for VTE prophylaxis and is being studied for VTE treatment, as well as apixaban and betrixaban, which are at earlier stages of clinical validation. These newer agents may represent viable options for prophylaxis and therapy as further clinical studies are performed.

Treatment of venous thromboembolism (VTE) should be continued until the reduction of recurrent VTE that anticoagulation is expected to achieve no longer outweighs the increase in bleeding associated with therapy, or until the patient wants to stop treatment even if treatment is expected to be of benefit. Reversibility of risk factors for VTE is the most important factor that influences risk of recurrence and duration of therapy. VTE associated with a reversible risk factor (eg, surgery) is treated for 3 months; unprovoked VTE often benefits from indefinite therapy provided patients do not have risk factors for bleeding; and cancer-associated VTE is usually treated indefinitely. A systematic approach to managing warfarin therapy improves its efficacy, safety, and acceptability.

In Western nations, venous thromboembolism (VTE) is an important cause of morbidity and the most common cause of maternal death during pregnancy and the puerperium. Pregnancy is a hypercoagulable state in which coagulation is activated and thrombolysis inhibited. This prothrombotic risk is compounded when hereditary and acquired thrombophilias and other prothrombotic risk factors are present. The risk of venous thrombotic events is increased fivefold during pregnancy and 60-fold in the first 3 months after delivery (postpartum period) compared with nonpregnant women. Many of the signs and symptoms of VTE overlap those of a normal pregnancy, which complicates the diagnosis. Patients with history of previous VTE should use graduated compression stockings throughout pregnancy and the puerperium, and should receive postpartum anticoagulant prophylaxis. The indications for antepartum anticoagulant prophylaxis are somewhat controversial. This article reviews the management of VTE during pregnancy and in the postpartum period.

Chronic thromboembolic pulmonary hypertension is one of the few forms of pulmonary hypertension that is surgically curable. It is likely underdiagnosed and must be considered in every patient presenting with pulmonary hypertension to avoid missing the opportunity to cure these patients. This article discusses the epidemiology, risk factors, natural history, diagnosis, and preoperative evaluation of patients with this disorder. Also covered are putative mechanisms for the conversion of acute emboli into fibrosed thrombembolic residua. Mechanical obstruction of the central pulmonary vasculature is rarely the sole cause of the pulmonary hypertension, and a discussion of the small vessel arteriopathy present in these patients is offered. Technical aspects of pulmonary endartectomy and the data supporting its role are discussed, as are the limited data on pulmonary arterial hypertension specific medical therapies for patients deemed noncandidates for the operation.

Acute venous thromboembolism remains a frequent disease, with an incidence ranging between 23 and 69 cases per 100,000 population per year. Of these patients, approximately one-third present with clinical symptoms of acute pulmonary embolism (PE) and two-thirds with deep venous thrombosis (DVT). Recent registries and cohort studies suggest that approximately 10% of all patients with acute PE die during the first 1 to 3 months after diagnosis. Overall, 1% of all patients admitted to hospitals die of acute PE, and 10% of all hospital deaths are PE-related. These facts emphasize the need to better implement our knowledge on the pathophysiology of the disease, recognize the determinants of death or major adverse events in the early phase of acute PE, and most importantly, identify those patients who necessitate prompt medical, surgical, or interventional treatment to restore the patency of the pulmonary vasculature.

Therapeutic strategies other than anticoagulation sometimes require consideration in the setting of acute venous thromboembolism. Vena caval filter placement is increasingly common, in part because of the availability of nonpermanent filter devices. Filter placement, surgical embolectomy, and catheter embolectomy have not been subjected to the same prospective, randomized clinical trial scrutiny as anticoagulation but seem appropriate in certain clinical settings. The indications, contraindications, and available data supporting these therapeutic methods are discussed.

Upper extremity deep vein thrombosis (UEDVT) is associated with significant morbidity and mortality. The susceptible populations and risk factors for UEDVT are well-known. The presenting symptoms can be subtle, and therefore objective testing is necessary for diagnosis. The optimal diagnostic strategy has not been determined, and more than one test may be required to exclude the diagnosis. Proper treatment reduces the occurrence of complications, and treatment should include long-term anticoagulation if the patient has no contraindications. This article discusses the risk factors, pathogenesis, diagnosis, complications, and management of UEDVT.

Clinics in Chest Medicine

ISSUES OF RELATED INTEREST

Cardiology Clinics Volume 26, Issue 2 (May 2008)
Thromboembolic Disease and Antithrombotic Agents in the Elderly
Edited by L.G. Jacobs

THE CLINICS ARE NOW AVAILABLE ONLINE!

Access your subscription at:
www.theclinics.com

Preface
Venous Thromboembolism

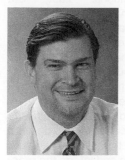 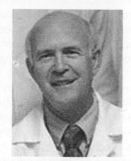

Terence K. Trow, MD   C. Gregory Elliott, MD
Guest Editors

Venous thromboembolism contributes to the death of 100,000 to 200,000 patients a year, and pulmonary embolism remains the third most common acute cardiovascular disease state behind myocardial infarction and stroke. Even for those surviving their acute thromboembolic event, morbidity remains significant with postphlebitic syndromes in approximately 30% of deep vein thrombosis survivors and with the development of chronic thromboembolic pulmonary hypertension in anywhere from 1%–4% of those surviving their acute pulmonary embolism. Clearly the need to properly diagnose and treat this entity, and just as importantly to prevent it altogether, in those at risk remains an important priority for our health care system. In fact it has recently been given the highest priority among 79 interventions detailed in a report by the Agency for Health Research and Quality.

In this issue of *Clinics in Chest Medicine*, experts from throughout the United States, Canada, and Europe with longstanding interest in this disease and its consequences offer the latest evidence-based approach to diagnosis and management. Dr Paul Stein and Dr Fadi Matta discuss the epidemiology and incidence of venous thromboembolism, with special attention to risk factors for its development. They estimate that 90% of pulmonary embolism cases have 1 or more such risk factors. The shift toward outpatient treatment of deep vein thrombosis with low molecular weight heparins is discussed, as is the exponential increase in the rates of pulmonary embolism and case fatality rates from such emboli with age. Next, Dr Phillip Wells and Dr Esteban Gandara review the use of diagnostic algorithms, including the Wells model, Geneva model, pulmonary embolism rule-out criteria, and the PISA-PED model, in the approach to the diagnosis of pulmonary embolism and deep vein thrombosis. Their discussion of these clinically validated models make a strong argument for safe and effective evaluation using clinical pretest probability assessment and the correct diagnostic techniques. Following up on this, Dr Greg Elliott, Dr Todd Lovelace, Dr Daniel Adams, and Dr Lynette Brown review what is known from the literature on diagnostic imaging techniques and limitations of the same including discussion of the role of chest roentgenography, ventilation-perfusion scanning, computerized tomography pulmonary angiography, and appraisal of the latest PIOPED III data on magnetic resonance imaging in this disease.

Although the mysteries of aberrant coagulation in patients with a tendency toward venous thromboembolism are far from fully understood, Dr Jeffrey Weitz and Dr Julia Anderson discuss what is known about heritable hypercoaguable states in their excellent article. Their cogent discussion underscores the interaction between genetic hypercoaguable states, acquired hypercoaguable states, and modification of risk by extrinsic or environmental factors. Their article identifies those patients who deserve laboratory evaluation for an underlying hypercoaguable state and outlines the treatment of patients with such states.

Sadly, recent studies suggest that opportunities to prevent this disease are being missed with alarming frequency. It is estimated that only 30%–40% of medical patients at increased risk of deep vein thrombosis actually receive the

Clin Chest Med 31 (2010) xi–xii
doi:10.1016/j.ccm.2010.07.007

chestmed.theclinics.com

recommended prophylaxis. It is also estimated that appropriate prophylaxis would prevent an additional 110,000 venous thromboembolic events annually. Dr Scott Stevens and Dr James Douketis discuss the very important issue of prophylaxis for those at risk of venous thrombosis, critically reviewing the data on risk factors and the recommended prophylaxis strategies. Next, Dr Robert Pendleton, Dr George Rogers, and Dr Russell Hull review the evidence for traditional therapies to treat venous thrombosis once established including heparin, low-molecular weight heparins, and vitamin K antagonists. They also offer a nice discussion on the important issue of heparin-induced thrombocytopenia and how to manage this increasingly recognized complication of heparin therapy. Dr Timothy Morris then reviews what is known about the newer therapeutic agents emerging in clinical trials including pentasaccharides, direct thrombin inhibitors, and direct Factor Xa inhibitors. Rounding out the topic of therapy for venous thrombosis, Dr Clive Kearon offers his thoughts on and experience with the all-important issue of how long to treat venous thrombosis once it has occurred.

The complication of venous thrombosis during or shortly after pregnancy is a frequently encountered clinical scenario, and Dr Paul Marik addresses some of the special issues surrounding diagnosis and management of these patients in his article in this issue of *Clinics of Chest Medicine*. This is followed by a review of the management of chronic thromboembolic pulmonary hypertension by Dr William Auger, Dr Terence Trow, and Dr Nick Kim with discussion of potential reasons for its development as well as surgical and medical therapies for this dreaded complication of acute pulmonary embolism. Although complex to evaluate, this remains one of the only curable forms of pulmonary hypertension and as such the authors appropriately emphasize the importance of not missing the opportunity for pulmonary thromboendarterectomy in suitable candidates.

Next, Dr Stavros Konstanides and Dr Mareike Lankeit discuss the controversial topic of thrombolysis for pulmonary embolism and the all important issue of risk assessment for this intervention for those at greatest risk of death. This is followed by a discussion of interventional techniques in the management of acute pulmonary

embolism by Dr Victor Tapson. His discussion includes a review of the literature on venal caval interruption, surgical embolectomy, and catheter-directed interventions. Last, but certainly not least, Dr Hilary Cain and Dr Peter Marshall discuss the special subset of patients who present with upper extremity deep vein thrombosis and nicely emphasize the importance of treatment beyond the outdated approach of warm soaks and arm elevation.

Although venous thromboembolism is common, the diagnosis is often missed and opportunities to prevent it frequently go unrecognized. We do hope the discussions offered in this *Clinics in Chest Medicine* will help to educate and inform the practice of clinicians throughout the world with an eye toward improving prevention for those at risk, and the care for those who do develop a venous thrombotic event. It is our hope that through heighted awareness and improved application of evidence-based prophylaxis the next issue of *Clinics in Chest Medicine* devoted to this topic will report marked improvement in our track record for preventing and treating this potentially fatal disease.

Terence K. Trow, MD
Pulmonary Vascular Disease Program
Department of Medicine
Yale University School of Medicine
Section of Pulmonary and Critical Care
LLCI 105D
333 Cedar Street, PO Box 208057
New Haven, CT 06520-8057, USA

C. Gregory Elliott, MD
Department of Medicine
Intermountain Medical Center
5121 South Cottonwood Street
Suite 307, Murray, UT 84107, USA

Department of Medicine
University of Utah School of Medicine
30 North 1900 East, Room 4C104
Salt Lake City, UT 84132-2406, USA

E-mail addresses:
terence.trow@yale.edu (T.K. Trow)
Greg.Elliott@imail.org (C.G. Elliott)

Epidemiology and Incidence: The Scope of the Problem and Risk Factors for Development of Venous Thromboembolism

Paul D. Stein, MD*, Fadi Matta, MD

KEYWORDS

- Epidemiology • Incidence • Venous thromboembolism
- Pulmonary embolism

PREVALENCE OF PULMONARY EMBOLISM

Pulmonary embolism (PE) is the third most common acute cardiovascular disease after myocardial infarction and stroke.[1] In 2006, 828,000 patients were hospitalized in short-stay non-Federal hospitals in the United States with acute myocardial infarction[2] and 564,000 with stroke (F. Matta and P.D. Stein, unpublished data from the National Hospital Discharge Survey, 2010). In 2006, 247,000 adults were hospitalized with acute PE.[2] The number and proportion of hospitalized patients with PE is increasing (**Figs. 1** and **2**).[3] As many as 25% may die before admission.[4] Patients with acute PE in 2006 represented 0.77% of hospitalized patients 18 years of age or older, and 110 patients/100,000 adult population.[2] In 2006, 467,000 patients were hospitalized with deep venous thrombosis (DVT).[2] This represented 1.5% of hospitalized adults and 208/100,000 adult population.[2]

The reported incidence of postthrombotic syndrome after symptomatic DVT varies and depends on the severity of the postthrombotic syndrome. Some reported that by the end of 1 month, among 347 patients with DVT, 34% developed mild postthrombotic syndrome, 10% moderate, and 4% severe.[5] Among patients with DVT who did not wear compression stockings, 20% to 82% developed postthrombotic syndrome of any severity.[6–10] There is no universal agreement on a definition of postthrombotic syndrome.[7] However, all definitions include chronic complaints of the legs following DVT.[11] Symptoms may include pain, heaviness, pruritus, and paresthesia, and signs may include pretibial edema, erythema, induration, hyperpigmentation, new venous ectasia, pain during calf compression, and ulceration.[11]

Support: none.

Conflicts of interest: neither of the authors has any financial or other potential conflicts of interest relative to the data in this manuscript.

Department of Internal Medicine and Research and Advanced Studies Program, College of Osteopathic Medicine, Michigan State University, MSU/COM Venous Thromboembolism Research Unit, 44405 Woodward Avenue, Pontiac, MI 48341-5023, USA

* Corresponding author. MSU/COM Venous Thromboembolism Research Unit, 44405 Woodward Avenue, Pontiac, MI 48341-5023.

E-mail address: steinp@trinity-health.org

Clin Chest Med 31 (2010) 611–628
doi:10.1016/j.ccm.2010.07.001
0272-5231/10/$ — see front matter © 2010 Elsevier Inc. All rights reserved.

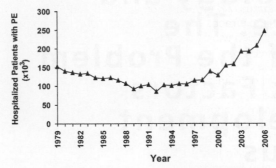

Fig. 1. Number of adults (aged ≥18 years) with PE hospitalized in short-stay hospitals in the United States from 1979 to 2006. Based on data from the National Hospital Discharge Survey.

GENDER

The risk of PE and DVT imparted by gender remains uncertain. PE has been reported to occur more frequently in women than in men because of estrogen use, childbearing, and a higher frequency of DVT.[12–16] The largest investigation was based on data from the National Hospital Discharge Survey, which reported on 139,000 patients who were discharged from short-stay hospitals in the United States in 1999 with a diagnosis of PE. The rate of diagnosis of PE in 1999, not adjusted for age, was higher in women (60 PE/100,000 women/y) than men (42 PE/100,000 men/y).[17] The age-adjusted rate of diagnosis of PE/ 100,000 population in men and women was similar.[17] The Worcester DVT Study showed higher rates of PE in men than women.[18] The French Multicenter Registry showed no differences between the sexes.[19] The Olmsted County study and the Minneapolis St Paul Metropolitan Area Study showed higher age-adjusted rates of PE among men.[20,21] The Tecumseh Community Health Study showed 4.5 PE/10,000 women/y compared with 1.75 PE/10,000 men/y.[15] In smaller investigations, results varied. Some showed

a higher prevalence among women[22] and others among men[1,23] and older men.[24] Postmortem study of PE showed PE in 11% of women and 7% of men.[25] On the other hand, the prevalence of PE among 61 patients at autopsy in the Framingham Study was also higher in men.[26] Data from the Prospective Investigation of Pulmonary Embolism Diagnosis (PIOPED) showed a higher prevalence of PE in men.[27]

Contrary to PE, both the unadjusted rate of diagnosis of DVT/100,000 population/y and the age-adjusted rate of diagnosis of DVT/100,000 population/y were higher in women.[17] In 1999, among 369,000 patients discharged from non-Federal short-stay hospitals with a diagnosis of DVT, the unadjusted rate of diagnosis was 115 DVT/100,000 men/y and 154 DVT/100,000 women/y.[17] Most previous literature[19,24,28] also showed higher rates of diagnosis of DVT in women, but objectively diagnosed rates of DVT also have been reported to be higher in men.[18]

RACE

The rate of diagnosis of PE/100,000 population, not adjusted for age, was comparable among blacks and whites.[29] In 1999, the rate of diagnosis among blacks was 41 PE/100,000 population/y and among whites it was 42 PE/100,000 population. In 1999, the age-adjusted rate of diagnosis of PE among blacks was 56/100,000/y and among whites it was 40/100,000/y.[29]

As with PE, the rate of diagnosis of DVT/100,000 population/y, not adjusted for age, was comparable among blacks and whites.[29] In 1999, the rate of diagnosis among blacks was 110 DVT/ 100,000 population and among whites it was 115 DVT/100,000 population. In 1999, the age-adjusted rate of diagnosis of DVT among blacks was146/100,000/y and among whites it was 111/100,000/y.[29] Caution has been recommended in the use of race as a variable when comparing blacks and whites. We must distinguish between

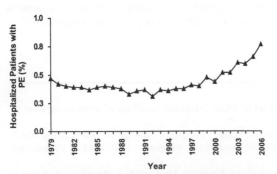

Fig. 2. Proportion of hospitalized adults (aged ≥18 years) with PE hospitalized in short-stay hospitals in the United States from 1979 to 2006. Based on data from the National Hospital Discharge Survey.

race and socioeconomic status. An emphasis on ethnic groups, rather than on race, implies an appreciation of cultural and behavioral attitudes, beliefs, lifestyle patterns, diet environmental living conditions, and other factors.[30]

The prevalence of PE in hospitalized patients was also lower among Asians/Pacific Islanders (0.1/100 hospitalizations) than among whites (0.4/100 hospitalizations) and African Americans (0.4/100 hospitalizations).[31] The prevalence of DVT among hospitalized Asians/Pacific Islanders (0.4/100 hospitalizations) was also lower than among African Americans (1.1/100 hospitalizations) and whites (1.1/100 hospitalizations).[31]

A lower prevalence of heritable predispositions to venous thromboembolism (VTE), such as factor V Leiden, has been speculated to contribute to the lower incidence of VTE in Asians.[32] Factor V Leiden is the most common genetic mutation predisposing to VTE.[33,34] It has been found in 4% to 5% of whites in North America and Europe,[35,36] 0.9% to 1.2% of African Americans, and in only 0% to 0.5% of Asians.[35–37] Blood levels of factor VIIc and factor VIIIc were also lower in rural and urban Japanese patients than in whites and Japanese Americans.[38] Some differences of coagulation factors between Asians and whites are attributable to environmental factors, especially diet and smoking, as well as genetic differences.[34,38] Asians may have a more efficient inactivation of coagulation by activated protein C or more fibrinolytic activity than non-Asians.[32] Asians also seem to be more sensitive to warfarin than whites.[39] The target range of the International Normalized Ratio for patients with nonvalvular atrial fibrillation is 1.5 to 2.1 in Japanese patients,[40] and for mechanical prosthetic heart valves it is 1.5 to 2.5 in Japanese patients.[41]

The incidence of PE and of DVT was also lower in American Indians and Alaskan Natives than in African Americans and whites.[42] Archaeological studies suggest that Native Americans may be descended from Asians who crossed the Bering Straits thousands of years ago. A lower prevalence of Factor V Leiden in American Indians/Alaskan Natives populations (1.25%) compared with whites (5.3%) has been observed.[35] From 1996 to 2001 the rate of diagnosis of VTE in American Indians/Alaskan Natives, based on combined data from the National Hospital Discharge Survey and the Indian Health Service, was 71/100,000/y, compared with 155/100,000/y in African Americans and 131/100,000 in whites.[42] The incidence of PE in American Indians/Alaskan Natives was too low to give an accurate estimate of the rate of diagnosis. Only 1 patient with PE was hospitalized in Indian Health Service hospitals between 1996 and 2001. During this interval, an estimated 420,000 patients were hospitalized.[42] The rate of diagnosis of VTE among patients discharged from Indian Health Service hospital care from 1980 to 1996 was reported as 33/100,000/y in American Indians/Alaskan Natives.[43]

AGE

The incidence of PE and DVT increases sharply with age, probably exponentially[18,21,44] (**Fig. 3**). The diagnosis of PE in patients 70 years or older was 6.2 times the rate in younger patients. DVT was diagnosed 12.7 times more frequently in patients aged 70 to 79 years than in younger patients aged 20 to 29 years.[44]

The data relating the incidence of PE to age fit a smooth exponential curve.[18,21,44] There is no cutoff age at which there is no risk of VTE. Even children may suffer a PE or DVT.[45] From 1979 to 2001, PE was diagnosed at discharge from short-stay non-Federal hospitals throughout the United States in 13,000 infants and children 17 years of age or younger and DVT was diagnosed in DVT in 64,000.[45] Rates of diagnosis were 0.9 PE/100,000 children/y, 4.2 DVT/100,000 children/y, and 4.9 VTE/100,000 children/y.[45]

A double peaked curve was shown, with the highest rates of diagnosis in infants less than 1 year old and a second peak in teenagers.[45,46] The rates in infants were comparable with the rates in teenagers. Teenage girls had twice the rates of DVT and VTE as teenage boys, although in younger children the frequencies were comparable in boys and girls.

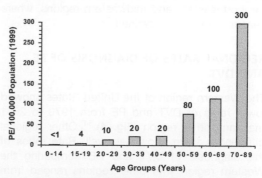

Fig. 3. PE/100,000 population, diagnosed at hospital discharge, shown according to age for the year 1999. (*Data from* Stein PD, Hull RD, Kayali F, et al. Venous thromboembolism according to age: the impact of an aging population. Arch Intern Med 2004;164:2260–5; Stein PD, Kayali F, Olson RE. Incidence of pulmonary thromboembolism in infants and children. J Pediatrics 2004;145:563–5.) (*Reproduced from* Stein PD. Pulmonary embolism. 2nd edition. Oxford (UK): Blackwell Future; 2007; with permission.)

Abortion and/or contraceptives were shown to be risk factors in 75% of female adolescents who had PE.[47] Teenage users of oral contraceptives did not seem to be at an increased risk of VTE compared with older users.[48] Teenage girls with DVT had an associated pregnancy in 27% of cases.[45] The rate of DVT in nonpregnant teenage girls was 10 DVT/100,000 teenage girls/y, and the rate of pregnancy-associated DVT was 109 DVT/100,000 teenage girls/y.[45] The rate of DVT in nonpregnant teenage girls did not differ significantly from the rate for teenage boys.

Indwelling catheter use was the most common predisposing factor for PE or DVT in children and adolescents, followed by surgery and trauma.[49] Neonatal thrombosis, with the exception of spontaneous renal vein thrombosis, was associated with indwelling catheters in 89%.[50] Lower-extremity DVT in children, when unrelated to venous catheterization or surgery, seemed to be related to local infection of the involved extremity, trauma, or immobilization.[51] One or more coagulopathies were reported in 65% of children with venous thrombosis who had an evaluation for a deficiency of protein C, protein S, or antithrombin III and assessment for a lupus anticoagulant.[52]

SEASON

An analysis of data from the National Hospital Discharge Survey based on 2,457,000 patients with PE and 5,767,000 patients with DVT obtained over 21 years showed no seasonal difference.[53] An absence of seasonal variation was shown in all regions of the United States, including the southern region, where winters are mild, and the northeastern and midwestern regions, where seasons are sharply defined.[53]

REGIONAL RATES OF DIAGNOSIS OF PE AND DVT

The Western region of the United States showed lower rates of DVT and PE from 1979 to 2001 than any other region (**Fig. 4**).[54] Other regional differences were shown as well. Rate ratios of the diagnosis of DVT and PE comparing the Western region with other regions ranged from 0.65 to 0.87.[54]

The mortality from PE was 40% to 45% lower in the Western region of the United States than any other region.[54] A younger population in the Western region does not explain the difference because lower rates were also observed in patients 65 years or older. A higher percentage of Asian Americans and/or Pacific Islanders living in the Western region might be considered to

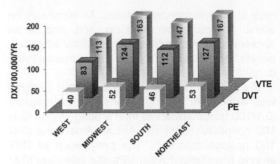

Fig. 4. Rates of diagnosis (Dx)/100,000 population/y of PE, DVT, and VTE according to region from 1979 to 2001. (*Reprinted from* Stein PD, Kayali F, Olson RE. Regional differences in rates of diagnosis and mortality of pulmonary thromboembolism. Am J Cardiol 2004;93:1194–7; with permission.)

explain the difference because incidences of PE and of DVT are lower in Asian Americans than in African Americans or whites.[31,55,56] However, lower rates of PE and DVT were also shown in whites in the Western region. The observed difference in regional rates of diagnosis of DVT and VTE is not likely to be related to differences in climate. No seasonal variation was observed in the rate of diagnosis of DVT, PE, or VTE in any of the regions, including the Southern region, where winters are mild, and the Northeastern and Midwestern regions, where seasons are sharply defined.[53]

POPULATION MORTALITY RATES FROM PE

The number of patients who died of PE in 1998 based on death certificates was 24,947.[57] This amounts to 9 PE deaths/100,000 population in 1 year. Assuming that death certificates are only 26.7% accurate for the diagnosis of fatal PE,[58] the estimated number of deaths from PE in 1998 may have been 93,000 and the death rate may have been 34 PE deaths/100,000 population.

In the last 2 decades the population mortality from PE (deaths from PE/100,000 population/y) decreased.[57,59] This finding could be a consequence of a declining incidence of PE (diagnoses of PE/100,000 population/y) or a declining case fatality rate from PE (deaths from PE/100 cases of PE) or the combination. From 1979 to 1989, there was no decline in the case fatality rate, which suggests that the declining population mortality from PE was largely due to a declining incidence of PE (**Fig. 5**). From 1979 to 1999 the incidence of diagnosis has decreased.[17]

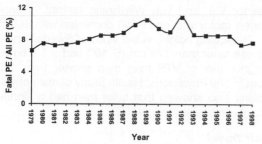

Fig. 5. Estimated case fatality rate for PE from 1979 to 1998. (*Reprinted from* Stein PD, Kayali F, Olson RE. Estimated case fatality rate of pulmonary embolism, 1979–1998. Am J Cardiol 2004;93:1197–9; with permission.)

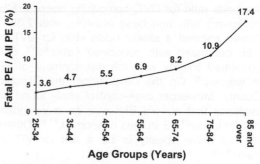

Fig. 6. Estimated case fatality rates for PE according to decades of age. The estimated case fatality rates are the average of yearly values over a 20-year period. (*Reprinted from* Stein PD, Kayali F, Olson RE. Estimated case fatality rate of pulmonary embolism, 1979–1998. Am J Cardiol 2004;93:1197–9; with permission.)

CASE FATALITY RATE

In untreated patients with clinically apparent DVT, the incidence of fatal PE was 37%.[60] In patients with clinically apparent PE, 37% died of the initial PE and an additional 36% died of a recurrent PE, total mortality being 73%.[61] The applicability of these results to the present era of early diagnosis of mild disease is questionable. The mortality from PE of patients with untreated silent DVT, found by radioactive fibrinogen scintiscans, was 5%.[62] Among patients with mild PE who inadvertently were untreated because the diagnosis was not made from the ventilation-perfusion (V/Q) lung scan, 1 of 20 (5%) died of the initial or recurrent PE.[63]

The estimated case fatality rate (deaths/100 cases of PE) between 1979 and 1998 ranged from 6.7% to 10.5% (see **Fig. 5**).[64] This rate is higher than has been reported in diagnostic trials and in pharmaceutical investigations. The case fatality rate in the PIOPED was 2.5%.[65] In PIOPED, which was an investigation of the accuracy of V/Q lung scans, patients were excluded if they were too ill to participate. In addition, most deaths from PE occur within the first 2.5 hours after the diagnosis is made,[66] thereby excluding another group of patients from such studies. For similar reasons, case fatality rates in trials of treatment with low-molecular-weight heparin (LMWH) were only 0.6% to 1.0%.[67,68] The case fatality rate from PE increased exponentially with age from 3.6% in patients aged 25 to 34 years to 17.4% in patients older than 85 years (**Fig. 6**).[64]

RISK FACTORS

Among all patients with PE in the PIOPED II trial 94% had 1 or more of the following assessed risk factors: bed rest within the last month of 3 days or more, travel within the last month of 4 hours or more, surgery within 3 months, malignancy, past history of DVT or PE, trauma of lower extremities or pelvis, central venous instrumentation within 3 months, stroke, paresis or paralysis, heart failure or chronic obstructive pulmonary disease (COPD).[69] Immobilization of only 1 or 2 days may predispose to PE, and 65% of those who were immobilized were immobilized for 2 weeks or less.[70]

Obesity and Height

Investigations that reported an increased risk for VTE caused by obesity have been criticized because they failed to control for hospital confinement or other risk factors.[71] High proportions of patients with VTE have been found to be obese,[18,72] but the importance of the association is diminished because of the high proportion of obesity in the general population.[73] Some investigations showed an increased risk ratio for DVT or PE in obese women,[26,74–76] but data in men were less compelling. The Nurses' Health Study showed that the age-adjusted risk ratio for PE women with a body mass index (BMI, calculated as weight in kilograms divided by the square of height in meters) 29.0 kg/m^2 or higher was 3.2 compared with the leanest category of less than 21.0 kg/m^2.[74] The Framingham Heart Study showed that metropolitan relative weight was significantly and independently associated with PE among women, but not men.[77] However, the Study of Men Born in 1913 showed that men in the highest decile of waist circumference (≥100 cm) had an adjusted relative risk for VTE of 3.92 compared with men with a waist circumference less than 100 cm.[78] Among 1272 outpatients (men and women), the odds ratio for DVT, comparing obese (BMI>30 kg/m^2) with nonobese patients, was 2.39.[79] Others showed a similar odds ratio for DVT of 2.26 compared with nonobese patients.[75] BMI correlated linearly with the development of PE in women.[80] On the other hand, the Olmsted County, Minnesota case-control study found no evidence that current BMI was an independent risk factor for VTE in men or women.[71,81] Others did not show obesity to be a risk for VTE in men.[26,76]

Analysis of the huge database of the National Hospital Discharge Survey[82] showed compelling evidence that obesity is a risk factor for VTE.[83] Among patients hospitalized in short-term hospitals throughout the United States, in whom obesity was coded among the discharge diagnoses but not defined, 91,000 of 12,015,000 (0.8%) had PE.[83] Among hospitalized patients who were not diagnosed with obesity, PE was diagnosed in 2,366,000 of 691,000,000 (0.3%). DVT was diagnosed in 243,000 of 12,015,000 (2.0%) of patients diagnosed with obesity, and in 5,524,000 of 691,000,000 (0.8%) who were not diagnosed with obesity.

The relative risk of PE, comparing obese patients with nonobese patients, was 2.18 and for DVT it was 2.50.[83] The relative risks for PE and DVT were age dependent. Obesity had the greatest effect on patients less than 40 years of age, in whom the relative risk for PE in obese patients was 5.19 and the relative risk for DVT was 5.20.[83] The higher relative risk of obesity in younger patients may have reflected that younger patients uncommonly have multiple confounding associated risk factors, which make the risk of obesity inapparent.

Previous investigators used several indices of obesity including a BMI greater than 35 kg/m^2 as well as BMI 30 to 35 kg/m^2,[84] BMI 29 kg/m^2 or greater,[74] weight more than 20% of median recommended weight for height,[18] and for men, waist circumference 100 cm or greater.[78] It is likely that all patients diagnosed with obesity in the National Hospital Discharge Survey database were obese, irrespective of the criteria used. However, some obese patients may not have had a listed discharge diagnosis of obesity, and they would have been included in the nonobese group. This situation would have tended to reduce the relative risk of obesity in VTE.

Various abnormalities of hemostasis have been described in obesity, in particular increased plasminogen activator inhibitor-1 (PAI-1).[85–87] Other abnormalities of coagulation have been reported as well,[87] including increased platelet activation,[77] increased levels of plasma fibrinogen, factor VII, factor VIII, and von Willebrand factor.[88] Fibrinogen, factor VIIc, and PAI-1 correlated with BMI.[89]

Regarding height, in the study of Swedish men, those taller than 179 cm (5' 10") had a 1.5 times higher risk of VTE than men shorter than 172 cm.[90] The Physicians' Health Study of male physicians also showed that taller men had a significantly increased risk of VTE.[91]

Air Travel

The possibility of VTE after travel is not unique to air travel.[92–94] Prolonged periods in cramped quarters, irrespective of travel, can lead to PE.[95] The term economy class syndrome was introduced in 1988,[96] but has since been replaced with flight-related DVT in recognition that all travelers are at risk, irrespective of the class of travel.[97]

Rates of development of PE with air travel lasting 12 to 18 hours have been calculated as 2.6 PE/million travelers.[98] With air travel of 8 hours or longer, 1.65/million passengers had acute PE on arrival.[99] With 6 to 8 hours of air travel the rate of acute PE on arrival was 0.25/million and among those who traveled for 6 hours or less none developed acute PE on arrival.[99] The trend showing increasing rates of PE with duration of travel is compelling, but the incidence of DVT was about 3000 times higher in a prospective investigation.[100] In a prospective investigation of travelers who traveled for 10 hours or longer, 4 of 878 (0.5%) developed PE and 5 of 878 (0.6%) developed DVT.[100]

Varicose Veins

Varicose veins were found by some to be an age-dependent risk factor for VTE.[81] Among patients aged 45 years the odds ratio for VTE was 4.2.[81] In patients aged 60 years the odds ratio was 1.9 and at aged 75 years, varicose veins were not associated with an increased risk of VTE.[81] However, others did not find varicose veins to be a risk factor for DVT[101] or PE found at autopsy.[26]

Oral Contraceptives

Although the risk of VTE is higher among users of oral estrogen-containing contraceptives than nonusers,[102,103] the absolute risk is low.[104] An absolute risk of VTE of less than 1/10,000 patients/y increased to only 3 to 4/10,000 patients/y during the time oral contraceptives were used.[104]

The relative risk for VTE in women using oral contraceptives containing 50 μg of estrogen, compared with users of oral contraceptives that contained less than 50 μg was 1.5.[105] The relative risk for VTE in women using oral contraceptives containing more than 50 µg of estrogen, compared with users of oral contraceptives that contained less than 50 µg was 1.7.[105] No difference in the risk of VTE was found with various levels of low doses of 20, 30, 40, and 50 µg/d.[106] With doses of estrogen of 50 µg/d, the rate of VTE was 7.0/10,000 contraceptive users/y and with more than 50 µg/d, the rate of VTE was 10.0/10,000 oral contraceptive users/y (**Fig. 7**).[105] However, some found no appreciable difference in the relative risk of VTE in relation to low or higher estrogen doses.[107]

Reports of the risk of VTE in relation to the duration of use of oral contraceptives are inconsistent. Some showed relative risks increased as the duration of use of estrogen-containing oral contraceptives increased.[108] The relative risks were 0.7 in women who used oral contraceptives for less than 1 year, 1.4 for those who used oral contraceptives for 1 to 4 years and 1.8 in those who used it for 5 years or longer.[108] Others showed the opposite effect, with a decreasing relative risk with duration of use.[106] The relative risk for DVT or PE was 5.1 with use for less than 1 year, 2.5 with use for 1 to 5 years, and 2.1 with use for longer than 5 years.[106] Some showed the risk to be unaffected by the duration of use.[107]

A synergistic effect of oral contraceptives with obesity has been shown.[109–111] The odds ratio of DVT in obese women (BMI $\geq$30 kg/m^2) who were users of oral contraceptives ranged from 5.2 to 7.8 compared with obese women who did not use oral contraceptives[75,109,110] and among women with a BMI 35 kg/m^2 or higher, the odds ratio was 3.1 compared with similarly obese nonusers of oral contraceptives.[111]

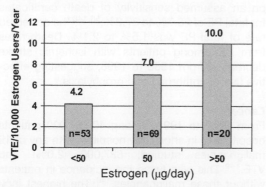

Fig. 7. VTE per 10,000 estrogen-using patients per year according to daily dose. (*Data from* Gerstman BB, Piper JM, Tomita DK, et al. Oral contraceptive estrogen dose and the risk of deep venous thromboembolic disease. Am J Epidemiol 1991;133:32–7.) (*Reproduced from* Stein PD. Pulmonary embolism. 2nd edition. Oxford (UK): Blackwell Future; 2007; with permission.)

Tamoxifen

Tamoxifen is a selective estrogen-receptor modulator used for treatment of breast cancer and for prevention of breast cancer in high-risk patients.[112–114] Among women with breast cancer currently being treated with tamoxifen, compared with previous users or those who never used it, the odds ratio was 7.1.[114] Others found a lower odds ratio of 2.7.[81] The odds ratio for VTE in women at high risk of breast cancer who received tamoxifen to prevent breast cancer was 2.1.[113] Others found a hazard ratio of 1.63.[112]

Hormonal Replacement Therapy

There is a 2- to 3-fold increased risk of VTE with the use of hormone replacement therapy in postmenopausal women.[115–119] Among postmenopausal women who had coronary artery disease and received estrogen plus progestin, the relative hazard of VTE was 2.7 compared with nonusers.[120] Review showed that the risk of VTE is highest in the first year of hormone replacement therapy.[121] The risk of VTE is increased for oral estrogen alone, oral estrogen combined with progestin, and probably for transdermal hormone replacement therapy.[121]

Hypercoagulable Syndrome

Hypercoagulable syndromes include inherited and acquired thrombophilias. The former is discussed in detail in the article by Weitz in this issue. The latter includes the antiphospholipid syndrome, heparin-induced thrombocytopenia, acquired dysfibrinogenemia, myeloproliferative disorders, and malignancy. Myeloproliferative disorders and malignancy are described elsewhere in this article.

Regarding the antiphospholipid syndrome, antiphospholipid antibodies are associated with both arterial and venous thrombosis.[122] The most commonly detected subgroups of antiphospholipid antibodies are lupus anticoagulant antibodies, anticardiolipin antibodies and anti-β_2-glycoprotein I antibodies.[123] DVT, the most common manifestation of the antiphospholipid syndrome, occurs in 29% to 55% of patients with the syndrome, and about half of these patients have pulmonary emboli.[124–126]

The risk of heparin-associated thrombocytopenia is more duration related than dose related. Heparin-associated thrombocytopenia occurs more frequently with unfractionated heparin when used for an extended duration than with LMWH used for an extended duration.[127] When used for prophylaxis, there was a higher prevalence of heparin-associated thrombocytopenia in those receiving unfractionated heparin (1.6%, 57 of 3463) than in those receiving LMWH (0.6%, 23 of 3714).[127] However, treatment resulted in only a small difference in the prevalence of heparin-associated thrombocytopenia comparing unfractionated heparin (0.9%, 22 of 2321) with LMWH (0.6%, 18 of 3126).[127]

Acquired dysfibrinogenemia occurs most often in patients with severe liver disease.[128] The impairment of the fibrinogen is a structural defect caused by an increased carbohydrate content impairing the polymerization of the fibrin, depending on the degree of abnormality of the fibrinogen molecule.[128]

Heart Failure

Congestive heart failure (CHF) is considered a major risk factor for VTE.[18,79,101,129–131] Among patients with established CHF, those with lower ejection fractions had a higher risk of thromboembolic event.[132,133] However, some investigators did not evaluate CHF among the risk factors for VTE.[134] The reported frequency of PE in patients with heart failure has ranged widely from 0.9% to 39% of patients.[18,132,133,135–138] The reported frequency of DVT in patients with CHF also ranged widely from 10% to 59%.[18,79,101] The largest investigation was from the National Hospital Discharge Survey.[139] Among 58,873,000 patients hospitalized with heart failure in short-stay hospitals from 1979 to 2003, 1.63% had VTE (relative risk = 1.47).[139] The relative risk for VTE was highest in patients less than 40 years old (relative risk = 6.91). Some showed the lower the ejection fraction, the greater the risk of VTE.[140] Among 755,807 adults older than 20 years with heart failure who died from 1980 to 1998, PE was listed as the cause of death in 20,387 (2.7%).[141] Assuming that the accuracy of death certificates was only 26.7%,[58] the rate of death from PE in these patients may have been as high as 10.1%. Therefore, the estimated death rate from PE in patients who died with heart failure was 3% to 10%. CHF seems to be a stronger risk factor in women. Dries and colleagues[132] reported a higher proportion of PE in women (24%) compared with men (14%). We too showed a higher relative risk of PE and of DVT in women with CHF than in men.[139] Although these data seem compelling, multivariate logistic analysis failed to identify CHF as an independent risk factor for DVT or PE.[81] However, it was a risk factor for postmortem VTE that was not a cause of death.[81]

COPD

Hospitalized patients with exacerbations of COPD, when routinely evaluated, showed PE in 25% to 29%.[142,143] From 1979 to 2003, 58,392,000 adults older than 20 years were hospitalized with COPD in short-stay hospitals in the United States.[144] PE was diagnosed in 381,000 (0.65%) and DVT in 632,000 (1.08%).[144] The relative risk for PE in adults hospitalized with COPD was 1.92 and for DVT it was 1.30. Among those aged 20 to 39 years with COPD, the relative risk for PE was 5.34. Among patients with COPD aged 40 to 59 years, the relative risk for PE decreased to 2.02, and among patients aged 60 to 79 years the relative risk for PE was 1.23.[144] The relative risk for DVT was also higher in patients with COPD aged 20 to 39 years (relative risk = 2.58) than in patients aged 40 years or older (relative risk 0.92–1.17, depending on age).[144] In young adults, other risk factors in combination with COPD are uncommon, so the contribution of COPD to the risk of PE becomes more apparent than in older patients. Although these data strongly suggest that COPD is a risk factor for PE and DVT, multivariate logistic analysis did not identify it as an independent risk factor.[81] Others, with univariate analysis, did not identify COPD as a risk factor.[101]

Stroke

Patients with stroke are at particular risk of developing DVT and PE because of limb paralysis, prolonged bed rest, and increased prothrombotic activity.[145] Among 14,109,000 patients with ischemic stroke hospitalized in short-stay hospitals from 1979 to 2003, VTE was diagnosed in 165,000 (1.17%).[146] Among 1,606,000 patients with hemorrhagic stroke, the incidence of VTE was higher (1.93%).

Among patients with ischemic stroke who died from 1980 to 1998, PE was the listed cause of death in 11,101 of 2,000,963 (0.55%).[147] Based on an assumed sensitivity of death certificates for fatal PE of 26.7% to 37.2%,[58,148] the corrected rate of fatal PE was 1.5% to 2.1%. Death rates from PE among patients with ischemic stroke decreased from 1980 to 1998, suggesting effective use of antithrombotic prophylaxis.

Cancer

From 1979 to 1999, among 40,787,000 patients hospitalized in short-stay hospitals with any of 19 malignancies studied, 827,000 (2.0%) had VTE.[149] This was twice the incidence in patients without these malignancies.[149] The highest incidence of VTE was in patients with carcinoma of the pancreas (4.3%) and the lowest incidences were in patients with carcinoma of the bladder and carcinoma of the lip, oral cavity, or pharynx (<0.6% to 1.0%). Incidences with cancer were not age dependent.[149] Myeloproliferative disease and lymphoma were associated with relative risks for VTE of 2.9 and 2.5, respectively (**Fig. 8**).[149] Leukemia was associated with a lower relative risk (1.7).

Based on death certificates from 1980 to 1998 among patients who died with cancer, PE was the listed cause of death in 0.21%.[150] Adjustment of the data for the frailty of the diagnosis of fatal PE based on death certificates indicated a likely range of 0.31% to 1.97%.[150]

Pregnancy

Pregnancy-associated DVT based on data from the National Hospital Discharge Survey was diagnosed in 93,000 of 80,798,000 women (0.12%) from 1979 to 1999.[151] The rate of pregnancy-associated DVT (vaginal delivery and cesarean section) increased from 1982 to 1999, although the rate of nonpregnancy-associated DVT decreased for most of this period (**Fig. 9**). Some showed the rate of pregnancy-associated DVT was twice the rate of nonpregnancy-associated DVT.[151] A 6-fold increase in the rate of thromboembolism during pregnancy and the puerperium compared with nonpregnant women has been reported by others.[152]

Although the rate of pregnancy-associated DVT was higher than the rate of nonpregnancy-associated DVT, the rate of pregnancy-associated PE was lower than the rate of nonpregnancy-associated PE.[151] The reason for this difference is unknown and could reflect difference of the natural history of DVT in pregnancy. It also could reflect a reluctance to expose pregnant women to ionizing radiation associated with imaging for PE, resulting in a decreased frequency of diagnosis of PE.

The rate of pregnancy-associated DVT was higher among women aged 35 to 44 years than in younger women. The rate of pregnancy-associated DVT among black women was higher than among white women.[151,153,154]

DVT was more frequent among women who underwent cesarean section (104/100,000/y) than those who underwent vaginal delivery (47/100,000/y).[151] VTE in pregnancy is discussed in detail in the article by Marik elsewhere in this issue.

Surgery and Trauma

In PIOPED, trauma of the lower extremities was a predisposing factor in 10% of patients with PE, and in PIOPED II trauma of the lower extremities or pelvis was a predisposing factor in 14%.[69,70] Surgery within 3 months of the acute PE was a predisposing factor in 54% in PIOPED and in 23% in PIOPED II.[69,70] The prevalence of VTE following various categories of surgery and trauma has been reviewed in detail by Geerts and colleagues[155]

UPPER-EXTREMITY DVT

As the use of central venous lines and pacemaker wires has increased, their role in the cause of upper-extremity DVT has become prominent.[156-160] The incidence of upper-extremity DVT in a community teaching general hospital in adults (>20 years) was 64 of 34,567 (0.19%).[161]

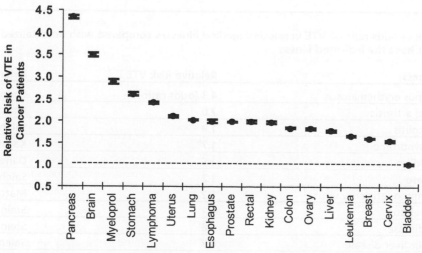

Fig. 8. Relative risks of VTE in patients hospitalized with cancer compared with those without cancer. The relative risk of VTE ranged from 1.02 to 4.34. (*Reprinted from* Stein PD, Beemath A, Meyers FA, et al. Incidence of venous thromboembolism in patients hospitalized with cancer. Am J Med 2006;119:60–8; with permission.)

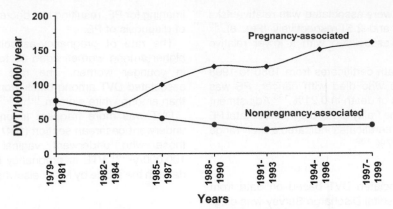

Fig. 9. Triennial rates of DVT in women aged 15 to 44 years. (*Reprinted from* Stein PD, Hull RD, Kayali F, et al. Venous thromboembolism in pregnancy: 21 year trends. Am J Med 2004;117:121–5; with permission.)

This prevalence of upper-extremity DVT was the same as reported by others (0.2%).[156]

All of the patients with upper-extremity DVT received therapy with anticoagulants.[161] None developed PE.[161] Others reported that 7% to 9% of patients with upper-extremity DVT had an acute PE.[162–164] Most PE (94%) in patients with upper-extremity DVT occurred in untreated patients.[165] Routine ventilation/perfusion lung scans in patients with upper-extremity DVT were high probability for PE in 13%.[164] Only 20% of patients with upper-extremity DVT who did not have a contraindication to anticoagulation were receiving anticoagulant prophylaxis at the time of diagnosis of upper-extremity DVT.[166]

MEDICAL ILLNESSES
Inflammatory Bowel Disease

The incidence of VTE among hospitalized medical patients with ulcerative colitis was 1.9% and the incidence with Crohn disease was lower (1.2%).[167] Among medical patients who had neither ulcerative colitis nor Crohn disease the incidence was 1.1%.[167] The relative risk of VTE among patients with ulcerative colitis compared with patients who did not have inflammatory bowel disease was 1.9 and with Crohn disease it was 1.2 (**Table 1**). Among patients younger than 40 years with ulcerative colitis, the relative risk of VTE compared with patients who did not have

Table 1
Relative risk or odds ratio of VTE in selected medical illnesses compared with hospitalized patients who do not have the indicated illness

Medical Illness	Relative Risk VTE	References
Systemic lupus erythematosus	4.3 (odds ratio)	Cogo et al[101]
Rheumatoid arthritis	2.0	Matta et al[175]
Ulcerative colitis	1.9	Saleh et al[167]
Nephrotic syndrome	1.7[a]	Kayali et al[178]
Hypothyroidism	1.6	Danescu et al[172]
Crohn disease	1.2	Saleh et al[167]
Human immunodeficiency virus	1.2	Matta et al[177]
Diabetes mellitus	1.1	Stein et al[176]
Sickle cell disease	0.8	Stein et al[179]
Nonalcoholic liver disease	0.7	Saleh et al[168]
Alcoholic liver disease	0.5	Saleh et al[168]

[a] Relative risk for DVT.

inflammatory bowel disease was 2.96 and in patients younger than 40 years with Crohn disease the relative risk was 2.23.[167]

Liver Disease

Patients with chronic liver disease (both alcoholic and nonalcoholic) seem to have a lower risk of PE than patients without liver disease,[81,168] but data are inconsistent.[169]

Chronic liver disease may result in impaired production of vitamin-K–dependent procoagulant factors.[170] However, decreased production of vitamin-K–dependent endogenous anticoagulants, such as protein C, protein S, and antithrombin III, may counter the hypocoagulability in such patients.[170] Other prothrombotic factors may counteract the impaired production of vitamin-K–dependent procoagulant factors including lupus anticoagulant, activated protein C resistance, PT20210A mutation, Factor V Leiden, MTHFR mutation, and increased levels of factor VIII.[171]

Based on data from the National Hospital Discharge Survey, among 4,927,000 hospitalized patients with chronic alcoholic liver disease from 1979 to 2006, the prevalence of VTE was 0.6% and among 4,565,000 hospitalized patients with chronic nonalcoholic liver disease it was 0.9%.[168] The prevalence of VTE was higher in those with chronic alcoholic liver disease than with nonalcoholic liver disease, but the difference was small and of no clinical consequence.[168] Both showed a lower prevalence of VTE than in hospitalized patients with most other medical diseases (see **Table 1**). It may be that both chronic alcoholic liver disease and chronic nonalcoholic liver disease have protective antithrombotic mechanisms although the mechanisms differ.

Hypothyroidism

Among 19,519,000 hospitalized patients with a diagnosis of hypothyroidism from 1979 to 2005, 119,000 (0.61%) had PE (relative risk = 1.64) (see **Table 1**).[172] DVT was diagnosed in 1.36% of hypothyroid patients (relative risk = 1.62).[172] The relative risk for PE in patients with hypothyroidism was highest in patients younger than 40 years (relative risk = 3.99) and the relative risk for DVT was also highest in patients younger than 40 years (relative risk = 2.25). Hyperthyroidism was not associated with an increased risk for VTE (relative risk = 0.98).

Rheumatoid arthritis

Rheumatoid arthritis is not generally considered a risk factor for VTE, although abnormalities of coagulation factors have been found in patients with rheumatoid arthritis.[173,174] Among 4,818,000 patients hospitalized in short-stay hospitals from 1979 to 2005 with rheumatoid arthritis who did not have joint surgery, the incidence of PE was 2.3%, and the relative risk of VTE compared with those who did not have rheumatoid arthritis was 1.99 (see **Table 1**).[175] Among patients younger than 50 years the relative risk was higher (2.13).[175]

Diabetes mellitus

Among 92,240,000 patients with diabetes mellitus hospitalized from 1979 to 2005, 1,267,000 (1.4%) had VTE.[176] The relative risk for VTE was increased only in patients younger than 50 years and was highest in patients aged 20 to 29 years (relative risk = 1.73). In patients with diabetes mellitus who did not have obesity, stroke, heart failure, or cancer, compared with those who did not have diabetes mellitus and did not have any of these comorbid conditions, the relative risk for VTE was 1.52 in patients aged 20 to 29 years and 1.19 in patients 30 to 39 years. In older patients, the relative risk of VTE in patients with diabetes mellitus was not increased.[176] Among all adults with diabetes mellitus, the relative risk of VTE was 1.05 (see **Table 1**).[176]

Human immunodeficiency virus

Among 2,429,000 patients older than 18 years hospitalized in short-stay hospitals from 1990 through 2005 with human immunodeficiency virus (HIV) infection; the prevalence of VTE was 1.7% (relative risk = 1.21) (see **Table 1**).[177] The prevalence of VTE in patients aged 30 to 49 years was also 1.7%, but the relative risk compared with patients who did not have HIV infection was higher (1.65).[177]

Nephrotic syndrome

From 1979 to 2005, 925,000 patients were discharged from short-stay hospitals with nephrotic syndrome and 14,000 (1.5%) had DVT (relative risk = 1.72) (see **Table 1**).[178] In patients aged 18 to 39 years the relative risk for DVT was 6.81.[178] Renal vein thrombosis was so uncommon that too few were reported to calculate its prevalence. Therefore, PE, if it occurs, is likely to be due to emboli from the lower extremities and not the renal vein.

Sickle cell disease

Sickle cell disease does not seem to be a risk factor for DVT.[179] Among 1,804,000 patients hospitalized in short-stay hospitals with sickle cell disease from 1979 to 2003, 11,000 (0.61%) had a discharge diagnosis of DVT, which was not more than in African Americans without sickle cell disease (0.81%).[179] Among patients with sickle cell disease, a discharge diagnosis of PE was made in 0.50% compared with 0.33% who did not have sickle cell disease. Regarding patients younger than 40 years, 0.44% had PE, whereas among patients who did not have sickle cell disease, 0.12% had PE.[179] The higher prevalence of apparent PE in patients with sickle cell disease compared with African American patients the same age who did not have sickle cell disease, and the comparable prevalence of DVT in both groups, is compatible with the concept that thrombosis in situ may be present in many.

Systemic lupus erythematosus
Systemic lupus erythematosus is believed to be independently associated with the risk of developing DVT.[101] The odds ratio for DVT in patients with systemic lupus erythematosus, compared with those without it, was 4.3 (see **Table 1**).[101]

Behçet disease
Behçet disease is a rare multisystem inflammatory disorder of unknown cause.[180] VTE occurs in about one-fifth of patients with Behçet disease.[181]

Paroxysmal nocturnal hemoglobinuria
Review of 13 retrospective studies of patients with paroxysmal nocturnal hemoglobinuria showed a 30% prevalence of venous thrombotic events in patients from Western nations.[182] The majority was within the hepatic and mesenteric veins.[182]

Buerger disease
PE associated with thromboangiitis obliterans (Buerger disease) is rare, and to our knowledge, limited to a case report.[183]

SUMMARY

One-quarter of a million patients are hospitalized yearly in the United States with acute PE. Home treatment of DVT has resulted in fewer hospital admissions for DVT than PE. The incidence of PE and of DVT is lower in Asian Americans, American Indians, and Alaskan Natives than in African Americans and whites. The incidence of PE increases exponentially with age, but PE can occur at any age. The estimated case fatality rate is 7% to 11%, and it too increases exponentially with age. More than 90% of patients with PE have 1 or more risk factors, including bed rest, travel, surgery, malignancy, history of DVT or PE, trauma of lower extremities or pelvis, central venous instrumentation, stroke, paresis or paralysis, heart failure, or COPD. Compelling evidence suggests that obesity is a risk factor for VTE. Although the risk of VTE is higher among users of oral estrogen-containing contraceptives than nonusers,

the absolute risk is low. There is a 2- to 3-fold increased risk of VTE with the use of hormone replacement therapy in postmenopausal women. DVT occurs in 29% to 55% of patients with the antiphospholipid syndrome, and about half of these patients have PE. Unfractionated heparin, when used for prophylaxis, was associated with a higher incidence of heparin-associated thrombocytopenia than when used for treatment. Pregnancy-associated DVT is 2 to 6 times the frequency of nonpregnancy-associated DVT. The rate of pregnancy-associated DVT has been increasing. Ulcerative colitis, rheumatoid arthritis, and nephrotic syndrome are associated with a nearly 2-fold risk of VTE. Patients with severe liver disease have about half the risk of VTE as patients without liver disease.

REFERENCES

1. Giuntini C, DiRicco G, Marini C, et al. Pulmonary embolism: epidemiology. Chest 1995;107(Suppl): 3S–9S.
2. Stein PD, Matta F. Acute pulmonary embolism. Curr Prob Cardiol 2010;35:314–76.
3. DeMonaco NA, Dang Q, Kapoor WN, et al. Pulmonary embolism incidence is increasing with use of spiral computed tomography. Am J Med 2008; 121:611–7.
4. Heit JA, Silverstein MD, Mohr DN, et al. Predictors of survival after deep vein thrombosis and pulmonary embolism: a population-based, cohort study. Arch Intern Med 1999;159:445–53.
5. Kahn SR, Shrier I, Julian JA, et al. Determinants and time course of the postthrombotic syndrome after acute deep venous thrombosis. Ann Intern Med 2008;149:698–707.
6. Brandjes DP, Büller HR, Heijboer H, et al. Randomized trial of effect of compression stockings in patients with symptomatic proximal-vein thrombosis. Lancet 1997;349:759–62.
7. Ginsberg JS, Hirsh J, Julian J, et al. Prevention and treatment of postphlebitic syndrome: results of a 3-part study. Arch Intern Med 2001;161:2105–9.
8. Partsch H, Kaulich M, Mayer W. Immediate mobilisation in acute vein thrombosis reduces post-thrombotic syndrome. Int Angiol 2004;23:206–12.
9. Prandoni P, Lensing AW, Prins MH, et al. Below-knee elastic compression stockings to prevent the post-thrombotic syndrome: a randomized, controlled trial. Ann Intern Med 2004;141:249–56.
10. Aschwanden M, Jeanneret C, Koller MT, et al. Effect of prolonged treatment with compression stockings to prevent post-thrombotic sequelae: a randomized controlled trial. J Vasc Surg 2008; 47:1015–21.

11. Kearon C, Kahn SR, Agnelli G, et al. American College of Chest Physicians. Antithrombotic therapy for venous thromboembolic disease: American College of chest physicians evidence-based clinical practice guidelines (8th edition). Chest 2008;133:454S–545S.

12. Palevsky HI. Pulmonary hypertension and thromboembolic disease in women. Cardiovasc Clin 1989;19:267–83.

13. Bernstein D, Goupey S, Schonberg SK. Pulmonary embolism in adolescents. AJDC 1986;140:667–71.

14. Coon W. Epidemiology of venous thromboembolism. Ann Surg 1977;186:149–64.

15. Coon WW, Willis PW III, Keller JB. Venous thrombosis and other venous disease in the Tecumseh Community Study. Circulation 1973;48:839–46.

16. Breckenridge RT, Ralnoff OD. Pulmonary embolism and unexpected death in supposedly normal persons. N Engl J Med 1964;270:298–9.

17. Stein PD, Hull RD, Patel KC, et al. Venous thromboembolic disease: comparison of the diagnostic process in men and women. Arch Intern Med 2003;163:1689–94.

18. Anderson FA Jr, Wheeler HB, Goldberg RJ, et al. A population-based perspective of the hospital incidence and case-fatality rates of deep vein thrombosis and pulmonary embolism. The Worcester DVT study. Arch Intern Med 1991;151:933–8.

19. Ferrari E, Baudouy M, Cerboni P, et al. Clinical epidemiology of venous thromboembolic disease. Results of a French multicentre registry. Eur Heart J 1997;18:685–91.

20. Lilienfeld DE, Godbold JH, Burke GL, et al. Hospitalization and case fatality for pulmonary embolism in the twin cities: 1979-1984. Am Heart J 1990;120:392–5.

21. Silverstein MD, Heit JA, Mohr DN, et al. Trends in the incidence of deep vein thrombosis and pulmonary embolism. A 25-year population-based study. Arch Intern Med 1998;158:585–93.

22. Stein PD, Huang H-L, Afzal A, et al. Incidence of acute pulmonary embolism in a general hospital: relation to age, sex, and race. Chest 1999;116:909–13.

23. Stein PD, Patel KC, Kalra NK, et al. Estimated incidence of acute pulmonary embolism in a community/teaching general hospital. Chest 2002;121:802–5.

24. Kniffin WD Jr, Baron JA, Barrett J, et al. The epidemiology of diagnosed pulmonary embolism and deep venous thrombosis in the elderly. Arch Intern Med 1994;154:861–6.

25. Karwinski B, Svendsen E. Comparison of clinical and postmortem diagnosis of pulmonary embolism. J Clin Pathol 1989;42:135–9.

26. Goldhaber SZ, Savage DD, Garrison RJ, et al. Risk factors for pulmonary embolism. The Framingham Study. Am J Med 1983;74:1023–8.

27. Quinn DA, Thompson BT, Terrin ML, et al. A prospective investigation of pulmonary embolism in women and men. JAMA 1992;268:1689–96.

28. Stein PD, Patel KC, Kalra NK, et al. Deep venous thrombosis in a general hospital. Chest 2002;122:960–2.

29. Stein PD, Hull RD, Patel KC, et al. Venous thromboembolic disease: comparison of the diagnostic process in blacks and whites. Arch Intern Med 2003;163:1843–8.

30. Haynes MA, Smedley BD, editors. The unequal burden of cancer: an assessment of NIH research and programs for ethnic minorities and the medically underserved. Washington, DC: National Academy Press; 1999. p. 19.

31. Stein PD, Kayali F, Olson RE, et al. Pulmonary thromboembolism in Asian-Pacific Islanders in the United States: analysis of data from the National Hospital Discharge Survey and the United States Bureau of the Census. Am J Med 2004;116:435–42.

32. White RH. The epidemiology of venous thromboembolism. Circulation 2003;107:I4–8.

33. Svensson PJ, Dahlback B. Resistance to activated protein C as a basis for venous thrombosis. N Engl J Med 1994;330:517–22.

34. Franco RF, Reitsma PH. Genetic risk factors of venous thrombosis. Hum Genet 2001;109:369–84.

35. Ridker PM, Miletich JP, Hennekens CH, et al. Ethnic distribution of factor V Leiden in 4047 men and women. Implications for venous thromboembolism screening. JAMA 1997;277:1305–7.

36. Rees DC, Cox M, Clegg JB. World distribution of factor V Leiden. Lancet 1995;346:1133–4.

37. Gregg JP, Yamane AJ, Grody WW. Prevalence of the factor V-Leiden mutation in four distinct American ethnic populations. Am J Med Genet 1997;73:334–6.

38. Iso H, Folsom AR, Wu KK, et al. Hemostatic variables in Japanese and Caucasian men. Plasma fibrinogen, factor VIIc, factor VIIIc, and von Willebrand factor and their relations to cardiovascular disease risk factors. Am J Epidemiol 1989;130:925–34.

39. Takahashi H, Echizen H. Pharmacogenetics of CYP2C9 and interindividual variability in anticoagulant response to warfarin. Pharmacogenomics J 2003;3:202–14.

40. Yamaguchi T. Optimal intensity of warfarin therapy for secondary prevention of stroke in patients with nonvalvular atrial fibrillation: a multicenter, prospective, randomized trial. Stroke 2000;31:817–21.

41. Matsuyama K, Matsumoto M, Sugita T, et al. Anticoagulant therapy in Japanese patients with mechanical mitral valves. Circulation 2002;66:668–70.

42. Stein PD, Kayali F, Olson RE, et al. Pulmonary thromboembolism in American Indians and Alaskan Natives. Arch Intern Med 2004;164:1804–6.

43. Hooper WC, Holman RC, Heit JA, et al. Venous thrombembolism hospitalizations among American Indians and Alaska Natives. Thromb Res 2003;108: 273–8.

44. Stein PD, Hull RD, Kayali F, et al. Venous thromboembolism according to age: the impact of an aging population. Arch Intern Med 2004;164:2260–5.

45. Stein PD, Kayali F, Olson RE. Incidence of pulmonary thromboembolism in infants and children. J Pediatr 2004;145:563–5.

46. Andrew M, David M, Adams M, et al. Venous thromboembolic complications (VTE) in children: first analyses of the Canadian Registry of VTE. Blood 1994;83:1251–7.

47. Bernstein D, Coupey S, Schonberg SK. Pulmonary embolism in adolescents. Am J Dis Child 1986;140: 667–71.

48. Royal College of General Practitioners' Oral Contraception Study. Oral contraceptives, venous thrombosis, and varicose veins. J R Coll Gen Pract 1978;28:393–9.

49. David M, Andrew M. Venous thromboembolic complications in children. J Pediatr 1993;123: 337–46.

50. Schmidt B, Andrew M. Neonatal thrombosis: report of a prospective Canadian and international registry. Pediatrics 1995;96:939–43.

51. Wise RC, Todd JK. Spontaneous, lower-extremity venous thrombosis in children. Am J Dis Child 1973;126:766–9.

52. Nuss R, Hays T, Manco-Johnson M. Childhood thrombosis. Pediatrics 1995;96:291–4.

53. Stein PD, Kayali F, Olson RE. Analysis of occurrence of venous thromboembolic disease in the four seasons. Am J Cardiol 2004;93:511–3.

54. Stein PD, Kayali F, Olson RE. Regional differences in rates of diagnosis and mortality of pulmonary thromboembolism. Am J Cardiol 2004;93:1194–7.

55. Klatsky AL, Armstrong MA, Poggi J. Risk of pulmonary embolism and/or deep venous thrombosis in Asian-Americans. Am J Cardiol 2000;85:1334–7.

56. White RH, Zhou H, Romano PS. Incidence of idiopathic deep venous thrombosis and secondary thromboembolism among ethnic groups in California. Ann Intern Med 1998;128:737–40.

57. Horlander KT, Mannino DM, Leeper KV. Pulmonary embolism mortality in the United States, 1979-1998: an analysis using multiple-cause mortality data. Arch Intern Med 2003;163:1711–7.

58. Attems J, Arbes S, Bohm G, et al. The clinical diagnostic accuracy rate regarding the immediate cause of death in a hospitalized geriatric population; an autopsy study of 1594 patients. Wien Med Wochenschr 2004;154:159–62.

59. Lilienfeld DE. Decreasing mortality from pulmonary embolism in the United States, 1979-1996. Int J Epidemiol 2000;29:465–9.

60. Byrne JJ. Phlebitis: a study of 748 cases at the Boston City Hospital. N Engl J Med 1955;253: 579–86.

61. Hermann RE, Davis JH, Holden WD. Pulmonary embolism: a clinical and pathologic study with emphasis on the effect of prophylactic therapy with anticoagulants. Am J Surg 1961;102:19–28.

62. Collins R, Scrimgeour A, Yusuf S, et al. Reduction in fatal pulmonary embolism and venous thrombosis by perioperative administration of subcutaneous heparin. Overview of results of randomized trials in general, orthopedic, and urologic surgery. N Engl J Med 1988;318:1162–73.

63. Stein PD, Henry JW, Relyea B. Untreated patients with pulmonary embolism: outcome, clinical and laboratory assessment. Chest 1995;107:931–5.

64. Stein PD, Kayali F, Olson RE. Estimated case fatality rate of pulmonary embolism, 1979–1998. Am J Cardiol 2004;93:1197–9.

65. Carson JL, Kelley MA, Duff A, et al. The clinical course of pulmonary embolism. N Engl J Med 1992;326:1240–5.

66. Stein PD, Henry JW. Prevalence of acute pulmonary embolism among patients in a general hospital and at autopsy. Chest 1995;108:978–81.

67. The Columbus Investigators. Low-molecular-weight heparin in the treatment of patients with venous thromboembolism. N Engl J Med 1997; 337:657–62.

68. Simonneau G, Sors H, Charbonnier B, et al. A comparison of low-molecular-weight heparin with unfractionated heparin for acute pulmonary embolism. The THESSE Study Group. N Engl J Med 1997;337:663–9.

69. Stein PD, Beemath A, Matta F, et al. Clinical characteristics of patient with acute pulmonary embolism: data from PIOPED II. Am J Med 2007;120:871–9.

70. Stein PD, Terrin ML, Hales CA, et al. Clinical, laboratory, roentgenographic and electrocardiographic findings in patients with acute pulmonary embolism and no pre-existing cardiac or pulmonary disease. Chest 1991;100:598–603.

71. Heit JA, Silverstein MD, Mohr DN, et al. The epidemiology of venous thromboembolism in the community. Thromb Haemost 2001;86:452–63.

72. Anderson FA Jr, Wheeler HB, Goldberg RJ, et al. The prevalence of risk factors for venous thromboembolism among hospital patients. Arch Intern Med 1992;152:1660–4.

73. Hedley AA, Ogden CL, Johnson CL, et al. Prevalence of overweight and obesity among US

children, adolescents, and adults, 1999–2002. JAMA 2004;291:2847–50.

74. Goldhaber SZ, Grodstein F, Stampfer MJ, et al. A prospective study of risk factors for pulmonary embolism in women. JAMA 1997;277:642–5.

75. Abdollahi M, Cushman M, Rosendaal FR. Obesity: risk of venous thrombosis and the interaction with coagulation factor levels and oral contraceptive use. Thromb Haemost 2003;89:493–8.

76. Coon WW, Coller FA. Some epidemiologic considerations of thromboembolism. Surg Gynecol Obstet 1959;109:487–501.

77. Basili S, Pacini G, Guagnano MT, et al. Insulin resistance as a determinant of platelet activation in obese women. J Am Coll Cardiol 2006;48:2531–8.

78. Hansson PO, Eriksson H, Welin L, et al. Smoking and abdominal obesity: risk factors for venous thromboembolism among middle-aged men: "the study of men born in 1913". Arch Intern Med 1999;159:1886–90.

79. Samama MM. An epidemiologic study of risk factors for deep vein thrombosis in medical outpatients: the Sirius study. Arch Intern Med 2000;160: 3415–20.

80. Kabrhel C, Varraso R, Goldhaber SZ, et al. Prospective study of BMI and the risk of pulmonary embolism in women. Obesity (Silver Spring) 2009; 17:2040–6.

81. Heit JA, Silverstein MD, Mohr DN, et al. Risk factors for deep vein thrombosis and pulmonary embolism: a population-based case-control study. Arch Intern Med 2000;160:809–15.

82. US Department of Health and Human Services. Public Health Service, National Center for Health Statistics National Hospital Discharge Survey 1979-2006 Multi-year Public-Use Data File Documentation. Available at: http://www.cdc.gov/nchs/about/major/hdasd/nhds.htm. Accessed April 28, 2010.

83. Stein PD, Beemath A, Olson RE. Obesity as a risk factor in venous thromboembolism. Am J Med 2005;118:978–80.

84. Farmer RD, Lawrenson RA, Todd JC, et al. A comparison of the risks of venous thromboembolic disease in association with different combined oral contraceptives. Br J Clin Pharmacol 2000;49:580–90.

85. Pannaciulli N, De Mitrio V, Marino R, et al. Effect of glucose tolerance status on PAI-1 plasma levels in overweight and obese subjects. Obes Res 2002; 10:717–25.

86. Juhan-Vague I, Alessi MC, Mavri A, et al. Plasminogen activator inhibitor-1, inflammation, obesity, insulin resistance and vascular risk. J Thromb Haemost 2003;1:1575–9.

87. De Pergola G, Pannacciulli N. Coagulation and fibrinolysis abnormalities in obesity. J Endocrinol Invest 2002;25:899–904.

88. Mertens I, Van Gaal LF. Obesity, haemostasis and the fibrinolytic system. Obes Rev 2002;3:85–101.

89. Bara L, Nicaud V, Tiret L, et al. Expression of a paternal history of premature myocardial infarction on fibrinogen, factor VIIC and PAI-1 in European offspring—the EARS study. European Atherosclerosis Research Study Group. Thromb Haemost 1994;71:434–40.

90. Rosengren A, Fredén M, Hansson PO, et al. Psychosocial factors and venous thromboembolism: a long-term follow-up study of Swedish men. J Thromb Haemost 2008;6:558–64.

91. Glynn RJ, Rosner B. Comparison of risk factors for the competing risks of coronary heart disease, stroke, and venous thromboembolism. Am J Epidemiol 2005;162:975–82.

92. Homans J. Thrombosis of the deep leg veins due to prolonged sitting. N Engl J Med 1954;250: 148–9.

93. Symington IS, Stack BH. Pulmonary thromboembolism after travel. Br J Dis Chest 1977;71:138–40.

94. Tardy B, Page Y, Zeni F, et al. Phlebitis following travel. Presse Med 1993;22:811–4.

95. Simpson K. Shelter deaths from pulmonary embolism. Lancet 1940;2:744.

96. Cruickshank JM, Gorlin R, Jennett B. Air travel and thrombotic episodes: the economy class syndrome. Lancet 1988;2:497–8.

97. Collins J. Thromboembolic disease related to air travel: what you need to know. Semin Roentgenol 2005;40:1–2.

98. Hertzberg SR, Roy S, Hollis G, et al. Acute symptomatic pulmonary embolism associated with long haul air travel to Sydney. Vasc Med 2003;8:21–3.

99. Perez-Rodriguez E, Jimenez D, Diaz G, et al. Incidence of air travel-related pulmonary embolism at the Madrid-Barajas airport. Arch Intern Med 2003; 163:2766–70.

100. Hughes RJ, Hopkins RJ, Hill S, et al. Frequency of venous thromboembolism in low to moderate risk long distance air travellers: the New Zealand Air Traveller's Thrombosis (NZATT) study. Lancet 2003;362:2039–44.

101. Cogo A, Bernardi E, Prandoni P, et al. Acquired risk factors for deep-vein thrombosis in symptomatic outpatients. Arch Intern Med 1994;154:164–8.

102. Lewis MA. The epidemiology of oral contraceptive use: a critical review of the studies on oral contraceptives and the health of young women. Am J Obstet Gynecol 1998;179:1086–97.

103. Realini JP, Goldzieher JW. Oral contraceptives and cardiovascular disease: a critique of the epidemiologic studies. Am J Obstet Gynecol 1985;152: 729–98.

104. Vandenbroucke JP, Rosing J, Bloemenkamp KW, et al. Oral contraceptives and the risk of venous thrombosis. N Engl J Med 2001;344:1527–35.

105. Gerstman BB, Piper JM, Tomita DK, et al. Oral contraceptive estrogen dose and the risk of deep venous thromboembolic disease. Am J Epidemiol 1991;133:32–7.

106. Lidegaard O, Edstrom B, Kreiner S. Oral contraceptives and venous thromboembolism. A case-control study. Contraception 1998;57:291–301.

107. World Health Organization Collaborative Study of Cardiovascular Disease and Steroid Hormone Contraception. Venous thromboembolic disease and combined oral contraceptives: results of international multicentre case-control study. Lancet 1995;346:1575–82.

108. Helmrich SP, Rosenberg L, Kaufman DW, et al. Venous thromboembolism in relation to oral contraceptive use. Obstet Gynecol 1987;69:91–5.

109. Pomp ER, le Cessie S, Rosendaal FR, et al. Risk of venous thrombosis: obesity and its joint effect with oral contraceptive use and prothrombotic mutations. Br J Haemotol 2007;139:289–96.

110. Lidegaard O, Edstrom B, Kreiner S. Oral contraceptives and venous thromboembolism: a five-year national case-control study. Contraception 2002;65:187–96.

111. Nightingale AL, Lawrenson RA, Simpson EL, et al. The effects of age, body mass index, smoking and general health on the risk of venous thromboembolism in users of combined oral contraceptives. Eur J Contracept Reprod Healthcare 2000;5:265–74.

112. Decensi A, Maisonneuve P, Rotmensz N, et al. Italian Tamoxifen Study Group. Effect of tamoxifen on venous thromboembolic events in a breast cancer prevention trial. Circulation 2005;111:650–6.

113. Duggan C, Marriott K, Edwards R, et al. Inherited and acquired risk factors for venous thromboembolic disease among women taking tamoxifen to prevent breast cancer. J Clin Oncol 2003;21:3588–93.

114. Meier CR, Jick H. Tamoxifen and risk of idiopathic venous thromboembolism. Br J Clin Pharmacol 1998;45:608–12.

115. Daly E, Vessey MP, Hawkins MM, et al. Risk of venous thromboembolism in users of hormone replacement therapy. Lancet 1996;348:977–80.

116. Jick H, Derby LE, Myers MW, et al. Risk of hospital admission for idiopathic venous thromboembolism among users of postmenopausal oestrogens. Lancet 1996;348:981–3.

117. Grodstein F, Stampfer MJ, Goldhaber SZ, et al. Prospective study of exogenous hormones and risk of pulmonary embolism in women. Lancet 1996;348:983–7.

118. Perez Gutthann S, García Rodriguez LA, Castellsague J, et al. Hormone replacement therapy and risk of venous thromboembolism: population based case-control study. BMJ 1997;314:796–800.

119. Varas-Lorenzo C, García-Rodriguez L, Cattaruzzi C, et al. Hormone replacement therapy and the risk of hospitalization for venous thromboembolism: a population-based study in southern Europe. Am J Epidemiol 1998;147:387–90.

120. Grady D, Wenger NK, Herrington D, et al. Postmenopausal hormone therapy increases risk for venous thromboembolic disease. The Heart and Estrogen/progestin Replacement Study. Ann Intern Med 2000;132:689–96.

121. Peverill RE. Hormone therapy and venous thromboembolism. Best Pract Res Clin Endocrinol Metab 2003;17:149–64.

122. Greaves M. Antiphospholipid antibodies and thrombosis. Lancet 1999;353:1348–53.

123. Levine JS, Branch DW, Rauch J. The antiphospholipid syndrome. N Engl J Med 2002;346:752–63.

124. Asherson RA, Khamashta MA, Ordi-Ros J, et al. The "primary" antiphospholipid syndrome: major clinical and serological features. Medicine (Baltimore) 1989;68:366–74.

125. Alarcon-Segovia D, Perez-Vazquez ME, Villa AR, et al. Preliminary classification criteria for the antiphospholipid syndrome within systemic lupus erythematosus. Semin Arthritis Rheum 1992;21:275–86.

126. Vianna JL, Khamashta MA, Ordi-Ros J, et al. Comparison of the primary and secondary antiphospholipid syndrome: a European Multicenter Study of 114 patients. Am J Med 1994;96:3–9.

127. Stein PD, Hull RD, Matta F, et al. Incidence of thrombocytopenia in hospitalized patients with venous thromboembolism. Am J Med 2009;122:919–30.

128. Brick W, Burgess R, Faguet GB. Dysfibrinogenemia. WebMD. Available at: www.webmd.com. Accessed March 19, 2010.

129. Shively BK. Deep venous thrombosis prophylaxis in patients with heart disease. Curr Cardiol Rep 2001;3:56–62.

130. Isnard R, Komajda M. Thromboembolism in heart failure, old ideas and new challenges. Eur J Heart Fail 2001;3:265–9.

131. Jafri SM, Ozawa T, Mammen E, et al. Platelet function, thrombin and fibrinolytic activity in patients with heart failure. Eur Heart J 1993;14:205–12.

132. Dries DL, Rosenberg YD, Waclawiw MA, et al. Ejection fraction and risk of thromboembolic events in patients with systolic dysfunction and sinus rhythm: evidence for gender differences in the studies of left ventricular dysfunction trials. J Am Coll Cardiol 1997;29:1074–80.

133. Kyrle PA, Korninger C, Gossinger H, et al. Prevention of arterial and pulmonary embolism by oral anticoagulants in patients with dilated cardiomyopathy. Thromb Haemost 1985;54:521–3.

134. Nordström M, Lindblad B, Bergqvist D, et al. A prospective study of the incidence of deep-vein thrombosis within a defined urban population. J Intern Med 1992;232:155–60.

135. Segal JP, Harvey WP, Gurel T. Diagnosis and treatment of primary myocardial disease. Circulation 1965;32:837–44.

136. Dunkman WB, Johnson GR, Carson PE, et al. Incidence of thromboembolic events in congestive heart failure. The V-HeFT VA Cooperative Studies Group. Circulation 1993;87(Suppl 6):VI94–101.

137. Kinsey D, White P. Fever in congestive heart failure. Arch Intern Med 1940;65:163–70.

138. Roberts WC, Siegel RJ, McManus BM. Idiopathic dilated cardiomyopathy: analysis of 152 necropsy patients. Am J Cardiol 1987;60:1340–55.

139. Beemath A, Stein PD, Skaf E, et al. Risk of venous thromboembolism in patients hospitalized with heart failure. Am J Cardiol 2006;98:793–5.

140. Howell MD, Geraci JM, Knowlton AA. Congestive heart failure and outpatient risk of venous thromboembolism: a retrospective, case-control study. J Clin Epidemiol 2001;54:810–8166.

141. Beemath A, Skaf E, Stein PD. Pulmonary embolism as a cause of death in adults who died with heart failure. Am J Cardiol 2006;98:1073–5.

142. Mispelaere D, Glerant JC, Audebert M, et al. Pulmonary embolism and sibilant types of chronic obstructive pulmonary disease decompensations. Rev Mal Respir 2002;19:415–23.

143. Tillie-Leblond I, Marquette CH, Perez T, et al. Pulmonary embolism in patients with unexplained exacerbation of chronic obstructive pulmonary disease: prevalence and risk factors. Ann Intern Med 2006;144:390–6.

144. Stein PD, Beemath A, Meyers FA, et al. Pulmonary embolism and deep venous thrombosis in patients hospitalized with chronic obstructive pulmonary disease. J Cardiovasc Med 2007;8:253–7.

145. Harvey RL. Prevention of venous thromboembolism after stroke. Topics Stroke Rehab 2003;10:61–9.

146. Skaf E, Stein PD, Beemath A, et al. Venous thromboembolism in patients with ischemic and hemorrhagic stroke. Am J Cardiol 2005;96:1731–3.

147. Skaf E, Stein PD, Beemath A, et al. Fatal pulmonary embolism and stroke. Am J Cardiol 2006;97:1776–7.

148. Dismuke SE, VanderZwaag R. Accuracy and epidemiological implications of the death certificate diagnosis of pulmonary embolism. J Chronic Dis 1984;37:67–73.

149. Stein PD, Beemath A, Meyers FA, et al. Incidence of venous thromboembolism in patients hospitalized with cancer. Am J Med 2006;119:60–8.

150. Stein PD, Beemath A, Meyers FA, et al. Pulmonary embolism as a cause of death in patients who died with cancer. Am J Med 2006;119:163–5.

151. Stein PD, Hull RD, Kayali F, et al. Venous thromboembolism in pregnancy: 21 year trends. Am J Med 2004;117:121–5.

152. Anonymous. Oral contraception and thromboembolic disease. J R Coll Gen Pract 1967;13:267–79.

153. Rochat RW, Koonin LM, Atrash HK, et al. Maternal mortality in the United States: report from the Maternal Mortality Collaborative. Obstet Gynecol 1988;72:91–7.

154. Buehler JW, Kaunitz AM, Hogue CJR, et al. Maternal mortality in women aged 35 years or older: United States. JAMA 1986;255:53–7.

155. Geerts WH, Bergqvist D, Pineo GF, et al. Preventive of venous thromboembolism. American College of Chest physicians evidence-based clinical practice guidelines (8th edition). Chest 2008;133:381S–453S.

156. Kroger K, Schelo C, Gocke C, et al. Colour Doppler sonographic diagnosis of upper limb venous thromboses. Clin Sci 1998;94:657–61.

157. Timsit JF, Farkas JC, Boyer JM, et al. Central vein catheter-related thrombosis in intensive care patients: incidence, risks factors, and relationship with catheter-related sepsis. Chest 1998;114:207–13.

158. Haire WD, Lieberman RP, Edney J, et al. Hickman catheter-induced thoracic vein thrombosis. Frequency and long-term sequelae in patients receiving high-dose chemotherapy and marrow transplantation. Cancer 1990;66:900–8.

159. Ryan JA Jr, Abel RM, Abbott WM, et al. Catheter complications in total parenteral nutrition. A prospective study of 200 consecutive patients. N Engl J Med 1974;290:757–61.

160. Dollery CM, Sullivan ID, Bauraind O, et al. Thrombosis and embolism in long-term central venous access for parenteral nutrition. Lancet 1994;344:1043–5.

161. Mustafa S, Stein PD, Patel KC, et al. Upper extremity deep venous thrombosis. Chest 2003;163:1213–9.

162. Hingorani A, Ascher E, Lorenson E, et al. Upper extremity deep venous thrombosis and its impact on morbidity and mortality rates in a hospital-based population. J Vasc Surg 1997;26:853–60.

163. Becker DM, Philbrick T, Walker FBIV. Axillary and subclavian venous thrombosis. Prognosis and treatment. Arch Intern Med 1991;151:1934–43.

164. Monreal M, Lafoz E, Ruiz J, et al. Upper-extremity deep venous thrombosis and pulmonary embolism. A prospective study. Chest 1991;99:280–3.

165. Horattas MC, Wright DJ, Fenton AH, et al. Changing concepts of deep venous thrombosis of the upper extremity—report of a series and review of the literature. Surgery 1988;104:561–7.

166. Joffe HV, Kucher N, Tapson VF, et al. Upper-extremity deep vein thrombosis: a prospective registry of 592 patients. Circulation 2004;110:1605—11.

167. Saleh T, Matta F, Yaekoub AY, et al. Risk of venous thromboembolism with inflammatory bowel disease. Clin Appl Thromb Hemost 2010. [Epub ahead of print].

168. Saleh T, Matta F, Alali F, et al. Liver disease and risk of venous thromboembolism. Submitted for publication.

169. Søgaard KK, Horváth-Puhó E, Grønbaek H, et al. Risk of venous thromboembolism in patients with liver disease: a nationwide population-based case-control study. Am J Gastroenterol 2009;104: 96—101.

170. Northup PG, McMahon MM, Ruhl AP, et al. Coagulopathy does not fully protect hospitalized cirrhosis patients from peripheral venous thromboembolism. Am J Gastroenterol 2006;101:1524—8.

171. Tripodi A, Primignani M, Chantarangkul V, et al. An imbalance of pro- vs anti-coagulation factors in plasma from patients with cirrhosis. Gastroenterology 2009;137:2105—11.

172. Danescu L, Badshah A, Danescu SC, et al. Venous thromboembolism in patients hospitalized with thyroid dysfunction. Clin Appl Thromb Hemost 2009;15:676—80.

173. Seriolo B, Accardo S, Garnero A, et al. Anticardiolipin antibodies, free protein S levels and thrombosis: a survey in a selected population of rheumatoid arthritis patients. Rheumatology 1999; 38:675—8.

174. McEntegart A, Capell HA, Creran D, et al. Cardiovascular risk factors, including thrombotic variables, in a population with rheumatoid arthritis. Rheumatology 2001;40:640—4.

175. Matta F, Singala R, Yaekoub AY, et al. Risk of venous thromboembolism with rheumatoid arthritis. Thromb Haemost 2009;101:134—8.

176. Stein PD, Goldman J, Matta F, et al. Diabetes mellitus and risk of venous thromboembolism. Am J Med Sic 2009;337:259—64.

177. Matta F, Yaekoub AY, Stein PD. Human immunodeficiency virus infection and risk of venous thromboembolism. Am J Med Sci 2008;336:402—6.

178. Kayali F, Najjar R, Aswad F, et al. Venous thromboembolism in patients hospitalized with nephrotic syndrome. Am J Med 2008;121:226—30.

179. Stein PD, Beemath A, Meyers FA, et al. Deep venous thrombosis and pulmonary embolism in patients hospitalized with sickle cell disease. Am J Med 2006;119:897—901.

180. Navarro S, Ricart JM, Medina P, et al. Activated protein C levels in Behçet's disease and risk of venous thrombosis. Br J Haematol 2004;126: 550—6.

181. Gül A, Ozbek U, Oztürk C, et al. Coagulation factor V gene mutation increases the risk of venous thrombosis in behçet's disease. Br J Rheumatol 1996;35:1178—80.

182. Ray JG, Burows RF, Ginsberg JS, et al. Paroxysmal nocturnal hemoglobinuria and the risk of venous thrombosis: review and recommendations for management of the pregnant and nonpregnant patient. Haemostasis 2000;30:103—17.

183. Fischer MD, Hopewell PC. Recurrent pulmonary emboli and Buerger's disease. West J Med 1981; 135:238—41.

Diagnosis: Use of Clinical Probability Algorithms

Esteban Gandara, MD[a,b], Philip S. Wells, MD, MSc[a,b],*

KEYWORDS

- Pulmonary embolism • Diagnosis • D-dimer
- Outcome assessment

Venous thromboembolism (VTE) is one of the most common cardiovascular diseases in industrialized countries, affecting 5% of the population during their lifetime.[1] If left undiagnosed, pulmonary embolism (PE) has a mortality ranging from 5% to 30%.[2,3] Approximately 22% of patients with PE die before a diagnosis is made.[1,4–6]

Evidence suggests that patients with suspected PE are managed better with a diagnostic strategy that includes clinical pretest probability assessment, D-dimer test, and/or imaging.[7,8] If algorithms are followed correctly, the chances of adverse events are extremely low (<1%) in patients in whom PE was ruled out.[8] The use of correct diagnostic approaches could affect mortality from PE, and the lack of an effect on mortality simply by the increased use of computed tomographic pulmonary angiography (CTPA) may speak further to the advantages of the algorithms.[7,9,10] Despite the overwhelming evidence, a recent study suggests that physicians prefer to use their clinical judgment and disregard the results of D-dimer test in favor of the use of CTPA.[11]

In this article, the authors explore the diagnostic issues faced by clinicians evaluating patients for suspected PE, concentrating on the role of initial clinical assessment and the use of clinical prediction rules combined with noninvasive testing for safely managing patients with suspected PE.

INITIAL ASSESSMENT

The initial assessment of a patient with a clinical picture suggestive of PE requires a careful medical history, physical examination, and in many cases a chest radiograph and electrocardiogram. The medical history should evaluate for risk factors and clinical symptoms of PE. A recent registry has shown that a constellation of 2 symptoms and 1 sign is typical in patients presenting with confirmed PE: chest pain, shortness of breath (SOB), and massive PE defined as shock or syncope.[12] The Prospective Investigative Study of Acute Pulmonary Embolism Diagnosis (PISA-PED) reported that 96% of the patients diagnosed with PE presented with acute SOB, chest pain, or fainting (alone or in combination) when compared with 59% of the patients without PE.[13] However, symptoms may be mild or even absent, particularly in patients with PE of only the segmental or subsegmental branches of the pulmonary artery.[14]

Risk factors have been reported in many studies, but a systematic review including data from 5997 patients reported that only cancer, recent surgery, and a history of deep vein thrombosis (DVT)/PE were associated with higher probabilities of having PE.[15] This study did not identify commonly considered risk factors (estrogen therapy, congestive heart failure, cardiac disease, major trauma, smoking, and pregnancy) as

a Thrombosis Program, Department of Medicine, Division of Hematology, The Ottawa Hospital and The University of Ottawa, Ottawa, Ontario, Canada
b Clinical Epidemiology Program, Ottawa Health Research Institute, Ottawa, Ontario, Canada
* Corresponding author. The Ottawa Hospital, General Campus LM 12, Box 206, 501 Smyth Road, Ottawa, Ontario K1H 8L6, Canada.
E-mail address: pwells@toh.on.ca

Clin Chest Med 31 (2010) 629–639
doi:10.1016/j.ccm.2010.07.002

significant risks, thus underscoring the importance of using tools that incorporate the interaction of several signs, symptoms, and risk factors as expanded in this article. Factors that are widely thought to be risks should be used in the overall clinical probability assessment, even though they are not individually predictive.

Physical examination is important despite the fact that it cannot confirm the diagnosis of PE, because it can help to identify other causes of the patient's symptoms and may provide a prognostic perspective if PE is confirmed.[16] Typical findings that were associated with an increased chance of PE included syncope, shock, leg swelling, and hemoptysis.[15,17] In one study, the presence of fever, crackles, and wheezes decreased the probability of PE.[17] Eliciting pain in the chest by palpation, without an obvious cause, is not associated with a lower prevalence of PE.[18] In patients older than 75 years, some risk factors, symptoms, and signs of VTE are less associated with PE, so caution is recommended when studying this group of patients.[19,20]

The role of chest radiography and electrocardiography in the diagnosis of PE is controversial because they have not shown specific diagnostic utility. However, these techniques can aid in the exclusion of other diagnostic findings (such as pneumonia, acute coronary syndrome, heart failure, septic shock, and atrial fibrillation) that can present with symptoms similar to PE. As such, the predominant role of chest radiography in the investigation of suspected PE is to exclude diagnostic findings that mimic PE and aid in the interpretation of the ventilation-perfusion (V/Q) scan.[21–24] The most common chest radiographic findings in patients with PE with no preexisting cardiac or pulmonary disease are atelectasis or parenchymal areas of increased opacity.[23] As discussed later, findings suggestive of other diagnoses reduce the chances of having PE when using the Wells criteria.

Electrocardiographic findings have not been proven to be directly useful in most clinical probability algorithms. The most common rhythm observed is the sinus rhythm. Abnormalities believed to be associated with PE, such as sinus tachycardia, incomplete right bundle branch block, complete right bundle branch block, $S_1Q_3T_3$ pattern, S_1Q_3 pattern, and extreme right axis deviation, occur with similar frequency in patients with or without PE.[25–27] Nonetheless, these findings present with PE and imply that PE should be part of the differential diagnosis. However, in general, electrocardiographic findings are most useful for suggesting an alternative diagnosis and indeed in some cases for suggesting a workup for PE, and

the application of a clinical probability algorithm should not be performed.[28–32]

CLINICAL PROBABILITY OF PE

Once the assessment is complete, clinicians should assign a pretest probability of PE to decide on the correct test to rule in or rule out PE. Bayes[33] theorem states that posttest odds equal the likelihood ratio of the test result multiplied by the pretest odds. The concept is that with a reasonably sensitive and specific test, the lower the pretest probability the more likely will a positive test result be falsely positive and with a high pretest probability the more likely will a negative test result be falsely negative. Concordant results (low probability and negative test result and positive test result with high pretest probability) are likely to be true. Hence, investigating patients with suspected PE requires an initial assessment of clinical probability to be made before diagnostic testing. The authors favor the use of clinical prediction rules over clinical gestalt as a tool for assigning a pretest probability. Clinical prediction rules are easy to use by less experienced physicians and allow a standardized approach to the diagnosis of the patient.[34]

CLINICAL PREDICTION RULES

To the authors' knowledge, several clinical prediction rules have been reported in the literature but only 4 have been validated prospectively. There are multiple differences between these rules, such as the ease of use, the requirements for complementary tests (chest radiography and measurement of blood gases and D dimer), the number of variables included, and the scoring systems used. All rules have limitations.

This review focuses on 4 of the rules that have been widely studied: the Geneva, the pulmonary embolism rule-out criteria (PERC), the PISA-PED, and the Wells models. Some of the clinical prediction rules and how they classify patients are presented in **Table 1**.

Geneva Model

The original model was derived from a sample of 1093 consecutive patients who presented with clinically suspected PE in an emergency department.[35] The prevalence of PE was 27%. The original rule, although effective, was complicated and required the evaluation of arterial blood gases. Two studies performed in emergency departments prospectively validated this rule combined with D-dimer measurement and imaging. When patients were stratified in the low- or intermediate-risk

Table 1
Most used clinical prediction rules and their variations

	Geneva Score	Modified/Simplified[a] Geneva Score	PERC	Traditional/Simplified[b] Wells Score
Variables	60–79 y (1 point) >80 y (2 points) Previous DVT or PE (2 points) Recent surgery, within 4 wk (3 points) HR>100 bpm (1 point) $Paco_2$ <35 mm Hg (2 points) 35–39 mm Hg (1 point) Pao_2 <49 mm Hg (4 points) 49–59 mm Hg (3 points) 60–71 mm Hg (2 points) 72–82 mm Hg (1 point) Chest radiograph findings Band atelectasis (1 point) Elevation of hemidiaphragm (1 point)	≥65 y (1 point) Previous DVT or PE (3 points) Surgery or fracture within 1 mo (2 points) Active malignant condition (2 points) Unilateral lower limb pain (3 points) Pain on deep palpation of lower limb and unilateral edema (4 points) Hemoptysis (2 points) HR 75 to 94 bpm (3 points) ≥95 bpm (5 points)	Hypoxia-Sao_2 <95% Unilateral leg swelling Hemoptysis Prior DVT or PE Recent surgery or trauma Age>50 y Hormone use Tachycardia	Clinically suspected DVT (3.0 points) Alternative diagnosis is less likely than PE (3.0 points) HR>100 bpm (1.5 points) Immobilization/surgery in previous 4 wk (1.5 points) History of DVT or PE (1.5 points) Hemoptysis (1.0 point) Malignancy (treatment within 6 mo, palliative, 1.0 point)
Categories	<5 points indicate a low probability of PE 5–8 points indicate a moderate probability of PE >8 points indicate a high probability of PE	Modified 0–3 points indicate low probability 4–10 points indicate intermediate probability 11 points or more indicate high probability Simplified <2 points, PE unlikely ≥3, PE likely	Absence of these variables classifies the patient as having a low risk of PE	Traditional interpretation Score >6.0, high 2.0–6.0, moderate <2.0, low Simplified Score >4, PE likely ≤4, PE unlikely Further simplified version[b] ≤1 point, PE unlikely

Abbreviations: bpm, beats per minute; HR, heart rate; Sao_2, arterial oxygen saturation.
[a] Simplified version assigns 1 point to each variable.
[b] Further simplified version assigns 1 point to each variable.

categories and had a negative result in a D-dimer test (nearly 30% of patients), no VTE events occurred in the 3-month follow-up period.[36,37]

Recently, the model was redesigned to avoid the need for evaluating arterial blood gases and chest radiography and to reduce the number of variables in the model. The score is composed of 8 variables (points): age more than 65 years (1 point), previous incidence of DVT or PE (3 points), surgery or fracture within 1 month (2 points), active malignant condition (2 points), unilateral lower limb pain (3 points), hemoptysis (2 points), heart rate of 75 to 94 beats per minute (3 points) or 95 beats per minute or more (5 points), and pain on lower-limb deep venous palpation and unilateral edema (4 points). In the validation set, the prevalence of PE was 8% in the low-probability category (0–3 points), 28% in the intermediate-probability category (4–10 points), and 74% in the high-probability category (>11 points). In a randomized controlled trial (RCT) that used this revised scoring scheme to stratify patients, 30% of the sample was included in the low-risk/intermediate-risk group and had a negative D-dimer test result. No VTE events occurred during 3 months of follow-up in these patients.[38] In patients with a positive D-dimer test result or a high probability of PE, a negative CTPA result ruled out PE with a VTE rate of 0.3% during follow-up.

In an effort to further simplify the model, a new scoring system has been evaluated retrospectively: 1 point is assigned to each variable. Patients with a score of 0 to 2 are categorized as unlikely to have PE and those with a score of 3 or more are categorized as likely to have PE. By this new scoring system, 64.9% of the patients were designated as unlikely with a 12.9% prevalence of PE and 35.1% were designated as likely with a 41.6% prevalence of PE. In this retrospective cohort analysis, none of the patients in the PE unlikely category with a negative D-dimer test result (30% of the sample) had a VTE event at 3 months of follow-up.[39]

Pulmonary Embolism Rule-out Criteria

PERC helps to assess patients in whom PE is suspected but is unlikely.[40,41] The PERC is designed to rule out the risk of PE when the physician has already stratified the patients into a low-risk category using a gestalt approach.

Patients in this low-risk category must have none of the following criteria to avoid further diagnostic tests for PE: (1) Sao_2 less than 95% at sea level, (2) unilateral leg swelling, (3) hemoptysis, (4) prior DVT or PE, (5) recent surgery or trauma, (6) age more than 50 years, (7) hormone use, and (8)

tachycardia.[42] The rule was prospectively validated in a cohort of 8138 patients from 13 emergency departments in the United States,[43] 85% of whom had a chief complaint of either dyspnea or chest pain. Clinicians reported a low suspicion for PE together with negative score in PERC in 20% of the sample. Within 45 days, 1% of the patients, in whom PE was ruled out and anticoagulant therapy was withheld, presented with VTE and only 1 patient died. The investigators concluded that clinicians could avoid ordering a D-dimer test on these patients but recommended that patients with risk factors, such as known thrombophilia or a strong family history of thrombosis, on β-blockers should undergo further diagnostic tests for acute PE.[43]

The PISA-PED Model

The PISA-PED rule was published in 2003, but this model does not seem to have been widely adopted perhaps because of its complexity and the 4 levels of probability of PE.[28,44] In this model, 15 variables are used: (1) male sex, (2) older age, (3) history of thrombophlebitis, (4) sudden-onset dyspnea, (5) chest pain, (6) hemoptysis, (7) electrocardiographic signs of acute right ventricular overload, (8) radiographic signs of oligemia, (9) amputation of the hilar artery, (10) pulmonary consolidation suggestive of infarction, (11) prior cardiovascular, (12) pulmonary disease, (13) high fever, (14) pulmonary consolidation other than infarction, and (15) pulmonary edema on the chest radiograph. With this model, 39% of the patients were rated as having a low probability of PE (4% prevalence of PE); 26%, intermediate probability (22% prevalence); 7%, moderately high probability (74% prevalence); and 28%, high probability (98% prevalence).[28,45] The same group of investigators has presented a new model derived mostly from an inpatient population with a PE prevalence of 41%. The model comprises 16 variables, of which 10 (older age, male sex, prolonged immobilization, history of DVT, sudden-onset dyspnea, chest pain, syncope, hemoptysis, unilateral leg swelling, and electrocardiographic signs of acute cor pulmonale) are positively associated and 6 (prior cardiovascular or pulmonary disease, orthopnea, high fever, wheezes, or crackles on chest auscultation) are negatively associated with PE.[17] Given the high prevalence of PE, which is not the norm in usual clinical practice, there is a concern that selection bias may affect the generalizability of this rule, and such prospective validation is required.

The Wells Model

The Wells model is one of the most validated and one of the easiest methods to use. This model uses only 7 clinical variables. The dichotomous version (PE likely or PE unlikely) has already been validated in 4 studies and has been shown to be as reliable as the original model.[46] More than 10,000 patients have been studied with the likely/unlikely version of the model (including randomized and outcomes studies). Less than 1% of the patients identified as PE unlikely who have a negative D-dimer test result and do not receive anticoagulants develop VTE within 90 days of evaluation. Patients with a positive D-dimer test result or classified as PE likely have a prevalence of PE ranging about 20%.[47–49] Moderate to substantial interrater agreement and reproducibility have been demonstrated in 3 studies.[50–52]

A recent meta-analysis that included 1660 consecutive patients (4 studies) determined the negative predictive value (NPV) of an "unlikely" score (≤ 4 points) combined with a negative D-dimer test result and the safety of withholding the use of anticoagulants based on these criteria.[46] The pooled 90-day incidence of VTE after initial exclusion of acute PE was 0.34%, resulting in an NPV of 99.7%. The risk for PE-related mortality was 0.06%. The investigators also reported that in up to 30% of the patients, no imaging would be needed.

The rule was further simplified by assigning 1 point to each variable and a cutoff of 1 point or less, providing a PE unlikely designation. The results showed that 30% of the patients could have PE ruled out by this score combined with a negative D-dimer test result.[53]

One objection raised about the Wells criteria is the need to consider an alternative diagnosis, with the criterion in the model being "PE is more likely than an alternative diagnosis." In one study, 61% of the patients were positive for this criterion, and this result was thought to be influenced by the presence of the other variables, with each point scored increasing the likelihood of scoring the "PE is more likely than an alternative diagnosis" variable by an odds ratio of 1.2. However, the same study demonstrated that this criterion had the second highest odds ratio, 4.6, of all the variables in the model.[54] It is clear that this variable plays a pivotal role in the assessment of PE, and as shown recently, having an alternative diagnosis reduces the chances of having a PE across all the categories of the Wells score.[54]

Comparison of Clinical Prediction Rules

At least 3 studies have compared the rules but none have performed a head-to-head comparison. In one retrospective comparison, the PERC rule, the unstructured assessment, and the Wells rule were found to perform similarly, but this result was derived retrospectively and the Wells rule was not applied in a prospective manner.[55] In a questionnaire survey, Iles and colleagues[56] published data suggesting that there might be better interrater agreement with the Geneva model than with the Wells model when they are used by inexperienced physicians. Another retrospective comparison suggested no predictive value for the original Geneva model and a reasonable predictive value for the Wells model, when they were predominantly used as a rule-out strategy.[45]

COMBINING CLINICAL PREDICTION RULES WITH DIAGNOSTIC TESTS

A negative D-dimer test result combined with a low- or intermediate-probability clinical assessment by clinical prediction rules excludes PE, if the D-dimer level is measured with an assay proved to have a sensitivity greater than 85%.[32,47,57–59] When the Wills rule is used, the 3-month risk of VTE is 0% to 0.5% in untreated patients with a negative D-dimer test result and an unlikely[46] or a low or intermediate clinical probability[37] Similar results have been reported with the Geneva rule and a gestalt approach, but data using gestalt approach are derived from very few patients and are limited as discussed later.[55,60] Exclusion by clinical probability assessment and D-dimer test spares the cost and radiation of an imaging evaluation in almost 30% to 40% of patients commonly evaluated for acute PE. However, the number needed to test with a D dimer, to rule out PE, is such that the utility and cost-effectiveness of D-dimer testing can be questioned in hospitalized patients, those older than 80 years, and patients with cancer.[20,61,62]

In patients with either a low or intermediate probability with an elevated D-dimer level or a high clinical probability, an imaging test should be performed. Currently acceptable approaches may include CTPA, V/Q scans, conventional pulmonary angiography, and bilateral lower extremity ultrasonography. If patients are hemodynamically stable and have no comorbidities that require hospitalization, imaging can be deferred safely for 24 hours, provided they are receiving therapeutic doses of low-molecular-weight heparin. This approach does not increase the risk of bleeding or death.[63,64] The authors follow this approach in most of the patients. The patients are seen at the authors' outpatient clinic within 24 hours, allowing them to decide between CTPA and V/Q scans.

The results of CTPA and V/Q scans are better interpreted in combination with clinical assessment based on a prediction rule. Positive results for intraluminal filling defects with high, intermediate or "likely" clinical pretest probability for PE have high positive predictive values for PE, and negative CTPA results have a high NPV.[65,66] Outcome studies that use pretest probability have shown that in patients categorized as PE unlikely with a positive D-dimer test result or as PE likely, the diagnosis of PE can be safely excluded by multi-row detector CTPA,[46,67,68] without the need of lower extremity ultrasonography when the CTPA result is negative.

However, the wide-scale adoption of CTPA has created new problems for physicians, such as overdiagnosis and false-positive studies.[69] A recent study of 322 patients with suspected PE assessed the influence of clinical probability on the false-positive rates for computed tomographic (CT) scans. Among the patients with a positive CT scan result who were treated for PE, 58% and 10% of the patients with low and moderate pretest probabilities, respectively, actually had false-positive results. Overall, up to 25% of all patients with a diagnosis of PE may have been treated inappropriately because of a false-positive result.[69] This mathematical fact is supported by a large accuracy study of CTPA (Prospective Investigation of Pulmonary Embolism Diagnosis

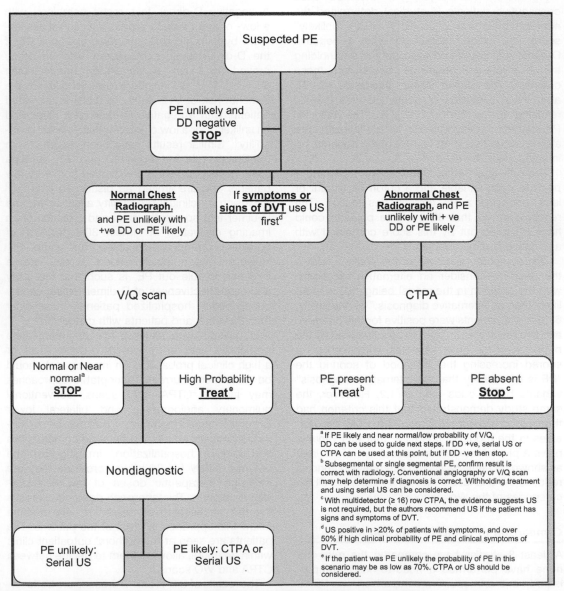

Fig. 1. Suggested approach combining clinical probabilities and diagnostic methods.

[PIOPED] II) that reported the positive predictive values for PE detected by CT scanners in the lobar, segmental, and subsegmental vessels to be 97%, 68%, and 25%, respectively.[66] The study used a composite end point as the reference standard to diagnose or rule out PE. The diagnosis of PE was confirmed by one of the following conditions: V/Q lung scanning showing a high probability of PE in a patient with no history of PE, abnormal findings on pulmonary digital subtraction angiography or on venous ultrasonography in a patient without previous DVT at that site, and nondiagnostic results on V/Q scanning. Furthermore, interobserver disagreement with pulmonary angiography was greatest for defects identified in subsegmental vessels, again raising doubt about the diagnosis if filling defects are limited to the subsegmental vessels on CTPA.[66,70]

Another noninvasive test that has been widely studied but does not seem to be widely used in clinical settings is alveolar dead space assessment. When combined with D-dimer test and clinical prediction rules, this noninvasive test may have merit.[29,71–75] In an RCT, a strategy composed of D-dimer test, alveolar dead space assessment, and the Wells model (in which PE is ruled out if 2 of the 3 tests are negative) was compared with V/Q scan.[29] The follow-up VTE event rate was 2.4% in the bedside test group versus 3.0% in the V/Q scan group (P = .76). PE was excluded in 34% of the bedside test group patients with at least 2 negative results on 3 bedside tests compared with 18% of the patients excluded using only the clinical model and the D-dimer test. In patients with an abnormal D-dimer test result, capnography alone does not exclude PE accurately, but in combination with a low clinical probability capnography can accurately exclude PE and could potentially avoid further testing in up to 30% of patients.[75] The main challenge for the adoption of this technique has been the need for specialized personnel to perform the measurements. New portable equipments using nose measurements of end-tidal CO_2 could make this technique widely available.

The implications are that the practicing physician has to consider the results of tests according to the clinical probability. As an example, high-probability V/Q scans or positive results on CTPA can be considered as diagnostic of PE if pretest probability is high or if the patient is categorized as PE likely but not when the pretest clinical probability is low or or the patient is PE unlikely (ie, single segmental or subsegmental findings on CTPA). In the latter case, the results should be reviewed with the radiologist to exclude a false-positive result. In this circumstance, confirmatory ultrasonography or conventional pulmonary angiography may be necessary or treatment may be withheld and serial lower extremity ultrasonography may be performed.[76]

The approach used by the authors in their clinical practice is presented in **Fig. 1**. Different use of methods or confirmation of results is based on the clinical probability assigned to each patient. However, when patients present with hypotension, the outlined approach in **Fig. 1** may not apply because of the need for urgent intervention. For considered approaches in this scenario, please see Fig. 2A in the article by Elliott and colleagues elsewhere in this issue.

SUMMARY

An effective and safe approach to the diagnosis of PE requires a clinical probability assessment and the correct diagnostic technique. Clinical probability assessment relies on medical history, careful physical examination, good-quality chest radiographs, and occasionally electrocardiograms. Physicians who are trained or experienced in the diagnosis of PE can decide the clinical probability based on their judgment. Some investigators advocate the use of a gestalt approach rather than the use of clinical prediction rules.[77,78] A systematic review showed that clinical gestalt approach and clinical prediction rules had a similar diagnostic accuracy.[34] It is advocated to use clinical prediction rules over gestalt approach because the rules can be used by less-experienced clinicians. The authors specifically recommend the use of the Geneva or Wells rules in their dichotomized versions. These 2 rules have been validated in randomized trials and outcomes studies and have been shown to be effective and safe to guide clinical decisions.

Some words of caution should be applied to the use of a gestalt approach for diagnosing PE:

1. Clinicians more often disagree on the pretest probability of PE.
2. Experience seems to influence the assessment.
3. Gestalt assessment tends to follow a middle road, often categorizing fewer patients in the useful categories such as high or low.
4. The methods used by each clinician are difficult to measure and categorize.
5. Most studies were conducted at centers with ample experience in the management of PE.
6. These centers use clinical prediction rules, making empirical judgment probably biased by the knowledge of clinical prediction rules, which may suggest that their judgment is not really gestalt. Other centers that have no

knowledge of, or experience with, prediction rules may perform less well but this has not been studied, making uncertain that the results of studies evaluating gestalt are widely applicable.

7. It is difficult or impossible to teach the gestalt approach.

There is evidence that physicians have difficulty complying with recommended diagnostic strategies and the lack of compliance results in worse outcomes.[7,11,79] A multicenter study showed that the diagnostic strategies used to diagnose PE were inappropriate in almost half of the cases studied, increasing the chances of missed VTE (7.7% vs 1.2%) and sudden death (5.7% vs 0.8%).[7] Furthermore, the D dimer–based strategies may be used incorrectly because the increased availability of rapid D-dimer assays might increase the number of patients tested for PE without showing an increasing number of patients diagnosed.[79] Emergency departments tend to perform better than inpatient services, diagnosing PE according to recommended guidelines.[80] Noncompliance with recommended diagnostic strategies might have other negative effects such as increase in cost, irradiation, or overdiagnosis of PE. Handheld clinical decision support tools may increase the safe use of diagnostic algorithms.[81]

To summarize, if a patient is categorized as low probability or PE unlikely and has a negative D-dimer test result, the chances of having subsequent VTE during 90 days of follow-up is approximately 0.5% and no imaging is needed. The remaining patients can be managed safely with a strategy based on CTPA or V/Q scans and serial ultrasonography as outlined in **Fig. 1**. If this stepwise approach is not used, physicians will overuse and misinterpret expensive diagnostic imaging tests, with a tendency to perform diagnostic tests for screening rather than for the diagnosis of PE.

REFERENCES

1. Spencer FA, Emery C, Lessard D, et al. A population-based study of the clinical epidemiology of venous thromboembolism. J Gen Intern Med 2006;21:722–7.

2. Stein PD, Henry JW, Relyea B. Untreated patients with pulmonary embolism. Outcome, clinical, and laboratory assessment. Chest 1995;107:931–5.

3. Dalen JE, Alpert JS. Natural history of pulmonary embolism. Prog Cardiovasc Dis 1975;17:259–70.

4. Heit JA, Silverstein MD, Mohr DN, et al. Risk factors for deep vein thrombosis and pulmonary embolism:

5. Heit JA, O'Fallon WM, Petterson TM, et al. Relative impact of risk factors for deep vein thrombosis and pulmonary embolism: a population-based study. Arch Intern Med 2002;162:1245–8.

6. Heit JA, Cohen AT, Anderson FA. Estimated annual number of incident and recurrent, non-fatal and fatal venous thromboembolism (VTE) events in the US [abstract]. Blood 2005;106:910.

7. Roy PM, Meyer G, Vielle B, et al. Appropriateness of diagnostic management and outcomes of suspected pulmonary embolism. Ann Intern Med 2006;144:157–64.

8. Roy PM, Colombet I, Durieux P, et al. Systematic review and meta-analysis of strategies for the diagnosis of suspected pulmonary embolism. BMJ 2005;331:259–68.

9. Park B, Messina L, Dargon P, et al. Recent trends in clinical outcomes and resource utilization for pulmonary embolism in the United States: findings from the nationwide inpatient sample. Chest 2009;136: 983–90.

10. Burge AJ, Freeman KD, Klapper PJ, et al. Increased diagnosis of pulmonary embolism without a corresponding decline in mortality during the CT era. Clin Radiol 2008;63:381–6.

11. Costantino MM, Randall G, Gosselin M, et al. CT angiography in the evaluation of acute pulmonary embolus. AJR Am J Roentgenol 2008;191:471–4.

12. Lobo JL, Zorrilla V, Aizpuru F, et al. Clinical syndromes and clinical outcome in patients with pulmonary embolism: findings from the RIETE registry. Chest 2006;130:1817–22.

13. Miniati M, Prediletto R, Formichi B, et al. Accuracy of clinical assessment in the diagnosis of pulmonary embolism. Am J Respir Crit Care Med 1999;159: 864–71.

14. Stein PD, Beemath A, Matta F, et al. Clinical characteristics of patients with acute pulmonary embolism: data from PIOPED II. Am J Med 2007;120:871–9.

15. West J, Goodacre S, Sampson F. The value of clinical features in the diagnosis of acute pulmonary embolism: systematic review and meta-analysis. QJM 2007;100:763–9.

16. Aujesky D, Roy PM, Le Manach CP, et al. Validation of a model to predict adverse outcomes in patients with pulmonary embolism. Eur Heart J 2006;27: 476–81.

17. Miniati M, Bottai M, Monti S, et al. Simple and accurate prediction of the clinical probability of pulmonary embolism. Am J Respir Crit Care Med 2008; 178:290–4.

18. Le Gal G, Testuz A, Righini M, et al. Reproduction of chest pain by palpitation: diagnostic accuracy in suspected pulmonary embolism. BMJ 2005; 330:452–3.

a population-based case-control study. Arch Intern Med 2000;160:809–15.

19. Righini M, Le Gal G, Perrier A, et al. The challenge of diagnosing pulmonary embolism in elderly patients: influence of age on commonly used diagnostic tests and strategies. J Am Geriatr Soc 2005;53:1039–45.

20. Righini M, Nendaz M, Le Gal G, et al. Influence of age on the cost-effectiveness of diagnostic strategies for suspected pulmonary embolism. J Thromb Haemost 2007;5:1869–77.

21. Bergus GR, Barloon TS, Kahn D. An approach to diagnostic imaging of suspected pulmonary embolism. Am Fam Physician 1996;53:1259–66.

22. Rissanen V, Suomalainen O, Karjalainen P, et al. Screening for postoperative pulmonary embolism on the basis of clinical symptomatology, routine electrocardiography and plain chest radiography. Acta Med Scand 1984;215:13–9.

23. Stein PD, Terrin ML, Hales CA, et al. Clinical, laboratory, roentgenographic, and electrocardiographic findings in patients with acute pulmonary embolism and no pre-existing cardiac or pulmonary disease. Chest 1991;100:598–603.

24. Stein PD, Alavi A, Gottschalk A, et al. Usefulness of noninvasive diagnostic tools for diagnosis of acute pulmonary embolism in patients with a normal chest radiograph. Am J Cardiol 1991;67:1117–20.

25. Fruergaard P, Launbjerg J, Hesse B. Frequency of pulmonary embolism in patients admitted with chest pain and suspicion of acute myocardial infarction but in whom this diagnosis is ruled out. Cardiology 1996;87:331–4.

26. Rodger MA, Makropoulos D, Turek M, et al. Diagnostic value of the electrocardiogram in suspected pulmonary embolism. Am J Cardiol 2000;86:807–9.

27. Stein PD, Dalen JE, McIntyre KM, et al. The electrocardiogram in acute pulmonary embolism. Prog Cardiovasc Dis 1975;17:247–57.

28. Miniati M, Monti S, Bauleo C, et al. A diagnostic strategy for pulmonary embolism based on standardised pretest probability and perfusion lung scanning: a management study. Eur J Nucl Med Mol Imaging 2003;30:1450–6.

29. Rodger MA, Bredeson CN, Jones G, et al. The bedside investigation of pulmonary embolism diagnosis study: a double-blind randomized controlled trial comparing combinations of 3 bedside tests vs ventilation-perfusion scan for the initial investigation of suspected pulmonary embolism. Arch Intern Med 2006;166:181–7.

30. Wells PS, Ginsberg JS, Anderson DR, et al. Use of a clinical model for safe management of patients with suspected pulmonary embolism. Ann Intern Med 1998;129:997–1005.

31. Wells PS, Hirsh J, Anderson DR, et al. A simple clinical model for the diagnosis of deep-vein thrombosis combined with impedance plethysmography: potential for an improvement in the diagnostic process. J Intern Med 1998;243:15–23.

32. Wells PS, Anderson DR, Rodger MA, et al. Derivation of a simple clinical model to categorize patients probability of pulmonary embolism: increasing the models utility with the SimpliRED D-dimer. Thromb Haemost 2000;83:416–20.

33. Bayes T. An essay towards solving a problem in the doctrine of chances. Philos Trans R Soc Lond 1763; 53:370–418.

34. Chunilal SD, Eikelboom JW, Attia J, et al. Does this patient have pulmonary embolism? JAMA 2003; 290:2849–58.

35. Wicki J, Perneger TV, Junod AF, et al. Assessing clinical probability of pulmonary embolism in the emergency ward: a simple score. Arch Intern Med 2001;161:92–7.

36. Perrier A, Roy P-M, Aujesky D, et al. Diagnosing pulmonary embolism in outpatients with clinical assessment, D-dimer measurement, venous ultrasound, and helical computed tomography: a multicenter management study. Am J Med 2004;116: 291–9.

37. Perrier A, Roy PM, Sanchez O, et al. Multidetector-row computed tomography in suspected pulmonary embolism. N Engl J Med 2005;352:1760–8.

38. Righini M, Le Gal G, Aujesky D, et al. Diagnosis of pulmonary embolism by multidetector CT alone or combined with venous ultrasonography of the leg: a randomised non-inferiority trial. Lancet 2008;371: 1343–52.

39. Klok FA, Mos IC, Nijkeuter M, et al. Simplification of the revised Geneva score for assessing clinical probability of pulmonary embolism. Arch Intern Med 2008;168:2131–6.

40. Kline JA, Mitchell AM, Kabrhel C, et al. Clinical criteria to prevent unnecessary diagnostic testing in emergency department patients with suspected pulmonary embolism. J Thromb Haemost 2004;2: 1247–55.

41. Kline JA, Nelson RD, Jackson RE, et al. Criteria for the safe use of D-dimer testing in emergency department patients with suspected pulmonary embolism: a multicenter US study. Ann Emerg Med 2002;39:144–52.

42. Hogg K, Dawson D, Kline J. Application of pulmonary embolism rule-out criteria to the UK Manchester Investigation of Pulmonary Embolism Diagnosis (MIOPED) study cohort. J Thromb Haemost 2005; 3:592–3.

43. Kline JA, Courtney DM, Kabhel C, et al. Prospective multicenter evaluation of the pulmonary embolism rule-out criteria. J Thromb Haemost 2008;6:772–80.

44. Miniati M, Monti S, Bottai M. A structured clinical model for predicting the probability of pulmonary embolism. Am J Med 2003;114:173–9.

45. Miniati M, Bottai M, Monti S. Comparison of 3 clinical models for predicting the probability of pulmonary embolism. Medicine (Baltimore) 2005;84:107–14.

46. Pasha SM, Klok FA, Snoep JD, et al. Safety of excluding acute pulmonary embolism based on an unlikely clinical probability by the Wells rule and normal D-dimer concentration: a meta-analysis. Thromb Res 2010;125:e123–7.

47. van Belle A, Buller HR, Huisman MV, et al. Effectiveness of managing suspected pulmonary embolism using an algorithm combining clinical probability, D-dimer testing, and computed tomography. JAMA 2006;295:172–9.

48. Goekoop RJ, Steeghs N, Niessen RW, et al. Simple and safe exclusion of pulmonary embolism in outpatients using quantitative D-dimer and Wells' simplified decision rule. Thromb Haemost 2007;97:146–50.

49. Anderson DR, Kahn SR, Rodger MA, et al. Computed tomographic pulmonary angiography vs ventilation-perfusion lung scanning in patients with suspected pulmonary embolism: a randomized controlled trial. JAMA 2007;298:2743–53.

50. Wolf SJ, McCubbin TR, Feldhaus KM, et al. Prospective validation of Wells Criteria in the evaluation of patients with suspected pulmonary embolism. Ann Emerg Med 2004;44:503–10.

51. Rodger MA, Maser E, Stiell I, et al. The interobserver reliability of pretest probability assessment in patients with suspected pulmonary embolism. Thromb Res 2005;116:101–7.

52. Penaloza A, Mélot C, Dochy E, et al. Assessment of pretest probability of pulmonary embolism in the emergency department by physicians in training using the Wells model. Thromb Res 2007;120:173–9.

53. Gibson NS, Sohne M, Gerdes VE, et al. Further validation and simplification of the Wells clinical decision rule in pulmonary embolism. Thromb Haemost 2008;99:229–34.

54. Testuz A, Le Gal G, Righini M, et al. Influence of specific alternative diagnoses on the probability of pulmonary embolism. Thromb Haemost 2006;95:958–62.

55. Kline JA, Runyon MS, Webb WB, et al. Prospective study of the diagnostic accuracy of the Simplify D-dimer assay for pulmonary embolism in emergency department patients. Chest 2006;129:1417–23.

56. Iles S, Hodges AM, Darley JR, et al. Clinical experience and pre-test probability scores in the diagnosis of pulmonary embolism. QJM 2003;96:211–5.

57. Wells PS, Anderson DR, Rodger MA, et al. Excluding pulmonary embolism at the bedside without diagnostic imaging: management of patients with suspected pulmonary embolism presenting to the emergency department by using a simple clinical model and D-dimer. Ann Intern Med 2001;135:98–107.

58. Stein PD, Hull RD, Patel KC, et al. D-dimer for the exclusion of acute venous thrombosis and pulmonary embolism. A systematic review. Ann Intern Med 2004;140:589–602.

59. Righini M, Aujesky D, Roy PM, et al. Clinical usefulness of D-dimer depending on clinical probability and cutoff value in outpatients with suspected pulmonary embolism. Arch Intern Med 2004;164:2483–7.

60. Carrier M, Righini M, Djurabi RK, et al. VIDAS D-dimer in combination with clinical pre-test probability to rule out pulmonary embolism. A systematic review of management outcome studies. Thromb Haemost 2009;101:886–92.

61. Le Gal G, Righini M, Roy PM, et al. Differential value of risk factors and clinical signs for diagnosing pulmonary embolism according to age. J Thromb Haemost 2005;3:2457–64.

62. Di Nisio M, Sohne M, Kamphuisen PW, et al. D-dimer test in cancer patients with suspected acute pulmonary embolism. J Thromb Haemost 2005;3:1239–42.

63. Siragusa S, Anastasio R, Porta C, et al. Deferment of objective assessment of deep vein thrombosis and pulmonary embolism without increased risk of thrombosis: a practical approach based on the pretest clinical model, D-dimer testing, and the use of low-molecular-weight heparins. Arch Intern Med 2004;164:2477–82.

64. Bauld DL, Kovacs MJ. Dalteparin in emergency patients to prevent admission prior to investigation for venous thromboembolism. Am J Emerg Med 1999;17:11–4.

65. Hayashino Y, Goto M, Noguchi Y, et al. Ventilation-perfusion scanning and helical CT in suspected pulmonary embolism: meta-analysis of diagnostic performance. Radiology 2005;234:740–8.

66. Stein PD, Fowler SE, Goodman LR, et al. Multidetector computed tomography for acute pulmonary embolism. N Engl J Med 2006;354:2317–27.

67. Ghanima W, Almaas V, Aballi S, et al. Management of suspected pulmonary embolism (PE) by D-dimer and multi-slice computed tomography in outpatients: an outcome study. J Thromb Haemost 2005;3:1926–32.

68. Stein PD, Sostman HD, Bounameaux H, et al. Challenges in the diagnosis acute pulmonary embolism. Am J Med 2008;121:565–71.

69. Ranji SR, Shojania KG, Trowbridge RL, et al. Impact of reliance on CT pulmonary angiography on diagnosis of pulmonary embolism: a Bayesian analysis. J Hosp Med 2006;1:81–7.

70. Stein PD, Henry JW, Gottschalk A. Reassessment of pulmonary angiography for the diagnosis of pulmonary embolism: relation of interpreter agreement to the order of the involved pulmonary arterial branch. Radiology 1999;210:689–91.

71. Rodger MA, Jones G, Raymond F, et al. Dead space ventilation parallels changes in scintigraphic

vascular obstruction at recurrence of pulmonary embolism and after thrombolytic therapy: a case report. Can Respir J 1998;5:215–8.

72. Rodger MA, Jones G, Djunaedi H, et al. Interobserver reliability of alveolar dead space measurements in suspected pulmonary embolism. Can J Respir Ther 2004;40:24–30.

73. Rodger MA, Jones G, Rasuli P, et al. Steady-state end-tidal alveolar dead space fraction and D-dimer: bedside tests to exclude pulmonary embolism. Chest 2001;120:115–9.

74. Kline JA, Israel EG, Michelson EA, et al. Diagnostic accuracy of a bedside D-dimer assay and alveolar dead-space measurement for rapid exclusion of pulmonary embolism: a multicenter study. JAMA 2001;285:761–8.

75. Sanchez O, Wermert D, Faisy C, et al. Clinical probability and alveolar dead space measurement for suspected pulmonary embolism in patients with an abnormal D-dimer test result. J Thromb Haemost 2006;4:1517–22.

76. Wells PS. Pulmonary embolism: a clinician's perspective. Semin Nucl Med 2008;38:404–11.

77. Kabrhel C, Camargo CA Jr, Goldhaber SZ. Clinical gestalt and the diagnosis of pulmonary embolism: does experience matter? Chest 2005;127: 1627–30.

78. Kabrhel C, McAfee AT, Goldhaber SZ. The contribution of the subjective component of the Canadian Pulmonary Embolism Score to the overall score in emergency department patients. Acad Emerg Med 2005;12:915–20.

79. Corwin MT, Donohoo JH, Partridge R, et al. Do emergency physicians use serum D-dimer effectively to determine the need for CT when evaluating patients for pulmonary embolism? Review of 5,344 consecutive patients. AJR Am J Roentgenol 2009;192: 1319–23.

80. Arnason T, Wells PS, Forster AJ. Appropriateness of diagnostic strategies for evaluating suspected venous thromboembolism. Thromb Haemost 2007; 97:195–201.

81. Roy PM, Durieux P, Gillaizeau F, et al. A computerized handheld decision-support system to improve pulmonary embolism diagnosis: a randomized trial. Ann Intern Med 2010;151:677–86.

Diagnosis: Imaging Techniques

C. Gregory Elliott, MD[a,b,*], Todd D. Lovelace, MD[c],
Lynette M. Brown, MD, PhD[a,b], Daniel Adams, MD[a]

KEYWORDS

- Deep vein thrombosis • Venous thromboembolism
- Pulmonary embolus • Computed tomography
- Ultrasonography • Radiation

The diagnostic evaluation of suspected acute deep vein thrombosis (DVT) (**Fig. 1**) or pulmonary embolism (PE) (**Fig. 2**) requires integration of clinical probability,[1–6] D-dimer test results (when appropriate), and the interpretation of imaging procedures.[7] Although this article focuses on imaging procedures, they are only the last step in an integrated diagnostic approach. For example, studies have shown that DVT can be excluded safely without imaging in approximately 1 of every 2 patients with a clinically suspected first episode of acute DVT, based on a low or moderate clinical probability score and a negative D-dimer test.[8] Similar outcome studies have shown that the diagnosis of acute PE can be excluded safely for approximately 1 of 3 patients based on a low clinical probability score and a negative D-dimer test result[9] (see article by Gandara and Wells in this issue). On the other hand, immediate imaging with either computed tomography pulmonary angiography (CTPA) or echocardiography is recommended for patients who present at high risk for death with shock or hypotension and possible acute PE.[10,11]

CHEST RADIOGRAPHY

Chest radiographs are basic imaging studies for the evaluation of cardiopulmonary disorders. Although chest radiographs have low sensitivity and specificity for the diagnosis of acute PE, they can be integral to the clinician's formulation of the probability that PE underlies cardiopulmonary symptoms.[12] Interpretation of the chest radiograph can influence the decision to perform additional diagnostic tests for PE.[6,13,14]

Patients with acute PE may have a normal chest radiograph or a variety of abnormalities (**Table 1**). Cardiomegaly is a common abnormality. However, findings of cardiomegaly and pulmonary artery enlargement on chest radiographs do not predict the echocardiographic finding of right ventricular

Funding: None.

Disclosure: Dr Elliott certifies that he has no relationship including consultation, paid speaking, grant support, equity, patents or royalties from any company that makes products relevant to this manuscript. Dr Lovelace certifies that he has no relationship including consultation, paid speaking, grant support, equity, patents or royalties from any company that makes products relevant to this manuscript. Dr Brown certifies that she has no relationship including consultation, paid speaking, grant support, equity, patents or royalties from any company that makes products relevant to this manuscript. Dr Adams certifies that he has no relationship including consultation, paid speaking, grant support, equity, patents or royalties from any company that makes products relevant to this manuscript.

[a] Department of Medicine, Intermountain Medical Center, 5121 South Cottonwood Street, Suite 307, Murray, UT 84107, USA
[b] Department of Medicine, University of Utah School of Medicine, 30 North 1900 East, Room 4C104, Salt Lake City, UT 84132-2406, USA
[c] Department of Radiology, Intermountain Medical Center, 5121 South Cottonwood Street, Suite 307, Murray, UT 84107, USA
* Corresponding author. Department of Medicine, Intermountain Medical Center, 5121 South Cottonwood Street, Suite 307, Murray, UT 84107.
E-mail address: Greg.Elliott@imail.org

Clin Chest Med 31 (2010) 641–657
doi:10.1016/j.ccm.2010.06.002

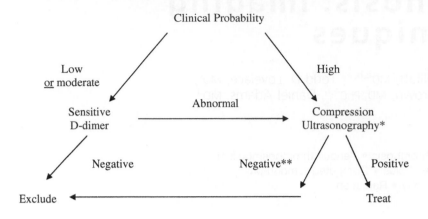

Fig. 1. One possible diagnostic algorithm for the evaluation of nonpregnant patients with a suspected first episode of DVT. The first step is an assessment of the clinical probability that the patient has DVT. The use of D-dimer tests and compression ultrasonography (CUS) follows. Anticoagulants can be withheld safely for most patients with low or moderate pretest probability and a negative sensitive D-dimer test, and for most patients with a negative whole-leg CUS examination or negative 2-point (groin and popliteal fossa) CUS examinations performed 5 to 7 days apart.

(RV) hypokinesis (**Table 2**),[15] a marker of increased mortality in the setting of acute PE.[16] Uncommon abnormalities include focal oligemia[17] or a homogeneous wedge-shaped density in a peripheral lung zone with a rounded apex pointed toward the hilum (**Fig. 3**).[18,19]

COMPRESSION ULTRASONOGRAPHY
Techniques

Compression ultrasonography (CUS) is the preferred technique to evaluate suspected acute DVT. CUS involves identification and compression of deep veins.[20] Noncompressibility of a venous segment strongly suggests the presence of venous thrombus, although false-positive tests may occur.[21] Acute venous thrombus is often associated with slight expansion of the involved vein. An absence of color flow Doppler signal and lack of venous spectral waveform are additional findings of venous thrombus (**Fig. 4**).

Investigators have applied 2 CUS techniques to assess suspected DVT.[22] The first, known as the 2-point technique, examines only proximal venous segments in the groin and the popliteal fossa. The second technique, whole-leg CUS, examines deep veins at 1- to 2-cm intervals from the groin

to the ankle.[20,23] The common femoral vein and the popliteal vein are imaged and compressed firmly in the 2-point technique. This technique relies on the high sensitivity and specificity of CUS for proximal DVT, but does not detect calf thrombi, which may propagate proximally when anticoagulants are withheld.[24] Therefore, clinical practice guidelines require a repeat 2-point examination 5 to 7 days after a negative 2-point examination, to exclude proximal propagation of undetected calf DVT.[25–27] Whole-leg CUS examines deep veins at 1- to 2-cm intervals from the iliac veins to the deep veins at the ankle and may exclude or confirm DVT with a single examination.[20,23–28]

Diagnostic Sensitivity and Specificity

Compression ultrasonography is highly sensitive (96%) and specific (98%) for diagnosing proximal DVT when applied to patients with symptoms and signs of acute DVT.[29–31] Compression ultrasonography is less sensitive (87%) for detecting symptomatic DVT limited to the calf veins.[31] In contrast, in asymptomatic high-risk patients (eg, patients who have had total hip or knee arthroplasty) CUS is insensitive (62%) for diagnosing proximal DVT[32–35] and is even less sensitive

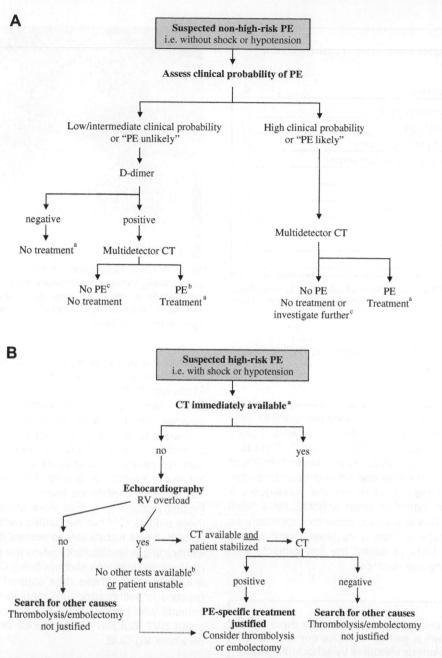

Fig. 2. (*A*) Proposed diagnostic algorithm for patients with suspected non–high-risk PE (ie, without shock and hypotension). Two alternative classification schemes may be used to assess clinical probability: a 3-level scheme (clinical probability low, intermediate, or high) or a 2-level scheme (PE unlikely or PE likely). When using a moderately sensitive assay, D-dimer measurement should be restricted to patients with a low clinical probability or a PE unlikely classification; highly sensitive assays may be used in patients with a low or intermediate clinical probability of PE. Plasma D-dimer measurement is of limited use in suspected PE occurring in postoperative or hospitalized patients. [a]Anticoagulant treatment of PE. [b]Multidetector CT is considered diagnostic of PE if the most proximal thrombosis is at least segmental. [c]If multidetector CT is negative in patients with high clinical probability, further investigation may be considered before withholding PE-specific treatment. (*Modified from* Torbicki A, Perrier A, Konstantinides S, et al. Guidelines on the diagnosis and management of acute pulmonary embolism: the Task Force for the Diagnosis and Management of Acute Pulmonary Embolism of the European Society of Cardiology (ESC). Eur Heart J 2008;29(18):2276–315.) (*B*) Proposed diagnostic algorithm for patients with suspected high-risk PE; ie, presenting with shock or hypotension. [a]CT is considered not immediately available if the critical condition of a patient allows only bedside diagnostic tests. [b]Transesophageal echocardiography may detect thrombi in the pulmonary arteries in many patients with RV overload; confirmation of DVT with bedside CUS may also guide decision making.

Table 1
Radiographic abnormalities associated with acute PE

Abnormalities	%
Cardiac enlargement	27
Pleural effusion	23
Elevated hemidiaphragm	20
Pulmonary artery enlargement	19
Atelectasis	18
Infiltrate	17
Pulmonary congestion	14
Oligemia	8
Pulmonary infarction	5
Overinflation	5

Data from Elliott CG, Goldhaber SZ, Visani L, et al. Chest radiographs in acute pulmonary embolism. Chest 2000;118(1):33–8.

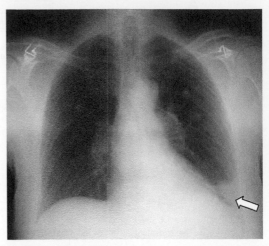

Fig. 3. A chest radiograph demonstrates a pleural-based, wedge-shaped pulmonary infarction (Hampton hump) at the left lung base (arrow). There was focal avascularity (Westermark lesion) in the right upper lung field.

(40%) in identifying asymptomatic DVT limited to the calf veins.[31]

Clinical Outcomes

Multiple studies have examined the safety of withholding anticoagulants after 2 negative 2-point CUS examinations 5 to 7 days apart.[36–38] In these studies, investigators found that fewer than 3% of consecutive patients had venous thromboembolism (VTE) diagnosed during the subsequent 3 months of follow-up when anticoagulants were withheld. This is a widely accepted approach; its disadvantage is that it requires many normal follow-up tests to detect the few patients with propagating calf thrombi.

Table 2
Cardiac enlargement identified by chest radiograph is neither sensitive nor specific for RV hypokinesis identified by echocardiography

Chest Radiograph[a]	RV Hypokinesis	No RV Hypokinesis
Cardiac enlargement, n	149	178
No cardiac enlargement, n	160	307

[a] Estimated sensitivity, 48% (95% CI 42%–54%); estimated specificity, 63% (95% CI 59%–67%); estimated positive predictive value, 46% (95% CI 40%–51%); estimated negative predictive value, 66% (95% CI 61%–70%).
Data from Elliott CG, Goldhaber SZ, Visani L, et al. Chest radiographs in acute pulmonary embolism. Chest 2000;118(1):33–8.

Several studies have examined the safety of withholding anticoagulants based on a negative whole-leg CUS.[22,23,39–43] A recent meta-analysis[28] reported 3-month outcomes for 4731 patients who had anticoagulants withheld after whole-leg CUS was performed for clinically suspected symptomatic DVT. Only 34 (0.7%) of these patients developed documented VTE during the follow-up period, a pooled incidence rate of 0.57% (95% confidence interval [CI] 0.25–0.89). Pretest probability scores were available in 2 of these studies,[23,42] but the pooled data from these 2 studies was insufficient to ensure the safety of withholding anticoagulants when the pretest clinical probability is high and whole-leg CUS is negative (Table 3).[28] These data support the current practice of withholding anticoagulants for most patients who present with symptoms or signs of acute DVT, but have no evidence of DVT found on whole-leg CUS.

COMPUTED TOMOGRAPHY

CTPA has replaced ventilation and perfusion lung scanning as the principal imaging modality for evaluating suspected PE.[10,44]

Techniques

CTPA combines high-speed intravenous iodinated contrast injection timed for pulmonary artery enhancement with helical CT acquisition of images through the thorax. During a typical CTPA, contrast material containing organically bound iodine is administered at a rate of 4 to 6 mL per

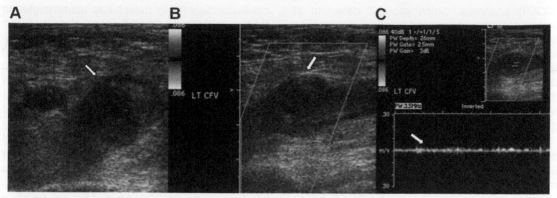

Fig. 4. Ultrasound findings of acute DVT. (*A*) Echogenic thrombus in the left common femoral vein (*arrow*). (*B*) Color Doppler image shows no color flow in the left common femoral vein (*arrow*). (*C*) Spectral waveform demonstrates lack of venous flow (*arrow*).

second through an 18- or 20-gauge intravenous line in the antecubital fossa. Depending on scanner technology and manufacturer, anywhere from 60 mL to 120 mL of intravenous contrast may be administered.

Matching the timing of the scan acquisition to peak pulmonary artery enhancement is critical to the quality of the examination and is achieved by one of several means. Many centers use a standard delay of approximately 15 seconds, theorizing this is an average time for contrast to opacify the pulmonary vessels before scan acquisitions. A more precise method of timing uses a timing bolus. A small bolus of 15 to 20 mL intravenous contrast is infused while cinegraphic imaging of the main pulmonary artery is performed, documenting the passage of contrast

through the pulmonary circulation. The information from the preprocedure timing bolus scan is used to calculate the specific time delay for the diagnostic CTPA. Use of bolus tracking software is a method whereby a nonenhanced image through the main pulmonary artery is obtained and a small region of interest is drawn within the pulmonary artery. During intravenous contrast infusion, cinegraphic imaging of the main pulmonary artery is performed and computer software tracks changes in pulmonary artery attenuation within this region. The CTPA scan is either manually or automatically triggered when pulmonary artery enhancement reaches an appropriate threshold. This procedure can be problematic for morbidly obese patients.

Helical CT technology improved substantially with the introduction of multidetector row CT

Table 3
Individual and pooled VTE incidence rates for pretest probability cohorts

Pretest Probability Cohort[a]	Stevens et al,[23] 2004			Sevestre et al,[42] 2009			Pooled VTE Incidence Rates[b]
	Patients (n)	VTE Events (n)	Incidence Rate % (95% CI)	Patients (n)	VTE Events (n)	Incidence Rate % (95% CI)	Incidence Rate % (95% CI)
Low	157	0	0.00 (0.00–2.32)	914	3	0.33 (0.07–0.96)	0.29 (0.00–0.70)
Moderate	180	2	1.11 (0.14–3.96)	287	2	0.70 (0.08–2.49)	0.82 (0.00–1.83)
High	38	1	2.63 (0.07–13.81)	42	1	2.38 (0.06–12.57)	2.49 (0.00–7.11)
Totals	375	3	NA	1243	6	NA	NA

Abbreviation: NA, not applicable.
[a] Pretest probability scores assessed by the method of Wells et al.[116]
[b] Calculated using the exact binomial method and random effects model.
Data from Johnson SA, Stevens SM, Woller SC, et al. Risk of deep vein thrombosis following a single negative whole-leg compression ultrasound: a systematic review and meta-analysis. JAMA 2010;303:438–45.

(MDCT) scanners, which allowed detection of emboli in the segmental and subsegmental branches of the pulmonary arterial tree with greater sensitivity, specificity, and overall accuracy.[7,45] MDCT scanners provide increased coverage of the thorax in fewer CT gantry rotations, thereby decreasing scan times and reducing motion artifacts. Current scanners using up to 320 rows of detectors can decrease radiation exposure.

Many current CT scanners cannot accommodate some morbidly obese patients. For example, both Toshiba Aquilon 64 and GE Light Speed models list a maximum patient weight of 205 kg. However, some scanners (eg, Aquilon Premium CT system, Toshiba) have increased capacity (300 kg maximum).

Interpretation

Interpretation of CTPA requires skill and experience, as multiple findings may be observed (**Fig. 5**).

Imaging findings documenting the presence of acute PE include a pulmonary artery filling defect that completely occludes the arterial branch, often resulting in slight expansion of the branch. A partial intraluminal filling defect may also be present, with one of several imaging appearances. When the vessel is imaged perpendicular to the lumen, a nonocclusive embolism may appear as a central low density surrounded by bright contrast resulting in the so-called polo mint sign, because of its close resemblance to a popular breath mint with a hole in the middle. If the partially occlusive central filling defect is imaged in the longitudinal plane, a railway track sign is noted as parallel lines of high density contrast surround the embolism. When an acute nonocclusive embolism is more eccentric within the vessel lumen, the corresponding filling defect has acute angles in relation to the vessel wall.[46]

Associated lung parenchymal and pleural findings, although not diagnostic, can raise suspicion for the presence of acute PE. Peripheral wedge-shaped areas of consolidation often represent areas of pulmonary infarction. If the opacity is more ground glass in appearance, an area of parenchymal hemorrhage or early infarction is suggested. Linear areas of atelectasis and pleural effusion may also be noted. The presence of a dilated right ventricle, reflux of contrast into the inferior vena cava and hepatic veins, and interventricular septum deviated toward the left ventricle are findings that indicate RV strain.[47]

CT scanning is subject to several potential artifacts and pitfalls that may mimic PE. Dense contrast in the superior vena cava may cause a beam-hardening artifact, which can result in an artificial low attenuation within the lumen of adjacent pulmonary artery branches. Respiratory motion and motion from left ventricular contraction can cause partial volume artifacts from imaging the pulmonary vessel and an adjacent structure of different density in the same voxel. Partial volume artifacts between pulmonary artery branches and adjacent bronchioles, lymph nodes, pulmonary veins, and mucus-plugged airways may simulate acute PE. Vascular flow-related phenomena, such as laminar flow (slower blood flow along the vessel wall compared with the central lumen) and transient interruption of the contrast bolus (nonopacified blood from the inferior vena cava mixes with opacified blood in the right heart during inspiration) can be mistaken for emboli.

Diagnostic Accuracy

Accuracy studies aim to establish the sensitivity and specificity of a test by comparing the test

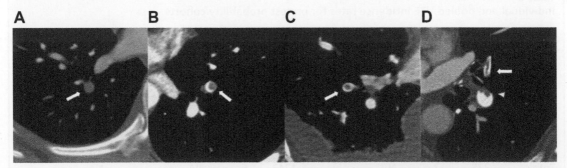

Fig. 5. Findings of acute PE on CTPA. (*A*) Occluded pulmonary artery with low attenuation filling defect slightly expanding the vessel (*arrow*). (*B*) Partially occluding eccentric low attenuation filling defect demonstrating acute angle with adjacent pulmonary artery wall (*arrow*). (*C*) Polo mint sign. Central low attenuation filling defect surrounded by contrast (*arrow*). (*D*) Railway car sign. Linear low attenuation filling defect surrounded by contrast (*arrow*). Also demonstrated is a partially occluding low attenuation filling defect having acute angles with adjacent vessel wall (*arrowhead*).

results with a diagnostic gold standard.[10] The second prospective investigation of PE diagnosis reported that MDCT pulmonary angiography (MDCTPA) had a sensitivity of 83% and a specificity of 96% for venous thromboembolism (including DVT found on ultrasound in the setting of a negative CTPA).[48,49] This study underscored the importance of combining the imaging results with the clinical assessment for management decisions (**Table 4**). The investigators concluded that additional testing was necessary when the clinical probability and the imaging results were discordant.

Contraindications

Relative contraindications to CTPA include reduced renal function or a history of iodine allergy. A recent multicenter study of CTPA for the diagnosis of acute PE excluded patients with abnormal serum creatinine levels.[48]

Risks: Radiation Exposure

Exposure to high-dose ionizing radiation is associated with the development of solid cancers and leukemia,[50] and recent evidence suggests that commonly performed medical imaging with ionizing radiation can expose patients to radiation levels that approach levels associated with increased risk for developing some cancers.[51,52] Radiation exposures ranging from 10 to 100 millisieverts (mSv) are associated with increased cancer risk.[53–56] Estimated CTPA exposure is 10 to 15 mSv[52,57] although there is considerable variation particularly between scanners using differing numbers of CT detector rows, as well as between scanner manufacturers. Smith-Bindman and colleagues[52] recently reported radiation exposures ranging from 2 to 30 mSv for CTPA examinations performed in a variety of San Francisco Bay area locations.

Risks: Contrast-induced Nephropathy

Contrast-induced nephropathy (CIN) remains one of the most common causes of acute renal failure in hospitalized patients.[58] Renal dysfunction before administration of contrast combined with diabetes, advanced age (>75 years), hypovolemia, heart failure, hypertension, proteinuria, gout, and/or use of nonsteroidal antiinflammatory medications increases the risk for this complication.[59] The risk of developing CIN increases with the number of risk factors in individual patients.[59] The risk of CIN is reduced by decreasing the volume of contrast medium[60,61] and by the infusion of isotonic saline.[62] The role of low-osmolar iodinated contrast mediums[63] or iso-osmolar contrast agents (eg, iodixanol) and antioxidants (eg, N-acetylcysteine) in reducing the risk of CIN following intravenous administration of contrast remains uncertain.[59,64]

Clinical Outcomes Related to CTPA

Rates of symptomatic venous thromboembolism during the 3 months after negative conventional pulmonary angiography provide a reference for clinical outcome studies.[10] Similar studies show that a negative single detector CTPA is not adequate to rule out PE and withhold anticoagulant treatment.[10] A combination of bilateral lower extremity CUS with single detector CTPA may allow anticoagulants to be withheld safely when neither test detects venous thrombi or pulmonary emboli.[65]

MDCTPA examinations have largely replaced single detector examinations because of the advanced quality of pulmonary artery opacification that they provide. Multiple studies have examined the safety of withholding anticoagulants from patients with clinically suspected acute PE after a negative MDCTPA.[9,66–68] In 1 rigorous study, all patients classified by a dichotomized Wells

Table 4
Positive and negative predictive values of CTPA differentiated by pretest clinical probability[a]

| | Clinical Probability | | |
| | High | Intermediate | Low |
Variable	Value (95% CI)	Value (95% CI)	Value (95% CI)
Positive predictive value, %	96 (78–99)	92 (84–96)	58 (40–73)
Negative predictive value, %	60 (32–83)	89 (82–93)	96 (92–98)

[a] The clinical probability of PE was based on the 3-category Wells score: less than 2.0, low probability; 2.0 to 6.0, intermediate probability; and more than 6.0, high probability.[1]

Data from Stein PD, Fowler SE, Goodman LR, et al. Multidetector computed tomography for acute pulmonary embolism. N Engl J Med 2006;354(22):2317–27.

score as likely to have PE, and all patients classified as unlikely to have PE who had an increased D-dimer level underwent MDCTPA.[9] In this study, 1505 patients had negative MDCTPA; anticoagulants were withheld in 1436 (the remaining 69 patients received anticoagulants for other indications, eg, atrial fibrillation). In the 3-month follow-up period, only 18 of the patients in whom anticoagulants were withheld (1.3%; 95% CI 0.7–2.0) subsequently developed symptomatic DVT or PE. Investigators in Canada and Europe have reported similar results.[67,68]

CT Venography Combined Routinely with CTPA

Combining routine CT venography (CTV) with MDCTPA adds a potential risk of additional radiation exposure without substantial added benefit for most patients with clinically suspected PE.[10,69] A recent report found that CTPA exposed patients to a mean effective radiation dose of 9 mSv, whereas CTPA combined with CTV of the pelvis and legs exposed patients to a mean effective dose of 21 mSv.[51] Compression ultrasonography can usually be substituted for CTV when the clinician opts for additional evaluation of patients with a high pretest probability for PE and negative or suboptimal MDCTPA.[70,71] However, routine use of CUS in combination with CTPA is not justifiable.[68,72,73] Data from a recent randomized trial that compared 2 diagnostic algorithms (MDCTPA alone vs MDCTPA and bilateral lower extremity CUS) found no difference in outcomes, underscoring the importance of limited use of additional testing such as CUS.[68]

MAGNETIC RESONANCE ANGIOGRAPHY

Gadolinium-enhanced magnetic resonance angiography (MRA) offers a potential alternative to CTPA or CTV to evaluate suspected PE or pelvic venous thrombosis in patients who have a history of contrast allergy, or when physicians seek to avoid exposing their patients to additional ionizing radiation.[74] MRA requires administration of high-dose gadolinium with the attendant risks of nephrogenic systemic fibrosis.[75–77] Early investigators reported that MRA has a sensitivity ranging from 77% to 100%, and a specificity ranging from 95% to 98% for acute PE.[74,78–80] Meaney and colleagues[78] also reported good interobserver agreement for detecting thromboemboli in lobar or segmental pulmonary artery branches. Earlier reports also suggested that magnetic resonance venography (MRV) has high sensitivity (95%) and specificity (91%) for detecting lower extremity DVT.[81] Fraser and colleagues[81] reported that the

sensitivity (88%) and specificity (95%) remained high for a small subgroup of patients with DVT limited to the calf.

In contrast, a recent report from the Prospective Investigation of Pulmonary Embolism Diagnosis III (PIOPED III) investigators indicates that MRA had low sensitivity for acute PE.[82] Almost one-third of 104 patients with acute PE had inadequate MRA or MRV, and 6 of these 104 had adequate MRA examinations, but false-negative results (overall sensitivity 63%, CI 53%–72%). There were 161 technically inadequate MR studies among 266 patients without PE, and 4 false-positive tests (overall specificity 38%, CI 32%–44%). The investigators also described how the risk of gadolinium-induced systemic and dermal fibrosis limited the use of MRA and MRV in patients with renal dysfunction,[83] Therefore, the use of MRA and MRV remains limited to settings where the patient's risk for allergic reaction to iodinated contrast and/or exposure to additional radiation is high, and where resources and expertise are available.

PERFUSION-VENTILATION LUNG SCANS

Recent evidence suggests that ventilation-perfusion scintigraphy remains useful for evaluating suspected acute PE when CTPA is contraindicated or the risk related to CTPA is increased.[11,84] In an analysis of PIOPED II images, investigators reported that more than 70% of PIOPED II patients had lung scans that allowed a definitive diagnostic interpretation, that is, PE present or PE absent.[84]

Techniques

Lung perfusion scans are performed by injecting albumin tagged with radionuclide particles (usually Tc 99m macroaggregated albumin) into a peripheral vein followed by imaging the lungs with a gamma camera.[85,86] The tagged particles are large enough (10–20 μm) to be trapped transiently in the pulmonary microcirculation. Thromboemboli obstruct blood flow to lung segments and produce defects on the perfusion lung scan. Perfusion defects are not specific for pulmonary emboli because other lung disorders, such as asthma or emphysema, may also result in perfusion defects. Therefore comparison of the perfusion scan with an accompanying ventilation scan and chest radiograph is essential. Lung ventilation scans are performed after inhalation of a radioactive gas (eg, xenon 131) or aerosol (eg, Tc 99m diethylenetriaminepentaacetic acid). Parenchymal lung diseases, such as emphysema, often result in defects on the ventilation scan. The diagnosis of PE becomes less likely when ventilation defects match the perfusion abnormalities and more likely when defects observed on perfusion scans are not matched by ventilation abnormalities (perfusion-ventilation mismatch).[87]

Sensitivity and Specificity

Perfusion lung scans offer high sensitivity for detecting clinically important PE.[14] However, in the first prospective investigation of PE diagnosis (PIOPED I), the investigators reported a low specificity of ventilation and perfusion lung scans for pulmonary emboli.[14] Criteria for interpreting ventilation and perfusion lung scans have been revised since this landmark study (**Box 1**).[88–93] The judgment of experienced readers is paramount.[94] Interpretation schemes based on high probability patterns (PE present), normal or nearly normal patterns (PE absent), with the remaining patterns

termed nondiagnostic, provide effective communication for clinicians.[95]

Outcome Studies

At least 2 studies have shown that it is safe to withhold anticoagulants when a technically satisfactory perfusion lung scan shows no perfusion defects.[96,97] In one large well-designed study, anticoagulants were withheld or discontinued following evaluation of 515 consecutive patients who had a normal perfusion lung scan and clinically suspected acute PE.[97] Only 1 of these patients suffered symptomatic PE during a 3-month follow-up.

CONVENTIONAL PULMONARY ANGIOGRAPHY

Until recently, conventional pulmonary angiography was the diagnostic reference standard for

---

Box 1
Revised criteria for the interpretation of ventilation and perfusion lung scans

High Probability

- ≥2 large (>75% of a segment) segmental perfusion defects without corresponding ventilation or chest radiograph abnormalities
- 1 large segmental perfusion defect and ≥2 moderate (25%–75% of a segment) segmental perfusion defects without corresponding ventilation or chest radiograph abnormalities
- ≥4 moderate segmental perfusion defects without corresponding ventilation or chest radiograph abnormalities

Immediate Probability

- 1 moderate to <2 large segmental perfusion defects without corresponding ventilation or chest radiograph abnormalities
- Corresponding ventilation-perfusion defects and chest radiograph parenchymal opacity in lower lung zone
- Single moderate matched ventilation-perfusion defects with normal chest radiograph findings
- Corresponding ventilation-perfusion defects and small pleural effusion
- Difficult to categorize as normal, low, or high probability

Low Probability

- Multiple matched ventilation-perfusion defects, regardless of size, with normal chest radiograph findings
- Corresponding ventilation-perfusion defects and chest radiograph parenchymal opacity in upper or middle lung zone
- Corresponding ventilation-perfusion defects and large pleural effusion
- Any perfusion defects with substantially larger chest radiograph abnormality
- Defects surrounded by normally perfused lung (stripe sign)
- >3 small (<25% of a segment) segmental perfusion defects with a normal chest radiograph
- Nonsegmental perfusion defects (cardiomegaly, aortic impression, enlarged hila)

Very Low

- ≤3 small (<25% of a segment) segmental perfusion defects with a normal chest radiograph

Normal

- No perfusion defects and perfusion outlines the shape of the lung seen on chest radiograph

From Worsley DF, Alavi A. Comprehensive analysis of the results of the PIOPED Study. Prospective Investigation of Pulmonary Embolism Diagnosis Study. J Nucl Med 1995;36(12):2380–7; with permission.

acute PE.[14] Diagnostic features of acute PE include the identification of an intraluminal filling defect or an abrupt cutoff of a pulmonary artery branch. Conventional pulmonary angiography allows identification of thromboemboli in subsegmental pulmonary arteries (1–2 mm in diameter), although interobserver agreement is low at this level.[14]

Conventional pulmonary angiography is invasive, and the mortality associated with this procedure is approximately 0.2%.[98] CTPA has largely replaced conventional pulmonary angiography for acute PE based on lower associated risks and costs, and outcome studies that show that MDCTPA interpretations guide management safely.[9,67,68] Conventional pulmonary angiography remains useful when MDCTPA is not diagnostic or when an intervention (eg, catheter embolectomy for acute PE or pulmonary endarterectomy (PEA) for chronic thromboembolic disease) is planned. It remains the procedure of choice for PEA preoperative evaluation (see article by Auger and colleagues in this issue).

ECHOCARDIOGRAPHY

Echocardiography has a limited role in the diagnostic evaluation of clinically suspected acute PE.[10] Specifically, echocardiography is not a recommended diagnostic imaging modality for evaluation of hemodynamically stable patients with suspected acute PE.[10,99] However, bedside echocardiography is recommended for evaluating critically ill patients who have shock or hypotension.[10,11,100] In this situation, the absence of echocardiographic signs of RV dysfunction excludes PE as the cause of hemodynamic instability or hypotension. Conversely, echocardiographic identification of thromboemboli in the right atrium, right ventricle, or central pulmonary arteries is diagnostic. Echocardiographic findings of RV overload, McConnell sign,[101] and the 60/60 sign (the 60/60 sign[102] is acceleration time of RV ejection <60 milliseconds in the presence of tricuspid insufficiency pressure gradient ≤60 mmHg) have varying sensitivities and specificities for acute PE, based on whether the patient has underlying chronic cardiorespiratory disease(s) (Table 5). RV free-wall hypokinesis caused by RV infarction may mimic the McConnell sign, but can be differentiated by the absence of echocardiographic findings of RV pressure overload.[103]

UNIQUE CLINICAL SETTINGS
Pregnancy

Pregnancy creates unique issues for diagnostic imaging in the evaluation of suspected venous thromboembolic disease (see also the article by Marik in this issue). Exposing the mother and the fetus to ionizing radiation is a major concern. A previous review suggested a small increase in the relative risk of childhood cancers after exposure of the fetus to low dose radiation.[104] Risks of subsequent fetal malformations and maternal and fetal malignancies must be balanced against

Table 5
Diagnostic value of 3 sets of echocardiographic signs suggesting the presence of acute PE in subgroups with and without known previous cardiorespiratory diseases

	Patients without Previous Cardiorespiratory Disease (n = 46)			Patients with Previous Cardiorespiratory Disease (n = 54)		
	RV Overload	60/60 Sign	McConnell Sign	RV Overload	60/60 Sign	McConnell Sign
Specificity (%)	78	100	100	21	89	100
Sensitivity (%)	81	25	19	80	26	20
PPV (%)	90	100	100	65	82	100
NPV (%)	64	37	35	36	40	40

The 60/60 sign[102] is acceleration time of RV ejection <60 milliseconds in the presence of tricuspid insufficiency pressure gradient ≤60 mmHg. The McConnell[101] sign is normokinesia and/or hyperkinesia of the apical segment of the RV free wall despite hypokinesia and/or akinesia of the remaining parts of the RV free wall. Concomitant echocardiographic signs of pressure overload are required to prevent false diagnosis of acute PE in patients with RV free-wall hypo/akinesis caused by RV infarction.[103] RV overload criteria: the presence of ≥ of 4 signs: (1) right-sided cardiac thrombus; (2) RV diastolic dimension (parasternal view) >30 mm or an RV/LV ratio >1; (3) systolic flattening of the interventricular septum; and (4) acceleration time <90 milliseconds or tricuspid insufficiency pressure gradient >30 mmHg in the absence of RV hypertrophy.

Abbreviations: NPV, negative predictive value; PPV, positive predictive value.

Data from Kurzyna M, Torbicki A, Pruszczyk P, et al. Disturbed right ventricular ejection pattern as a new Doppler echocardiographic sign of acute pulmonary embolism. Am J Cardiol 2002;90:507–11.

risks of undiagnosed venous thromboembolic disease, and the risk of maternal and fetal mortality. Investigators have estimated that approximately 1 of every 1000 pregnancies is complicated by PE,[105] and undiagnosed PE is the most common cause of maternal mortality. Concern for radiation exposure must be balanced against concern of missing a potentially fatal diagnosis.[106]

A diagnostic approach that limits radiation exposure is warranted. Signs and symptoms suggestive of both DVT and PE are common during pregnancy. The need for diagnostic testing increases with new symptoms, particularly changes in the degree of breathlessness or asymmetric (more than 2 cm difference in circumference) swelling of the left leg.[107] Normal D-dimer levels identify pregnant patients for whom VTE is unlikely.[10]

CUS of the deep veins of the lower extremities is the first imaging test for suspected DVT or PE (unless the pregnant patient presents in shock). Negative 2-point CUS should be repeated in 5 to 7 days. If deep vein thrombi are present, treatment should be instituted, thus allowing the physician to avoid imaging procedures that expose the fetus and mother to ionizing radiation. However, additional testing is necessary if CUS is negative because of the possibility of isolated iliac vein thrombosis or PE. MRV has the advantage of not exposing the mother or fetus to radiation,[10] and investigators have reported that MRV has a high sensitivity for isolated iliac DVT.[108] Pelvic MRV suggests a high rate of pelvic vein thrombosis after cesarean section.[108]

Unfortunately, the use of imaging modalities that deliver ionizing radiation is often necessary to confirm or exclude VTE during pregnancy. **Table 6** provides estimates of radiation absorbed by the fetus for imaging procedures used in the assessment of suspected VTE. Radiologists can alter both CTPA and lung scan procedures to reduce the radiation exposure.[109] Common practices include altering CT acquisition parameters, use of shields, and a 50% reduction in the radionuclide used for perfusion scans.

During the first or second trimester, CTPA may deliver less radiation to the fetus than a perfusion lung scan.[110] However, CTPA delivers more radiation to proliferating breast tissue than perfusion and ventilation lung scans.[111] Therefore, physicians may choose to order perfusion lung scans for pregnant women at increased risk for breast cancer. If the diagnosis of PE cannot be excluded or confirmed by ventilation and perfusion lung scanning, then MDCTPA is preferable to conventional

Table 6
Estimated radiation absorbed by fetus in procedures for diagnosing PE

Test	Estimated Radiation (mSv)
Chest radiograph	0.01
Perfusion lung scan with technetium 99m–labeled albumin (1–2 mCi)	0.06–0.12
Ventilation lung scan	0.2
CT angiography:	
First trimester	0.003–0.02
Second trimester	0.008–0.08
Third trimester	0.051–0.13
Pulmonary angiography by femoral access	2.2–3.7
Pulmonary angiography by brachial access	<0.5

Data from Torbicki A, Perrier A, Konstantinides S, et al. Guidelines on the diagnosis and management of acute pulmonary embolism: the Task Force for the Diagnosis and Management of Acute Pulmonary Embolism of the European Society of Cardiology (ESC). Eur Heart J 2008;29(18):2276–315.

pulmonary angiography because conventional pulmonary angiography delivers more radiation to the fetus. The use of CTPA requires attention to physiologic changes in the respiratory rate and cardiac output that accompany pregnancy. Failure to adapt contrast injection protocols may lead to poor bolus tracking of contrast and therefore poor-quality images.[112]

Previous PE

Patients who have a past history of PE may present challenges in interpreting diagnostic imaging. Lung perfusion scan defects may represent previous PE. Interpretation of lung perfusion scans should include comparison with previous studies; if they are not available, the interpretation should acknowledge that the distinction between acute and chronic PE cannot be made reliably.

In contrast to lung perfusion scans, the appearance of chronic thromboemboli can be distinguished by CTPA or conventional pulmonary angiography (**Fig. 6**). Conventional pulmonary arteriography may show any of 5 abnormal patterns when chronic thromboemboli are present: (1) pouching, (2) webs or bands, (3) intimal irregularity giving a scalloped appearance to the pulmonary arterial wall, (4) abrupt narrowing of

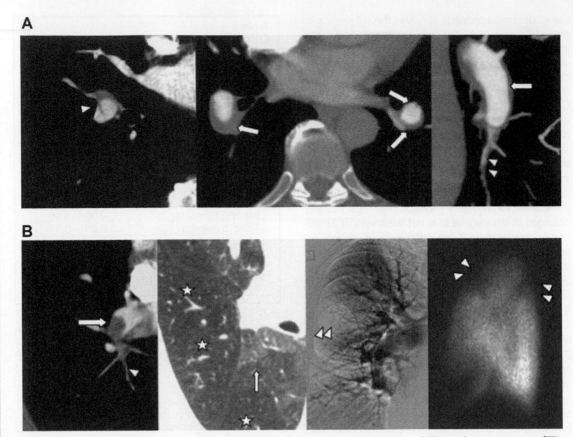

Fig. 6. Findings of chronic thromboembolic disease on CTPA. (*A*) Curvilinear weblike pulmonary artery filling defect (*arrowhead*), mural thrombus (*arrows*), and attenuated, irregular vessels (*double arrowhead*) are common findings readily demonstrated by CTPA. (*B*) Peripheral clot (*arrow*) associated with chronically occluded and attenuated arterial branches (*arrowhead*) results in mosaic perfusion with areas of normal parenchymal flow showing increased density (*arrow*) and areas of poor parenchymal flow because of chronic vessel occlusion having decreased density (*stars*). The finding of mosaic perfusion is also demonstrated on the parenchymal phase of conventional pulmonary arteriography and on perfusion scintigraphy, which demonstrate corresponding geographic perfusion defects (*double arrowheads*) secondary to chronic vessel occlusion.

a pulmonary artery, and (5) obstruction of a lobar vessel.[113] MDCTPA shows these same patterns accompanied by mosaic patterns of variable attenuation and marked disparity in the size of segmental vessels for most patients with chronic thromboemboli.[114]

Clinicians who evaluate patients with pulmonary hypertension should rely on perfusion lung scans to screen for chronic thromboemboli.[115] A normal perfusion scan excludes operable chronic thromboemboli. When perfusion scintigraphy is abnormal, use of both CTPA and conventional pulmonary arteriography can provide complementary information in determining patients who may benefit from PEA. However, interpretations of CTPA and/or conventional pulmonary angiography require considerable experience and expertise for diagnosis and management of patients with chronic thromboembolic pulmonary hypertension (CTEPH).[115]

SUMMARY

Imaging techniques are essential for the investigation of suspected VTE. Selection of specific imaging techniques requires individualization based on such factors as renal function, contrast allergies, risk of radiation exposure, and whether acute or chronic thromboembolic disease is suspected. A substantial body of clinical science provides a strong foundation for the application and interpretation of imaging techniques, and the science consistently underscores the importance of combining the clinical pretest probability with the interpretation of diagnostic images to determine the likelihood that VTE is present.

REFERENCES

1. Wells PS, Anderson DR, Rodger M, et al. Excluding pulmonary embolism at the bedside without diagnostic

imaging: management of patients with suspected pulmonary embolism presenting to the emergency department by using a simple clinical model and D-dimer. Ann Intern Med 2001;135(2):98—107.

2. Le Gal G, Righini M, Roy PM, et al. Prediction of pulmonary embolism in the emergency department: the revised Geneva score. Ann Intern Med 2006;144(3):165—71.

3. Kline JA, Nelson RD, Jackson RE, et al. Criteria for the safe use of D-dimer testing in emergency department patients with suspected pulmonary embolism: a multicenter US study. Ann Emerg Med 2002;39(2):144—52.

4. Wells PS, Anderson DR, Rodger M, et al. Derivation of a simple clinical model to categorize patients probability of pulmonary embolism: increasing the models utility with the SimpliRED D-dimer. Thromb Haemost 2000;83(3):416—20.

5. Goekoop RJ, Steeghs N, Niessen RW, et al. Simple and safe exclusion of pulmonary embolism in outpatients using quantitative D-dimer and Wells' simplified decision rule. Thromb Haemost 2007; 97(1):146—50.

6. Miniati M, Monti S, Bottai M. A structured clinical model for predicting the probability of pulmonary embolism. Am J Med 2003;114(3):173—9.

7. Remy-Jardin M, Pistolesi M, Goodman LR, et al. Management of suspected acute pulmonary embolism in the era of CT angiography: a statement from the Fleischner Society. Radiology 2007;245 (2):315—29.

8. Bates SM, Kearon C, Crowther M, et al. A diagnostic strategy involving a quantitative latex D-dimer assay reliably excludes deep venous thrombosis. Ann Intern Med 2003;138(10):787—94.

9. van Belle A, Buller HR, Huisman MV, et al. Effectiveness of managing suspected pulmonary embolism using an algorithm combining clinical probability, D-dimer testing, and computed tomography. JAMA 2006;295(2):172—9.

10. Torbicki A, Perrier A, Konstantinides S, et al. Guidelines on the diagnosis and management of acute pulmonary embolism: the Task Force for the Diagnosis and Management of Acute Pulmonary Embolism of the European Society of Cardiology (ESC). Eur Heart J 2008;29(18):2276—315.

11. Konstantinides S. Clinical practice. Acute pulmonary embolism. N Engl J Med 2008;359(26): 2804—13.

12. Wells PS, Ginsberg JS, Anderson DR, et al. Use of a clinical model for safe management of patients with suspected pulmonary embolism. Ann Intern Med 1998;129(12):997—1005.

13. Miniati M, Pistolesi M, Marini C, et al. Value of perfusion lung scan in the diagnosis of pulmonary embolism: results of the Prospective Investigative Study of Acute Pulmonary Embolism Diagnosis (PISA-PED). Am J Respir Crit Care Med 1996;154 (5):1387—93.

14. Value of the ventilation/perfusion scan in acute pulmonary embolism. Results of the prospective investigation of pulmonary embolism diagnosis (PIOPED). The PIOPED Investigators. JAMA 1990;263(20):2753—9.

15. Elliott CG, Goldhaber SZ, Visani L, et al. Chest radiographs in acute pulmonary embolism. Chest 2000;118(1):33—8.

16. ten Wolde M, Sohne M, Quak E, et al. Prognostic value of echocardiographically assessed right ventricular dysfunction in patients with pulmonary embolism. Arch Intern Med 2004;164(15):1685—9.

17. Westermark N. On the roentgen diagnosis of lung embolism. Acta Radiol Diagn (Stockh) 1938;19:357.

18. Hampton AO, Castleman B. Correlation of post-mortem chest teleroentgenograms with autopsy findings with special reference to pulmonary embolism and infarction. AJR Am J Roentgenol 1940;43:305.

19. Sokolove PE, Offerman SR. Images in clinical medicine. pulmonary embolism. N Engl J Med 2001;345(18):1311.

20. Talbot SR. B-mode evaluation of peripheral veins. Semin Ultrasound CT MR 1988;9(4):295—319.

21. Birdwell BG, Raskob GE, Whitsett TL, et al. Predictive value of compression ultrasonography for deep vein thrombosis in symptomatic outpatients: clinical implications of the site of vein noncompressibility. Arch Intern Med 2000;160(3):309—13.

22. Bernardi E, Camporese G, Buller HR, et al. Serial 2-point ultrasonography plus D-dimer vs whole-leg color-coded Doppler ultrasonography for diagnosing suspected symptomatic deep vein thrombosis: a randomized controlled trial. JAMA 2008; 300(14):1653—9.

23. Stevens SM, Elliott CG, Chan KJ, et al. Withholding anticoagulation after a negative result on duplex ultrasonography for suspected symptomatic deep venous thrombosis. Ann Intern Med 2004;140(12): 985—91.

24. Lagerstedt CI, Olsson CG, Fagher BO, et al. Need for long-term anticoagulant treatment in symptomatic calf-vein thrombosis. Lancet 1985;2(8454):515—8.

25. Kearon C, Julian JA, Newman TE, et al. Noninvasive diagnosis of deep venous thrombosis. McMaster Diagnostic Imaging Practice Guidelines Initiative. Ann Intern Med 1998;128(8):663—77.

26. Qaseem A, Snow V, Barry P, et al. Current diagnosis of venous thromboembolism in primary care: a clinical practice guideline from the American Academy of Family Physicians and the American College of Physicians. Ann Intern Med 2007; 146(6):454—8.

27. Polak JF, Yucel EK, Bettmann MA, et al. Suspected lower extremity deep vein thrombosis. J Am Coll Radiol 2005;1—5. [Online].

28. Johnson SA, Stevens SM, Woller SC, et al. Risk of deep vein thrombosis following a single negative whole-leg compression ultrasound: a systematic review and meta-analysis. JAMA 2010;303: 438–45.

29. Lensing AW, Prandoni P, Brandjes D, et al. Detection of deep-vein thrombosis by real-time B-mode ultrasonography. N Engl J Med 1989;320(6): 342–5.

30. Rose SC, Zwiebel WJ, Nelson BD, et al. Symptomatic lower extremity deep venous thrombosis: accuracy, limitations, and role of color duplex flow imaging in diagnosis. Radiology 1990;175(3): 639–44.

31. Lensing AW, Büller HR. Objective tests for the diagnosis of venous thrombosis. In: Hull R, Pineo GF, editors. Disorders of thrombosis. Philadelphia: WB Saunders; 1996. p. 244–50.

32. Borris LC, Christiansen HM, Lassen MR, et al. Comparison of real-time B-mode ultrasonography and bilateral ascending phlebography for detection of postoperative deep vein thrombosis following elective hip surgery. The Venous Thrombosis Group. Thromb Haemost 1989;61 (3):363–5.

33. Ginsberg JS, Caco CC, Brill-Edwards PA, et al. Venous thrombosis in patients who have undergone major hip or knee surgery: detection with compression US and impedance plethysmography. Radiology 1991;181(3):651–4.

34. Davidson BL, Elliott CG, Lensing AW. Low accuracy of color Doppler ultrasound in the detection of proximal leg vein thrombosis in asymptomatic high-risk patients. The RD Heparin Arthroplasty Group. Ann Intern Med 1992;117(9):735–8.

35. Elliott CG, Suchyta M, Rose SC, et al. Duplex ultrasonography for the detection of deep vein thrombi after total hip or knee arthroplasty. Angiology 1993; 44(1):26–33.

36. Heijboer H, Buller HR, Lensing AW, et al. A comparison of real-time compression ultrasonography with impedance plethysmography for the diagnosis of deep-vein thrombosis in symptomatic outpatients. N Engl J Med 1993;329(19):1365–9.

37. Cogo A, Lensing AW, Koopman MM, et al. Compression ultrasonography for diagnostic management of patients with clinically suspected deep vein thrombosis: prospective cohort study. BMJ 1998;316(7124):17–20.

38. Birdwell BG, Raskob GE, Whitsett TL, et al. The clinical validity of normal compression ultrasonography in outpatients suspected of having deep venous thrombosis. Ann Intern Med 1998;128(1):1–7.

39. Elias A, Mallard L, Elias M, et al. A single complete ultrasound investigation of the venous network for the diagnostic management of patients with a clinically suspected first episode of deep venous thrombosis of the lower limbs. Thromb Haemost 2003;89(2):221–7.

40. Schellong SM, Schwarz T, Halbritter K, et al. Complete compression ultrasonography of the leg veins as a single test for the diagnosis of deep vein thrombosis. Thromb Haemost 2003;89(2):228–34.

41. Subramaniam RM, Heath R, Chou T, et al. Deep venous thrombosis: withholding anticoagulation therapy after negative complete lower limb US findings. Radiology 2005;237(1):348–52.

42. Sevestre MA, Labarere J, Casez P, et al. Accuracy of complete compression ultrasound in ruling out suspected deep venous thrombosis in the ambulatory setting. A prospective cohort study. Thromb Haemost 2009;102(1):166–72.

43. Sevestre MA, Labarere J, Casez P, et al. Outcomes for inpatients with normal findings on whole-leg ultrasonography. A multicenter prospective cohort study. Am J Med 2010;123(2):158–65.

44. Stein PD, Kayali F, Olson RE. Trends in the use of diagnostic imaging in patients hospitalized with acute pulmonary embolism. Am J Cardiol 2004;93 (10):1316–7.

45. Rubin GD, Shiau MC, Schmidt AJ, et al. Computed tomographic angiography: historical perspective and new state-of-the-art using multi detector-row helical computed tomography. J Comput Assist Tomogr 1999;23(Suppl 1):S83–90.

46. Castaner E, Gallardo X, Ballesteros E, et al. CT diagnosis of chronic pulmonary thromboembolism. Radiographics 2009;29(1):31–50 [discussion: 50–3].

47. Wittram C, Maher MM, Yoo AJ, et al. CT angiography of pulmonary embolism: diagnostic criteria and causes of misdiagnosis. Radiographics 2004; 24(5):1219–38.

48. Stein PD, Fowler SE, Goodman LR, et al. Multidetector computed tomography for acute pulmonary embolism. N Engl J Med 2006;354(22):2317–27.

49. Perrier A, Bounameaux H. Accuracy or outcome in suspected pulmonary embolism. N Engl J Med 2006;354(22):2383–5.

50. National Research Council. Health risks from exposure to low levels of ionizing radiation: BEIR VII phase 2. Washington, DC: National Academies Press; 2006.

51. Fazel R, Krumholz HM, Wang Y, et al. Exposure to low-dose ionizing radiation from medical imaging procedures. N Engl J Med 2009;361(9):849–57.

52. Smith-Bindman R, Lipson J, Marcus R, et al. Radiation dose associated with common computed tomography examinations and the associated lifetime attributable risk of cancer. Arch Intern Med 2009;169(22):2078–86.

53. Pierce DA, Preston DL. Radiation-related cancer risks at low doses among atomic bomb survivors. Radiat Res 2000;154(2):178–86.

54. Preston DL, Ron E, Tokuoka S, et al. Solid cancer incidence in atomic bomb survivors: 1958–1998. Radiat Res 2007;168(1):1–64.

55. Preston DL, Pierce DA, Shimizu Y, et al. Dose response and temporal patterns of radiation-associated solid cancer risks. Health Phys 2003; 85(1):43–6.

56. Brenner DJ, Doll R, Goodhead DT, et al. Cancer risks attributable to low doses of ionizing radiation: assessing what we really know. Proc Natl Acad Sci U S A 2003;100(24):13761–6.

57. Mettler FA, Huda W, Yoshizumi TT, et al. Effective doses in radiology and diagnostic nuclear medicine: a catalog. Radiology 2008;248(1):254–63.

58. Nash K, Hafeez A, Hou S. Hospital-acquired renal insufficiency. Am J Kidney Dis 2002;39(5): 930–6.

59. Barrett BJ, Parfrey PS. Clinical practice. Preventing nephropathy induced by contrast medium. N Engl J Med 2006;354(4):379–86.

60. Cigarroa RG, Lange RA, Williams RH, et al. Dosing of contrast material to prevent contrast nephropathy in patients with renal disease. Am J Med 1989;86(6 Pt 1):649–52.

61. Freeman RV, O'Donnell M, Share D, et al. Nephropathy requiring dialysis after percutaneous coronary intervention and the critical role of an adjusted contrast dose. Am J Cardiol 2002;90(10):1068–73.

62. Mueller C, Buerkle G, Buettner HJ, et al. Prevention of contrast media-associated nephropathy: randomized comparison of 2 hydration regimens in 1620 patients undergoing coronary angioplasty. Arch Intern Med 2002;162(3):329–36.

63. Barrett BJ, Carlisle EJ. Metaanalysis of the relative nephrotoxicity of high- and low-osmolality iodinated contrast media. Radiology 1993;188(1): 171–8.

64. Sandler CM. Contrast-agent-induced acute renal dysfunction—is iodixanol the answer? N Engl J Med 2003;348(6):551–3.

65. Perrier A, Howarth N, Didier D, et al. Performance of helical computed tomography in unselected outpatients with suspected pulmonary embolism. Ann Intern Med 2001;135(2):88–97.

66. Perrier A, Roy PM, Sanchez O, et al. Multidetector-row computed tomography in suspected pulmonary embolism. N Engl J Med 2005;352(17): 1760–8.

67. Anderson DR, Kahn SR, Rodger MA, et al. Computed tomographic pulmonary angiography vs ventilation-perfusion lung scanning in patients with suspected pulmonary embolism: a randomized controlled trial. JAMA 2007;298(23):2743–53.

68. Righini M, Le Gal G, Aujesky D, et al. Diagnosis of pulmonary embolism by multidetector CT alone or combined with venous ultrasonography of the leg: a randomised non-inferiority trial. Lancet 2008; 371(9621):1343–52.

69. Kalva SP, Jagannathan JP, Hahn PF, et al. Venous thromboembolism: indirect CT venography during CT pulmonary angiography—should the pelvis be imaged? Radiology 2008;246(2):605–11.

70. Elias A, Colombier D, Victor G, et al. Diagnostic performance of complete lower limb venous ultrasound in patients with clinically suspected acute pulmonary embolism. Thromb Haemost 2004;91 (1):187–95.

71. Goodman LR, Stein PD, Matta F, et al. CT venography and compression sonography are diagnostically equivalent: data from PIOPED II. AJR Am J Roentgenol 2007;189(5):1071–6.

72. Turkstra F, Kuijer PM, van Beek EJ, et al. Diagnostic utility of ultrasonography of leg veins in patients suspected of having pulmonary embolism. Ann Intern Med 1997;126(10):775–81.

73. Anderson DR, Kovacs MJ, Dennie C, et al. Use of spiral computed tomography contrast angiography and ultrasonography to exclude the diagnosis of pulmonary embolism in the emergency department. J Emerg Med 2005;29(4):399–404.

74. Stein PD, Woodard PK, Hull RD, et al. Gadolinium-enhanced magnetic resonance angiography for detection of acute pulmonary embolism: an in-depth review. Chest 2003;124(6):2324–8.

75. Ledneva E, Karie S, Launay-Vacher V, et al. Renal safety of gadolinium-based contrast media in patients with chronic renal insufficiency. Radiology 2009;250(3):618–28.

76. Bridges MD, St Amant BS, McNeil RB, et al. High-dose gadodiamide for catheter angiography and CT in patients with varying degrees of renal insufficiency: prevalence of subsequent nephrogenic systemic fibrosis and decline in renal function. AJR Am J Roentgenol 2009;192(6):1538–43.

77. Perazella MA. Gadolinium-contrast toxicity in patients with kidney disease: nephrotoxicity and nephrogenic systemic fibrosis. Curr Drug Saf 2008;3(1):67–75.

78. Meaney JF, Weg JG, Chenevert TL, et al. Diagnosis of pulmonary embolism with magnetic resonance angiography. N Engl J Med 1997;336(20):1422–7.

79. Oudkerk M, van Beek EJ, Wielopolski P, et al. Comparison of contrast-enhanced magnetic resonance angiography and conventional pulmonary angiography for the diagnosis of pulmonary embolism: a prospective study. Lancet 2002;359(9318): 1643–7.

80. Gupta A, Frazer CK, Ferguson JM, et al. Acute pulmonary embolism: diagnosis with MR angiography. Radiology 1999;210(2):353–9.

81. Fraser DG, Moody AR, Morgan PS, et al. Diagnosis of lower-limb deep venous thrombosis: a prospective blinded study of magnetic resonance direct

thrombus imaging. Ann Intern Med 2002;136(2):
89–98.

82. Stein PD, Chenevert TL, Fowler SE, et al. Gadolinium-enhanced magnetic resonance angiography for pulmonary embolism: a multicenter prospective study (PIOPED III). Ann Intern Med 2010;152(7): 434–43, W142–3.

83. Stein PD, Gottschalk A, Sostman HD, et al. Methods of Prospective Investigation of Pulmonary Embolism Diagnosis III (PIOPED III). Semin Nucl Med 2008;38(6):462–70.

84. Sostman HD, Stein PD, Gottschalk A, et al. Acute pulmonary embolism: sensitivity and specificity of ventilation-perfusion scintigraphy in PIOPED II study. Radiology 2008;246(3):941–6.

85. Wagner HN Jr, Sabiston DC Jr, Iio M, et al. Regional pulmonary blood flow in man by radioisotope scanning. JAMA 1964;187:601–3.

86. Taplin GV, Johnson DE, Dore EK, et al. Lung photoscans with macroaggregates of human serum radioalbumin. Experimental basis and initial clinical trials. Health Phys 1964;10:1219–27.

87. Alderson PO. Scintigraphic evaluation of pulmonary embolism. Eur J Nucl Med 1987;13(Suppl):S6–10.

88. Gottschalk A, Sostman HD, Coleman RE, et al. Ventilation-perfusion scintigraphy in the PIOPED study. Part II. Evaluation of the scintigraphic criteria and interpretations. J Nucl Med 1993;34(7): 1119–26.

89. Gottschalk A, Stein PD, Henry JW, et al. Matched ventilation, perfusion and chest radiographic abnormalities in acute pulmonary embolism. J Nucl Med 1996;37(10):1636–8.

90. Stein PD, Henry JW, Gottschalk A. Mismatched vascular defects. An easy alternative to mismatched segmental equivalent defects for the interpretation of ventilation/perfusion lung scans in pulmonary embolism. Chest 1993;104(5):1468–71.

91. Stein PD, Henry JW, Gottschalk A. Small perfusion defects in suspected pulmonary embolism. J Nucl Med 1996;37(8):1313–6.

92. Stein PD, Terrin ML, Gottschalk A, et al. Value of ventilation/perfusion scans versus perfusion scans alone in acute pulmonary embolism. Am J Cardiol 1992;69(14):1239–41.

93. Worsley DF, Alavi A. Comprehensive analysis of the results of the PIOPED Study. Prospective Investigation of Pulmonary Embolism Diagnosis Study. J Nucl Med 1995;36(12):2380–7.

94. Sostman HD, Coleman RE, DeLong DM, et al. Evaluation of revised criteria for ventilation-perfusion scintigraphy in patients with suspected pulmonary embolism. Radiology 1994;193(1):103–7.

95. Hull RD, Raskob GE, Pineo GF, et al. The low-probability lung scan. A need for change in nomenclature. Arch Intern Med 1995;155(17): 1845–51.

96. Kipper MS, Moser KM, Kortman KE, et al. Longterm follow-up of patients with suspected pulmonary embolism and a normal lung scan. Perfusion scans in embolic suspects. Chest 1982;82(4):411–5.

97. Hull RD, Raskob GE, Coates G, et al. Clinical validity of a normal perfusion lung scan in patients with suspected pulmonary embolism. Chest 1990;97 (1):23–6.

98. Perrier A, Bounmeaux H. Acute pulmonary embolism: diagnosis. In: Peacock AJ, Rubin L, editors. Pulmonary circulation. London: Arnold; 2004. p. 414–28.

99. Roy PM, Colombet I, Durieux P, et al. Systematic review and meta-analysis of strategies for the diagnosis of suspected pulmonary embolism. BMJ 2005;331(7511):259.

100. British Thoracic Society Standards of Care Committee Pulmonary Embolism Guideline Development Group. British Thoracic Society guidelines for the management of suspected acute pulmonary embolism. Thorax 2003;58(6):470–83.

101. McConnell MV, Solomon SD, Rayan ME, et al. Regional right ventricular dysfunction detected by echocardiography in acute pulmonary embolism. Am J Cardiol 1996;78(4):469–73.

102. Kurzyna M, Torbicki A, Pruszczyk P, et al. Disturbed right ventricular ejection pattern as a new Doppler echocardiographic sign of acute pulmonary embolism. Am J Cardiol 2002;90(5):507–11.

103. Casazza F, Bongarzoni A, Capozi A, et al. Regional right ventricular dysfunction in acute pulmonary embolism and right ventricular infarction. Eur J Echocardiogr 2005;6(1):11–4.

104. Ginsberg JS, Hirsh J, Rainbow AJ, et al. Risks to the fetus of radiologic procedures used in the diagnosis of maternal venous thromboembolic disease. Thromb Haemost 1989;61(2):189–96.

105. Rutherford SE, Phelan JP. Deep venous thrombosis and pulmonary embolism in pregnancy. Obstet Gynecol Clin North Am 1991;18(2):345–70.

106. Toglia MR, Weg JG. Venous thromboembolism during pregnancy. N Engl J Med 1996;335(2): 108–14.

107. Merhi Z, Awonuga A. Acute abdominal pain as the presenting symptom of isolated iliac vein thrombosis in pregnancy. Obstet Gynecol 2006;107 (2 Pt 2):468–70.

108. Rodger MA, Avruch LI, Howley HE, et al. Pelvic magnetic resonance venography reveals high rate of pelvic vein thrombosis after cesarean section. Am J Obstet Gynecol 2006;194(2):436–7.

109. Pahade JK, Litmanovich D, Pedrosa I, et al. Quality initiatives: imaging pregnant patients with suspected pulmonary embolism: what the radiologist needs to know. Radiographics 2009;29(3):639–54.

110. Winer-Muram HT, Boone JM, Brown HL, et al. Pulmonary embolism in pregnant patients: fetal

radiation dose with helical CT. Radiology 2002;224 (2):487–92.

111. Cook JV, Kyriou J. Radiation from CT and perfusion scanning in pregnancy. BMJ 2005;331 (7512):350.

112. Schaefer-Prokop C, Prokop M. CTPA for the diagnosis of acute pulmonary embolism during pregnancy. Eur Radiol 2008;18(12):2705–8.

113. Auger WR, Fedullo PF, Moser KM, et al. Chronic major-vessel thromboembolic pulmonary artery obstruction: appearance at angiography. Radiology 1992;182(2):393–8.

114. Bergin CJ, Rios G, King MA, et al. Accuracy of high-resolution CT in identifying chronic pulmonary thromboembolic disease. Am J Roentgenol 1996; 166(6):1371–7.

115. Simonneau G, Robbins IM, Beghetti M, et al. Updated clinical classification of pulmonary hypertension. J Am Coll Cardiol 2009;54(Suppl 1): S43–54.

116. Wells PS, Anderson DR, Bormanis J, et al. Value of assessment of pretest probability of deep-vein thrombosis in clinical management. Lancet 1997; 350(9094):1795–8.

Hypercoagulable States

Julia A.M. Anderson, MD[a,b], Jeffrey I. Weitz, MD[c,d],*

KEYWORDS

- Thrombophilia • Hypercoagulable state • Thrombosis
- Thromboprophylaxis • Anticoagulation

Arterial thrombosis and venous thrombosis are common problems facing clinicians. Some patients with thrombosis have an underlying hypercoagulable state. These states can be divided into 3 categories: inherited disorders, acquired disorders, and those that are mixed in origin.[1,2]

Inherited hypercoagulable states, also known as thrombophilic disorders, can be caused by loss of function of natural anticoagulant pathways or gain of function in procoagulant pathways (**Table 1**). Acquired hypercoagulable states represent a heterogeneous group of disorders in which the risk of thrombosis is higher than that in the general population. The spectrum covers such diverse risk factors as a prior history of thrombosis, obesity, pregnancy, cancer and its treatment, antiphospholipid antibody syndrome, heparin-induced thrombocytopenia, and myeloproliferative disorders. The pathogenesis of thrombosis in these situations is largely unknown and, in many cases, is likely multifactorial in origin. Finally, mixed disorders are those with both an inherited and an acquired component such as hyperhomocysteinemia.[2]

Genetic hypercoagulable states and acquired risk factors combine to establish an intrinsic risk of thrombosis for each individual.[3,4] This risk can be modified by extrinsic or environmental factors such as surgery, immobilization, or hormonal therapy, all of which increase the risk of thrombosis. When the intrinsic and extrinsic forces exceed a critical threshold, thrombosis occurs (**Fig. 1**). Appropriate thromboprophylaxis can prevent the thrombotic risk from exceeding this critical threshold, but breakthrough thrombosis can occur if procoagulant stimuli overwhelm protective mechanisms.

Focusing on hypercoagulable states, this article (a) details the inherited, acquired, and mixed hypercoagulable states, (b) explains how these disorders trigger thrombosis, (c) discusses the laboratory evaluation of hypercoagulable states, (d) identifies those patients who deserve laboratory evaluation for an underlying hypercoagulable state, and (e) outlines the treatment of patients with hypercoagulable states.

INHERITED HYPERCOAGULABLE STATES

Inherited disorders are found in up to half of the patients who present with venous thromboembolism before the age of 45 years, particularly those whose event occurred in the absence of well-recognized risk factors, such as surgery or immobilization, or with minimal provocation, such as after a long-distance flight or after taking estrogens. Patients with inherited thrombophilic disorders often have a family history of thrombosis. Of greatest significance is a family history of sudden death due to pulmonary embolism or a history of multiple family members requiring long-term anticoagulation therapy because of recurrent

a Department of Clinical and Laboratory Hematology, Royal Infirmary of Edinburgh, Scotland EH16 4SA, UK
b Department of Medicine, McMaster University, Hamilton, Ontario L8N 3Z5, Canada
c Department of Medicine, Thrombosis & Atherosclerosis Research Institute, McMaster University, Hamilton, Ontario L8L 2X2, Canada
d Department of Biochemistry and Biomedical Sciences, Thrombosis & Atherosclerosis Research Institute, McMaster University, Hamilton, Ontario L8N 3Z5, Canada
* Corresponding author. Thrombosis & Atherosclerosis Research Institute, Hamilton General Hospital, 237 Barton Street East, Hamilton, ON L8L 2X2, Canada.
E-mail address: weitzj@taari.ca

Clin Chest Med 31 (2010) 659–673
doi:10.1016/j.ccm.2010.07.004

Table 1
Classification of hypercoagulable states

Hereditary	Mixed	Acquired
Loss of Function		
Antithrombin deficiency	Hyperhomocysteinemia	Previous venous thromboembolism
Protein C deficiency		Obesity
Protein S deficiency		Cancer
		Pregnancy, puerperium
		Drug-induced:
		Heparin-induced thrombocytopenia
		Prothrombin complex concentrates
		L-Asparaginase
		Hormonal therapy
Gain of Function		
Factor V Leiden		Postoperative
Prothrombin F11G20210A		Myeloproliferative disorders
Elevated factor VIII, IX, or XI		

thrombosis. Patients who present with venous thrombosis in unusual sites, such as the cerebral venous sinuses or mesenteric veins, those with recurrent thrombosis, and patients who develop skin necrosis on initiation of warfarin therapy also should be suspected of having an inherited hypercoagulable state.[5,6]

Loss of Function of Endogenous Anticoagulants

This group of disorders includes deficiency of antithrombin, protein C, or protein S.

Antithrombin deficiency

Antithrombin, a member of the serine protease inhibitor (serpin) superfamily, is synthesized in the liver. Antithrombin plays a critical role in regulating coagulation by forming a 1:1 covalent complex with thrombin, factor Xa, and other activated clotting factors. The rate of antithrombin interaction with its target proteases is accelerated by heparin.[7]

Antithrombin deficiency can be inherited or acquired. Acquired antithrombin deficiency can reflect decreased antithrombin synthesis,

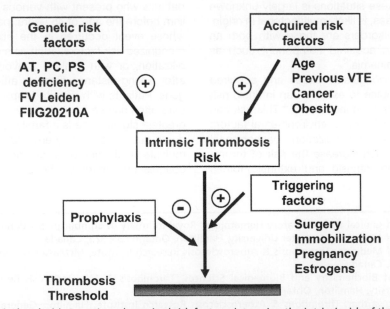

Fig. 1. Thrombosis threshold. Genetic and acquired risk factors determine the intrinsic risk of thrombosis for each individual. This risk is increased by extrinsic triggering factors and decreased by thromboprophylaxis. If the intrinsic and extrinsic forces exceed a critical threshold where thrombin generation overwhelms the protective mechanisms, thrombosis will result. AT, antithrombin; PC, protein C; PS, protein S.

Table 2
Causes of acquired antithrombin deficiency

Decreased Synthesis	Increased Consumption	Enhanced Clearance
Hepatic cirrhosis	Major surgery	Heparin
Severe liver disease	Acute thrombosis	Nephrotic syndrome
L-Asparaginase	Disseminated intravascular coagulation	
	Severe sepsis	
	Multiple trauma	
	Malignancy	
	Prolonged extracorporeal circulation	

increased consumption, or enhanced clearance (**Table 2**). Inherited antithrombin deficiency is relatively rare, occurring in about 1 in 2000, and can be one of two types (**Table 3**), both of which are inherited in an autosomal dominant fashion.[8,9] Type I deficiency is the result of reduced synthesis of biologically normal antithrombin.[10] More than 250 mutations have been identified as causes of Type I antithrombin deficiency, including nonsense mutations, small deletions, insertions, single base deletions, and gene deletions.[8]

Type II antithrombin deficiencies are characterized by normal levels of antithrombin with reduced functional activity. This condition is caused by missense mutations that result in single amino acid substitutions. The clinical consequences of Type II antithrombin deficiency depend on the location of the mutation.[11]

Protein C deficiency
The protein C pathway is a natural anticoagulant "on demand" pathway that is activated when thrombin is generated (**Fig. 2**). Protein C deficiency can be inherited or acquired. Like antithrombin deficiency, protein C deficiency is inherited in an autosomal dominant fashion.[12] Heterozygous protein C deficiency can be found in up to 1 in 200 of the adult population,[13] but many of these individuals do not have a history of thrombosis. Thus, the phenotypic expression of hereditary protein C deficiency is highly variable and may depend on other, as yet unrecognized, modifying factors. In contrast to antithrombin deficiency where the homozygous state is embryonic lethal, homozygous or doubly heterozygous protein C

deficiency can occur. Newborns with these disorders often present with purpura fulminans characterized by widespread thrombosis. Individuals with heterozygous protein C deficiency can develop skin necrosis on initiation of warfarin therapy.[14–16]

As outlined in **Table 4**, hereditary protein C deficiency can be further delineated into 2 subtypes using immunologic and functional assays.[17] The most common form of hereditary protein C deficiency is the classic or type I deficiency state. This disorder reflects reduced synthesis of a normal protein, and is characterized by a parallel reduction in protein C antigen and activity. Type II protein C deficiency, which reflects synthesis of a dysfunctional protein, is characterized by normal protein C antigen with reduced functional activity. Most Type II protein C deficiency states are caused by point mutations.[6,18]

Acquired protein C deficiency can be caused by decreased synthesis or increased consumption. Decreased synthesis can occur in patients with liver disease or in those given warfarin.[19] Warfarin decreases functional activity more than immunologic activity. Newborns have protein C levels 20% to 40% lower than those of adults, and premature infants have even lower levels.[20] Protein C consumption can occur with severe sepsis, with disseminated intravascular coagulation, or after surgery.

Protein S deficiency
Protein S serves as a cofactor for activated protein C (APC) and enhances its capacity to inactivate factors Va and VIIIa. In addition, protein S may have direct anticoagulant activity by inhibiting

Table 3
Types of inherited antithrombin deficiency

Type	Antigen	Activity (No Heparin)	Activity (With Heparin)
I (decreased protein)	Low	Low	Low
II (active site defect)	Normal	Low	Low
II (heparin-binding site defect)	Normal	Normal	Low

Protein C Pathway

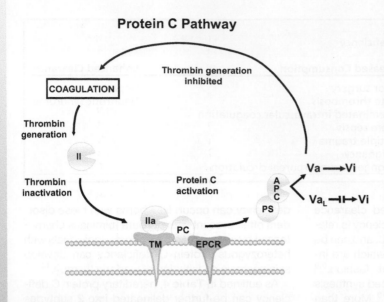

Fig. 2. Protein C pathway. Activation of coagulation triggers thrombin (IIa) generation. Excess thrombin binds to thrombomodulin (TM) on the endothelial cell surface. Once bound, the substrate specificity of thrombin is altered so that it no longer acts as a procoagulant but becomes a potent activator of protein C (PC). Endothelial protein C receptor (EPCR) binds protein C and presents it to thrombomodulin-bound thrombin where it is activated. Activated protein C (APC), together with its cofactor, protein S (PS), binds to the activated platelet-surface and protolytically degrades factor Va (Va) into inactive fragments (Vi). Because factor Va is a critical component of the prothrombinase complex, factor Va inactivation by activated protein C attenuates thrombin generation. Factor Va$_{Leiden}$ (FVa$_L$) is resistant to inactivation by activated protein C. Consequently, patients with the factor V$_{Leiden}$ mutation have reduced capacity to regulate thrombin generation.

prothrombin activation through its capacity to bind factor Va or factor Xa, components of the pro-thrombinase complex. The importance of the direct anticoagulant activity of protein S is uncertain.[12] In the circulation, about 60% of total protein S is bound to C4b-binding protein, a complement component. Only the 40% of the protein S that is free is functionally active.[6] Diagnosis of protein S deficiency, therefore, requires measurement of both free and bound forms of protein S.[21,22]

Protein S deficiency can be inherited or acquired. As outlined in **Table 5**, based on measurements of total and free protein S antigen and protein S activity, 3 types of inherited protein S deficiency have been identified. Type I or classic deficiency results from decreased synthesis of a normal protein, and is characterized by reduced levels of total and free protein S antigen together with reduced protein S functional activity. Type II protein S deficiency is characterized by normal levels of total and free protein S, associated with reduced protein S activity. Type III protein S

deficiency is characterized by normal levels of total protein S, but low levels of free protein S associated with reduced protein S activity. The molecular basis of Type III deficiency appears to be similar to that of Type I deficiency states, and the 2 types are likely part of the spectrum of the same disorder.

Acquired protein S deficiency can be caused by decreased synthesis, increased consumption, and loss or shift of free protein S to the bound form. Patients with nephrotic syndrome can lose free protein S in their urine, causing decreased protein S activity.[23] Total protein S levels in these patients are often normal because the levels of C4b-binding protein increase, shifting more protein S to the bound form. C4b-binding protein levels also increase in pregnancy and with the use of oral contraceptives. This process shifts more protein S to the bound form, and lowers the levels of free protein S and protein S activity.[24] The path-ophysiological consequences of this phenomenon are uncertain.

Table 4
Types of inherited protein C deficiency

Type	Antigen	Activity
I	Low	Low
II	Normal	Low

Table 5
Types of inherited protein S deficiency

Type	Total Protein S	Free Protein S	Protein S Activity
I	Low	Low	Low
II	Normal	Normal	Low
III	Normal	Low	Low

Gain of Function Mutations

Gain of function mutations include factor V Leiden, FIIG20210A, and elevated levels of procoagulant proteins.

Factor V Leiden

In 1993, Dahlbäck and colleagues[25,26] described 3 families with a history of venous thromboembolism. Affected family members exhibited limited prolongation of the activated partial thromboplastin time (aPTT) when APC was added to their plasma. Accordingly, this phenotype was designated APC resistance (APCR). Bertina and colleagues[27] demonstrated that APCR cosegregated with the factor V gene and was caused by a single base substitution, guanine to adenine at position 1691, that produced an Arg 506 Gln mutation at one of the APC cleavage sites on factor Va.[27–29] This mutation, which is designated Factor V_{Leiden}, endows activated Factor V_{Leiden} with a 10-fold longer half-life in the presence of APC than its wild-type counterpart.

The Factor V_{Leiden} mutation is responsible for most cases of APCR.[30] Other causes are mutations at Arg 306, another APC cleavage site. Arg 306 is replaced by a Gly residue in $FV_{Hong Kong}$[31] and by a Thr residue in $FV_{Cambridge}$[32]; neither mutation is associated with thrombosis.

The Factor V_{Leiden} mutation is inherited in an autosomal dominant fashion. The prevalence of the mutation ranges from 2% to 5% in Caucasians, but is rare in Asians and Africans. The prevalence of Factor V_{Leiden} homozygosity is about 1 in 2500.[6] Patients with Factor V Leiden are at lower risk for thrombotic complications than those with deficiencies of antithrombin, protein C, or protein S.[33–35] Heterozygotes with the Factor V_{Leiden} mutation have an annual risk of thrombosis of 0.1% to 0.3%, whereas the risk with deficiencies of antithrombin, protein C, or protein S ranges from 0.5% to 1.5% per year.

A diagnosis of APCR is established using a functional assay based on the ratio of the aPTT after APC addition divided by that determined before APC addition.[36] The use of Factor V–deficient plasma renders the test more specific, but questionable results can be confirmed with a genetic test for the Factor V_{Leiden} mutation.[37]

Prothrombin Gene Mutation

After extensive screening of 28 families with unexplained venous thromboembolism, Poort and colleagues[38] identified a heterozygous G to A nucleotide transition at position 20210 in the 3'-untranslated region of the prothrombin gene in 5 of the probands. This mutation, FIIG20210A, results in elevated levels of prothrombin. Elevated levels of prothrombin, in turn, may increase the risk of thrombosis by enhancing thrombin generation[39,40] or by inhibiting factor Va inactivation by APC.[41]

FIIG20210A is found in 1% to 6% of Caucasians. The mutation is more common in southern than in northern Europe, a gradient opposite to that of Factor V_{Leiden}.[42] Rare individuals homozygous for the FIIG20210A mutation have been identified.[43,44] Laboratory diagnosis of FIIG20210A depends on genetic screening after polymerase chain reaction (PCR) amplification of the 3'-untranslated region of the FII gene. Although FIIG20210A heterozygotes have 30% higher levels of prothrombin than noncarriers, the wide range of prothrombin levels in healthy individuals precludes the use of this phenotype to identify carriers.

Elevated Levels of Procoagulant Proteins

Elevated levels of factor VIII and other coagulation factors, including factors XI and IX, have been implicated as independent risk factors for thrombosis.[45–47] Although the molecular bases for the high levels of these coagulation factors have yet to be identified, genetic mechanisms are likely responsible because of the high heritability of these quantitative abnormalities.

ACQUIRED HYPERCOAGULABLE STATES

Acquired hypercoagulable states include antiphospholipid antibody syndrome, cancer, heparin-induced thrombocytopenia, pregnancy and estrogen therapy (oral contraception or hormone replacement therapy), and a prior history of venous thromboembolism.

Antiphospholipid Antibody Syndrome

Antiphospholipid antibodies are a heterogeneous group of autoantibodies directed against proteins that bind phospholipid.[48] Antibodies can be categorized into those that prolong phospholipid-dependent coagulation assays, known as lupus anticoagulants (LA), or anticardiolipin antibodies (ACL), that target cardiolipin. A subset of ACL recognizes other phospholipid-bound proteins, particularly β_2-glycoprotein I.

Patients with thrombosis in association with an LA and/or ACL are diagnosed with antiphospholipid antibody syndrome (APS). APS is considered primary when it occurs in isolation and secondary when it is associated with autoimmune disorders, such as systemic lupus erythematosus or other connective tissue diseases. Thrombosis in APS patients can be arterial, venous, or placental.

Placental thrombosis is hypothesized to be the cause of the pregnancy-related complications that characterize APS. These complications include fetal loss before 10 weeks' gestation and unexplained fetal death after 10 weeks' gestation.[49] Intrauterine growth retardation, preeclampsia, and eclampsia also have been associated with APS.

Laboratory diagnosis of APS requires the presence of LA or ACL on at least 2 assays with a period of at least 6 weeks between each test. LA are detected using phospholipid-dependent clotting tests. Most screening assays are based on the aPTT. aPTT reagents differ in their sensitivity for detection of LA, and many laboratories have adopted less sensitive aPTT reagents for routine aPTT testing. LA is suspected when the aPTT is prolonged and fails to correct after mixing with normal plasma. The diagnosis is confirmed by demonstrating that addition of excess hexagonal phase phospholipid normalizes the aPTT, thereby documenting the phospholipid dependence of the abnormal test result. In addition to the aPTT, a battery of phospholipid-dependent clotting tests is often used for diagnosis of LA. These tests include the dilute Russell viper venom time and kaolin clotting time.[50]

ACL antibodies are detected using immunoassays.[51] Only ACL antibodies of medium to high titer and of the IgG or IgM subclass are associated with thrombosis. Lack of standardization of ACL assays makes it difficult to compare results between laboratories. ACL antibodies are found in 3% to 10% of healthy individuals and with infections such as mycobacterial pneumonia, malaria, or parasitic disorders, and after exposure to some medications. Often, these antibodies are of low titer and are transient. ACL antibodies are detected in about 30 to 50% of patients with systemic lupus erythematosus.[52] Of these, 10% to 20% also have LA. In contrast to most hypercoagulable states, APS can be associated with spontaneous arterial thrombosis as well as with venous thromboembolism. Arterial thrombosis can manifest as a stroke or transient ischemic attack.[53,54] Thrombosis of the sagittal sinus, a form of venous thrombosis, also can cause stroke in these patients.[55]

Heparin-Induced Thrombocytopenia

Heparin-induced thrombocytopenia (HIT) is diagnosed on the basis of clinical features (**Table 6**) and laboratory detection of HIT antibodies. The risk of HIT is higher with unfractionated heparin than with low molecular weight heparin (LMWH), is more common in surgical patients than medical

Table 6
Features of heparin-induced thrombocytopenia

Feature	Details
Thrombocytopenia	Platelet count of 100,000/μL or less or a decrease in platelet count of 50% or more
Timing	Platelet count falls 5–10 days after starting heparin
Type of heparin	More common with unfractionated heparin than LMWH. Rare with fondaparinux
Type of patient	More common in surgical patients than medical patients. More common in women than in men
Thrombosis	Venous thrombosis more common than arterial thrombosis

patients, and more common in women than in men.[56]

Typical clinical features of HIT include thrombocytopenia and thrombosis (arterial or venous). Less common features include necrotic skin lesions at the sites of subcutaneous heparin injection, acute systemic reactions to heparin and, rarely, disseminated intravascular coagulation.[56,57] Thrombocytopenia is the most common finding, occurring in 90% of patients. The platelet count typically decreases 5 to 10 days after heparin is started. However, thrombocytopenia can occur earlier if the patient has been exposed to heparin in the past 3 months. Rarely, the onset of HIT can be delayed and occurs several days after stopping heparin.[58]

HIT is an autoimmune-like disorder and is caused by heparin-dependent, platelet-activating antibodies of the IgG subclass. These antibodies are directed against neoantigens exposed on platelet factor 4 (PF4) when it is complexed by heparin. By binding to Fcγll receptors on platelets, these antibodies trigger platelet activation. Activated platelets and platelet-derived microparticles provide an anionic phospholipid surface on which coagulation factors assemble and promote thrombin generation. This process produces a hypercoagulable state and explains why 30% to 70% of HIT patients develop thrombosis.[59,60]

The diagnosis of HIT is supported by assays that capitalize on the platelet-activating properties of HIT antibodies. The platelet serotonin release assay is the gold standard for the diagnosis of HIT.[61] Enzyme immunoassays for detection of antibodies against PF4 are more sensitive, but are less specific than the serotonin release assay.[62]

When the diagnosis of HIT is established, heparin must be stopped and an alternative anticoagulant should be given (**Box 1**). Options include direct thrombin inhibitors, such as lepirudin, argatroban, or bivalirudin. Factor Xa inhibitors, such as fondaparinux, have also been used successfully, but have yet to receive regulatory approval for this indication. Treatment with these agents should be continued until the platelet count returns to baseline levels, at which point low-dose warfarin can be initiated.

Cancer

About 25% of patients who present with venous thromboembolism have cancer.[63] Cancer patients who develop venous thromboembolism have reduced survival compared with those who do not develop venous thromboembolism. Patients with brain tumors and advanced ovarian or prostate cancer have particularly high rates of venous thromboembolism.[64] Treatment with chemotherapy, hormonal therapy, and biologic agents, such as erythropoietin and antiangiogenic drugs, further increases the risk of venous thromboembolism.

The pathogenesis of thrombosis in cancer patients is multifactorial in origin and represents a complex interplay between the tumor, characteristics of the patient, and the hemostatic system. Tumor cells often express tissue factor or other procoagulants that can initiate coagulation.[65,66] In addition to its role in coagulation, tissue factor also acts as a cell-signaling molecule that promotes tumor proliferation and spread. Patient-related factors that contribute to venous thromboembolism include immobility and venous stasis secondary to extrinsic compression of major veins by tumor. Surgical procedures, indwelling central venous catheters, and chemotherapy can produce vessel wall injury.[67] In addition, tamoxifen and selective estrogen receptor modulators (SERM) induce an acquired hypercoagulable state by reducing the levels of natural anticoagulant proteins.[68]

Some patients who present with unprovoked venous thromboembolism have occult cancer. This observation has prompted some experts to recommend extensive screening for cancer in such patients. Any benefits of this approach, however, are offset by potential harms, including procedure-related morbidity, the psychological impact of false-positive tests, and the cost of screening. Furthermore, early detection of cancer is only of benefit if there is potentially curative therapy and only screening for breast, cervical, and possibly colon cancer has been shown to reduce mortality.[69] Small studies comparing extensive cancer screening with no screening in patients with unprovoked venous thromboembolism have yet to demonstrate that extensive screening reduces cancer-related mortality. Therefore, it is difficult to recommend extensive screening at this time. Instead, a careful history should be taken to identify any symptoms suggestive of underlying cancer. If there are no symptoms suggestive of underlying cancer, patients should be encouraged to undergo age-appropriate screening tests for breast, cervical, or colon cancer.

Pregnancy

Venous thromboembolic disease is the leading cause of maternal morbidity and mortality. About 1 in 1000 pregnancies are complicated by venous thromboembolism and about 1 in 1000 women develop venous thromboembolism in the postpartum period.[70] The individual risk of venous thromboembolism in pregnancy and the puerperium is influenced by patient-related factors; these include age older than 35 years, body mass index greater than 29 (calculated as the weight in kilograms divided by height in meters squared), Cesarean delivery, and thrombophilia, or family history of venous thromboembolism.[70,71] A personal history of venous thromboembolism, ovarian hyperstimulation, and multiparity are other risk factors.

More than 90% of deep vein thrombosis in pregnancy occurs in the left leg because the enlarged uterus further compresses the left iliac vein by

---

Box 1
Management of heparin-induced thrombocytopenia

Stop all heparin

Give an alternative anticoagulant, such as lepirudin, argatroban, bivalirudin, or fondaparinux

Do not give platelet transfusions

Do not give warfarin until the platelet count returns to its baseline level. If warfarin was administered, give vitamin K to restore the international normalized ratio (INR) to normal

Evaluate for thrombosis, particularly deep vein thrombosis

placing pressure on the overlying right iliac and ovarian arteries.[72,73] A similar mechanism likely explains the isolated left iliofemoral thrombosis that can occur in pregnancy.

Hypercoagulability of the blood occurs in pregnancy, and reflects a combination of venous stasis and changes in the hemostatic system. The enlarging uterus reduces venous blood flow from the lower extremities. However, this is not the only mechanism responsible for venous stasis because blood flow from the lower extremities begins to decrease by the end of the first trimester, likely reflecting hormonally induced venous dilatation. Systemic factors also contribute to hypercoagulability. Thus, the levels of circulating procoagulant proteins, such as factor VIII, fibrinogen, and von Willebrand protein, increase in the third trimester of pregnancy.[74,75] Coincidentally, there is suppression of natural anticoagulant pathways. Thus, there is an acquired resistance to activated protein C related, at least in part, to reduced levels of free protein S.[76,77] The net effect of these changes is enhanced thrombin generation as evidenced by elevated levels of prothrombin fragments and thrombin/antithrombin complexes.[78,79]

About half of the episodes of venous thromboembolism in pregnancy occur in women with thrombophilia.[80,81] The risk of venous thromboembolism in women with thrombophilic defects depends on the type of abnormality and the presence of other risk factors The risk appears to be highest in women with antithrombin, protein C, or protein S deficiency, and lower in those with Factor V_{Leiden} or the prothrombin gene mutation.[82,83] In general, the daily risk of venous thromboembolism in these women is higher in the postpartum period than it is during pregnancy. The risk during pregnancy is similar in all 3 trimesters. Therefore, if thromboprophylaxis is given during pregnancy, it must be administered throughout the pregnancy and continued for at least 6 weeks postpartum.[84]

Hormonal Therapy

Oral contraceptives, estrogen replacement therapy, and SERM are all associated with an increased risk of thrombosis.[85,86] The relatively high risk of venous thromboembolism associated with early oral contraceptives prompted development of low-dose formulations containing reduced doses of estrogen and progestin. Currently available low-estrogen combination oral contraceptives contain 20 to 50 μg of ethinylestradiol and one of several different progestins. Even these low-dose combination contraceptives are associated with a 3- to 4-fold increased risk of venous

thromboembolism compared with the risk in nonusers. In absolute terms, this translates to an incidence of 3 to 4 per 10,000 compared with 5 to 10 per 100,000 in nonusers of reproductive age.[87]

Case-control studies suggest that the risk of venous thromboembolism is 20- to 30-fold higher in women with inherited thrombophilia who use oral contraceptives than it is in nonusers with thrombophilia or users without these defects. Despite the increased risk, however, routine screening for thrombophilia is not indicated in women considering the use of oral contraceptives. Based on the estimated incidence and case fatality rate of thrombotic events, it is estimated that 400,000 women would need to be screened to detect 20,000 carriers of Factor V_{Leiden}. Oral contraceptives would need to be withheld in all of these women to prevent a single death.[88] For less prevalent thrombophilic defects, even large numbers of women would need to be screened. Based on these considerations, routine screening cannot be recommended. There is mounting evidence that hormonal replacement therapy with conjugated equine estrogen, with or without a progestin, increases the risk of myocardial infarction, ischemic stroke, and venous thromboembolism. Consequently, the use of hormone replacement therapy has markedly decreased.

Prior History of Venous Thromboembolism

A history of previous venous thromboembolism places patients at risk for recurrence.[89,90] Those with unprovoked venous thromboembolism have a particularly high risk of recurrence when anticoagulant treatment is stopped[91]; 10% at 1 year and 30% at 5 years. This risk appears to be independent of whether or not there is an underlying thrombophilic defect, such as Factor V_{Leiden} or the prothrombin gene mutation.

The risk of recurrent venous thromboembolism is lower in patients whose incident event occurs in association with a well-recognized and transient risk factor, such as major surgery or prolonged immobilization. These patients have a risk of recurrence of about 4% at 1 year and 10% at 5 years. Patients whose venous thromboembolic event occurred against the background of minor risk factors, such as oral contraceptive use or a long-distance flight, likely have an intermediate risk of recurrence. Patients at highest risk for recurrence are those with inherited deficiencies of antithrombin, protein C or protein S, antiphospholipid antibody syndrome, advanced malignancy, or those homozygous for Factor V_{Leiden} or the prothrombin gene mutation. Their risk of recurrence is likely to be at least 15% at 1 year and up to 50% at 5 years.

COMBINED INHERITED AND ACQUIRED HYPERCOAGULABLE STATES

Hyperhomocysteinemia is the prototypical hypercoagulable state that occurs due to a combination of inherited and acquired factors.[92,93] Homocysteine is an intermediate sulfur-containing amino acid that acts as a methyl group donor during the metabolism of methionine, an essential amino acid derived from the diet. The interconversion of methionine and homocysteine depends on the availability of 5-methyltetrahydrofolate, a methyl group donor, vitamin B12 and folate, cofactors in the interconversion, and the enzyme methionine synthase.[94] Increased levels of homocysteine can be the result of increased production or reduced metabolism. Severe hyperhomocysteinemia and cysteinuria are rare and are usually caused by deficiency in the enzyme, cystathione β-synthetase. More common is mild to moderate hyperhomocysteinemia, which can be caused by genetic mutations in methyltetrahydrofolate reductase (MTHFR) when they are accompanied by nutritional deficiency of folate, vitamin B12, or vitamin B6.[95] The cofactor requirements are therefore increased with these mutations.[96]

A fasting serum homocysteine level greater than 15 mmol/L is considered elevated. Although elevated levels were a common finding, routine fortification of flour with folic acid has resulted in lower homocysteine levels in the general population.[96,97] Elevated serum levels of homocysteine have been associated with an increased risk of arterial thrombosis (myocardial infarction, stroke, and peripheral arterial disease) and venous thromboembolism.

Administration of folate, along with vitamin B12 and vitamin B6, will reduce homocysteine levels.[98] Recent randomized trials, however, have shown that such therapy does not reduce the risk of recurrent cardiovascular events in patients with coronary artery disease or stroke,[99] nor does it lower the risk of recurrent venous thromboembolism. Based on these negative trials and the declining incidence of hyperhomocysteinemia, the enthusiasm for screening for hyperhomocysteinemia has rapidly declined.

TREATMENT OF THROMBOSIS IN PATIENTS WITH HYPERCOAGULABLE STATES
Initial Treatment

With few exceptions, management of initial thrombotic events in patients with hypercoagulable states is no different from the management of these events in patients without underlying hypercoagulable disorders. The exceptions are purpura fulminans in newborns with homozygous protein C or protein S deficiency and thrombosis in patients with severe antithrombin deficiency. Newborns with purpura fulminans require protein C or protein S concentrates or sufficient amounts of plasma to increase the levels of protein C or protein S.[100,101] Patients with severe antithrombin deficiency require antithrombin concentrates to increase plasma levels of antithrombin to a point where heparin or LMWH can be used for treatment.[102]

Extended Therapy

Extended treatment of thrombosis in patients with hypercoagulable states is similar to that in those without these underlying disorders. Caution is needed when starting patients with protein C or protein S deficiency on warfarin or other vitamin K antagonists to prevent skin necrosis. Warfarin should not be started in these patients until therapeutic anticoagulation has been achieved with heparin or LMWH. Once started, low doses of warfarin should be given to prevent precipitous decreases in the levels of protein C or protein S.

Recent randomized trials have shown that usual-intensity warfarin (target INR of 2.0–3.0) is as effective as higher-intensity warfarin in patients with antiphospholipid antibody syndrome. The risk of major bleeding is lower with usual-intensity warfarin than it is with higher-intensity regimens.[103,104] A target INR of 2.0 to 3.0 is appropriate for patients with other hypercoagulable states as well.

Patients with thrombosis against a background of metastatic cancer do better with extended treatment with LMWH than with warfarin. Randomized clinical trials have shown that compared with warfarin, LMWH reduces the risk of recurrent venous thromboembolism without increasing bleeding.[105] Furthermore, LMWH simplifies treatment because it can be given subcutaneously once daily without coagulation monitoring. The drug can be held before invasive procedures and the dose reduced if there is thrombocytopenia. The major drawback of LMWH is cost, although the drug has been shown to be cost-effective in patients at high risk for recurrent venous thromboembolism.[106]

Duration of Treatment

The presence of a hypercoagulable state has no influence on the duration of anticoagulant treatment in patients whose venous thromboembolic event has occurred in the setting of a well-recognized and transient risk factor, such as major surgery or prolonged immobilization due to medical illness. These patients are treated with anticoagulants for at least 3 months.[107] For those with unprovoked venous thromboembolism, life-long anticoagulation treatment is often recommended provided that patients are not at high risk for bleeding.[91,108] An elevated D-dimer 1 month after stopping anticoagulant therapy and persistent abnormalities on compression ultrasonography may identify patients at highest risk for recurrence. Heterozygosity for Factor V_{Leiden} or the prothrombin gene mutation does not influence the risk of recurrence. In contrast, patients with deficiency of antithrombin, protein C or protein S, or those homozygous for Factor V_{Leiden} or the prothrombin gene mutation appear to be at higher risk for recurrence and likely require lifelong anticoagulation treatment.[109–111] Likewise, patients with APS with a persistently positive LA also are at high risk for recurrence and require lifelong treatment.

Treatment and Prevention of Thrombosis During Pregnancy

Thrombophilic disorders have no influence on the treatment of venous thrombosis during pregnancy. These women require therapeutic doses of subcutaneous heparin, LMWH, or fondaparinux throughout pregnancy.[84,112] Heparin is given once daily with the dose titrated to achieve a therapeutic mid-interval aPTT. LMWH can be given once or twice daily in a weight-adjusted fashion. Monitoring with anti–factor Xa levels is recommended,

particularly in the third trimester. Fondaparinux is given once daily. It is uncertain whether monitoring is required. After delivery, LMWH or warfarin should be given for at least 4 to 6 weeks. In total, treatment should be given for 6 months from the time of diagnosis. Warfarin should be avoided in pregnancy because it crosses the placenta and can cause bone and central nervous system abnormalities, fetal hemorrhage, or placental abruption. Warfarin can be safely administered in nursing mothers, with no detectable anticoagulant effect in breast milk.[113] (See the article by Marik elsewhere in this issue).

Women with a history of unprovoked or recurrent venous thromboembolism, those with deficiencies of antithrombin, protein C, or protein S, and those homozygous for Factor V_{Leiden} or the prothrombin gene mutation should receive antepartum prophylaxis with heparin or LMWH.[84] Postpartum, LMWH or warfarin should be given for 4 to 6 weeks. Postpartum treatment with LMWH or warfarin for 4 to 6 weeks is likely adequate for women with a history of venous thrombosis secondary to a well-defined risk factor.[114] Prophylaxis during pregnancy, as well as postpartum, should be considered for women who have developed venous thromboembolism after taking oral contraceptives, particularly if they have underlying thrombophilia. Women with thrombophilic defects and no prior history of venous thromboembolism likely do not require antepartum prophylaxis or postpartum treatment, but definitive data are lacking.[84] A summary of these recommendations is provided in **Table 7**.

Table 7
Management of women with a history of venous thrombosis during pregnancy and the puerperium

Clinical History	Thrombophilia	Antepartum	Postpartum[a]
Prior venous thrombosis secondary to a transient risk factor	No	Surveillance	Yes
Prior venous thrombosis secondary to pregnancy or estrogens	Yes or no	Prophylactic heparin or LMWH	Yes
Prior idiopathic venous thrombosis	Yes or no	Prophylactic heparin or LMWH	Yes
Recurrent venous thrombosis	Yes or no	Treatment-dose heparin or LMWH	Resume long-term anticoagulation
No prior venous thrombosis	Antithrombin deficiency; *FIIG20210A* or factor V Leiden	Prophylactic heparin or LMWH	Yes

[a] Postpartum prophylaxis involves a 4- to 6-week course of warfarin with the dose adjusted to achieve an INR of 2.0 to 3.0. Prophylactic doses of LMWH can be used as an alternative.

THROMBOPHILIA SCREENING

The indications for thrombophilia screening remain controversial.[115,116] For patients with a first episode of venous thromboembolism, thrombophilia screening is indicated if the results influence the duration of treatment or impact on family counseling regarding use of estrogen-containing compounds. It is reasonable to screen patients whose first episode of thrombosis has occurred before the age of 45 years, those with recurrent thrombosis, particularly if unprovoked, and patients with thrombosis in an unusual site,[117] such as cerebral or mesenteric veins and those with 2 or more first-degree relatives with thrombosis. It may also be reasonable to screen women with a history of 3 or more second-trimester pregnancy losses or an intrauterine death for LA and ACL.[6]

Screening should include functional assays for antithrombin and protein C, a free protein S level, testing for activated protein C resistance using the modified APC sensitivity ratio with DNA testing for the Factor V_{Leiden} mutation if the screening test is equivocal, DNA testing for the prothrombin gene mutation, phospholipid-based clotting tests to detect LA, and enzyme immunoassay for ACL identification.

SUMMARY AND FUTURE DIRECTIONS

With increased understanding of the regulation of coagulation, inherited or acquired hypercoagulable states can now be identified in up to 50% of patients with venous thromboembolism. The role of these disorders in the pathogenesis of arterial thrombosis is less clear. Therefore, more work is needed to identify patients who are vulnerable to arterial thrombosis after plaque rupture.

Although our ability to diagnose hypercoagulable states has improved, the impact of this information on clinical decisions remains limited. Common congenital hypercoagulable states increase the risk of a first thrombotic episode, but have little impact on the risk of recurrence. Identification of patients at risk for recurrent thrombosis and elucidation of new hypercoagulable states are goals for the future.

REFERENCES

1. Crowther MA, Kelton JG. Congenital thrombophilic states associated with venous thrombosis: a qualitative overview and proposed classification system. Ann Intern Med 2003;138(2):128–34.
2. Jacques PF, Bostom AG, Williams RR, et al. Relation between folate status, a common mutation in methylenetetrahydrofolate reductase, and plasma homocysteine concentrations. Circulation 1996; 93(1):7–9.
3. Salomon O, Steinberg DM, Zivelin A, et al. Single and combined prothrombotic factors in patients with idiopathic venous thromboembolism: prevalence and risk assessment. Arterioscler Thromb Vasc Biol 1999;19(3):511–8.
4. Vandenbroucke JP, Koster T, Briët E, et al. Increased risk of venous thrombosis in oral-contraceptive users who are carriers of factor V Leiden mutation. Lancet 1994;3449(8935):1453–7.
5. Kitchens CS. Thrombophilia and thrombosis in unusual sites. In: Colman RW, Hirsh J, Marder VJ, editors. Hemostasis and thrombosis. Basic principles and clinical practice. Philadelphia: J.B.Lippincott Company; 1994. p. 1255–73.
6. Aiach M, Emmerich J. Thrombophilia genetics. In: Colman RW, Marder VJ, Clowes AW, et al, editors. Hemostasis and thrombosis basic principles and clinical practice. 5th edition. Philadelphia: Lippincott, Williams and Wilkins; 2006. p. 779–93.
7. Olson ST, Björk I. Regulation of thrombin activity by antithrombin and heparin. Semin Thromb Hemost 1994;20(4):373–409.
8. Perry D, Carrell R. Molecular genetics of human antithrombin deficiency. Hum Mutat 1996;7(1): 7–22.
9. Perry DJ. Antithrombin and its inherited deficiencies. Blood Rev 1994;8(1):37–55.
10. Ambruso DR, Leonard BD, Bies RD. Antithrombin III deficiency: decreased synthesis of a biochemically normal molecule. Blood 1982;60(1):78–83.
11. van Boven H, Lane D. Antithrombin and its inherited deficiency states. Semin Hematol 1997; 34(3):188–204.
12. Griffin JH, Evatt B, Zimmerman TS. Deficiency of protein C in congenital thrombotic disease. J Clin Invest 1981;68(5):1370–3.
13. Tait RC, Walker ID, Reitsma PH, et al. Prevalence of protein C deficiency in the healthy population. Thromb Haemost 1995;73(1):87–93.
14. Monagle P, Andrew M, Halton J, et al. Homozygous protein C deficiency: description of a new mutation and successful treatment with low molecular weight heparin. Thromb Haemost 1998;79(4): 756–61.
15. Alhenc-Gelas M, Emmerich J, Gandrille S, et al. Protein C infusion in a patient with inherited protein C deficiency caused by two missense mutations: Arg 178 to Gln and Arg-1 to His. Blood Coagul Fibrinolysis 1995;6(1):35–41.
16. Pescatore P, Horellou HM, Conard J, et al. Problems of oral anticoagulation in an adult with homozygous protein C deficiency and late onset of thrombosis. Thromb Haemost 1993;69(4):311–5.
17. Miletich JP. Laboratory diagnosis of protein C deficiency. Semin Throm Haemost 1990;16(2):169–76.

18. Broze GJ, Warren LA, Novotny WF, et al. The lipoprotein-associated coagulation inhibitor that inhibits the factor VII-tissue factor complex also inhibits factor Xa: insight into its possible mechanism of action. Blood 1988;71(2):335–43.

19. Weiss P, Soff GA, Halkin H, et al. Decline of protein C and S and Factors II, VII, IX and X during the initiation of warfarin therapy. Thromb Res 1987;45(6):783–90.

20. Manco-Johnson MJ, Marlar RA, Jacobson LY, et al. Severe protein C deficiency in newborn infants. J Pediatr 1988;113(2):359–63.

21. Wolf M, Boyer-Neumann C, Martinoli JL, et al. A new functional assay for human protein S activity using activated factor V as substrate. Thromb Haemost 1989;62(4):1144–5.

22. Tripodi A. A review of the clinical and diagnostic utility of laboratory tests for the detection of congenital thrombophilia. Semin Thromb Hemost 2005;31(1):25–32.

23. Vigano-D'Angelo S, d'Angelo A, Kaufman CE Jr, et al. Protein S deficiency occurs in the nephrotic syndrome. Ann Intern Med 1987;107(1):42–7.

24. Malm J, Laurell M, Dahlbäck B. Changes in the plasma levels of vitamin K-dependent proteins C and S and of C4b-binding protein during pregnancy and oral contraception. Br J Haematol 1988;68(4):437–43.

25. Dahlbäck B, Carlsson M, Svensson PJ. Familial thrombophilia due to a previously unrecognized mechanism characterized by poor anticoagulant response to activated protein C: prediction of a cofactor to activated protein C. Proc Natl Acad Sci U S A 1993;90(3):1004–8.

26. Dahlbäck B. The discovery of activated protein C resistance. J Thromb Haemost 2003;1(1):3–9.

27. Bertina RM, Koeleman BP, Koster T, et al. Mutation in blood coagulation factor V association with resistance to activated protein C. Nature 1994;369(6475):64–7.

28. Kalafatis M, Bertina RM, Rand MD, et al. Characterisation of the molecular defect in factor VR506Q. J Biol Chem 1995;270(8):4053–7.

29. Camire RM, Kalafatis M, Cushman M, et al. The mechanism of inactivation of human platelet factor Va from normal and activated protein C-resistant individuals. J Biol Chem 1995;270(35):20794–800.

30. Nicolaes G, Dahlbäck B. Activated protein C resistance (FV Leiden) and thrombosis: factor V mutations causing hypercoagulable states. Hematol Oncol Clin North Am 2003;17(1):37–61.

31. Chan WP, Lee CK, Kwong YL, et al. A novel mutation of Arg306 of factor V gene in Hong Kong Chinese. Blood 1998;91(4):1135–9.

32. Williamson D, Brown K, Luddington R, et al. Factor V: Cambridge: a new mutation (Arg306-Thr) associated with resistance to activated protein C. Blood 1998;91(4):1140–4.

33. Rodegheiro F, Tosetto A. Activated protein C resistance and factor V Leiden mutation are independent risk factors for venous thromboembolism. Ann Intern Med 1999;130(8):643–50.

34. Martinelli I, Mannucci PM, De Stefano V, et al. Different risks of thrombosis in four coagulation defects associated with inherited thrombophilia: a study of 150 families. Blood 1998;92(7):2353–8.

35. Bucciarelli P, Rosendaal FR, Tripodi A, et al. Risks of venous thromboembolism and clinical manifestations in carriers of antithrombin, protein C, protein S deficiency, or activated protein C resistance: a multicenter collaborative family study. Arterioscler Thromb Vasc Biol 1999;19(4):1026–33.

36. Dahlback B, Hildebrand B. Inherited resistance to activated protein C is corrected by anticoagulant cofactor activity found to be a property of factor V. Proc Natl Acad Sci U S A 1994;91(4):1396–400.

37. Hertzberg MS. Genetic testing for thrombophilia mutations. Semin Thromb Hemost 2005;31(1):33–8.

38. Poort SR, Rosendaal FR, Reitsma PH, et al. A common genetic variation in the 3′-untranslated region of the prothrombin gene is associated with elevated plasma prothrombin levels and an increase in venous thrombosis. Blood 1996;88(10):3698–703.

39. Wolberg AS, Monroe DM, Roberts HR, et al. Elevated prothrombin results in clots with an altered fiber structure: a possible mechanism of the increased thrombotic risk. Blood 2003;101(8):3008–13.

40. Kyrle PA, Mannhalter C, Beguin S, et al. Clinical studies and thrombin generation in patients homozygous or heterozygous for the G20210A mutation in the prothrombin gene. Arterioscler Thromb Vasc Biol 1998;18(8):1287–91.

41. Smirnov MD, Safa O, Esmon NL, et al. Inhibition of activated protein C anticoagulant activity by prothrombin. Blood 1999;94(11):3839–46.

42. Bauer K. Hypercoagulable states. In: Hoffman R, Benz EJ Jr, Shattil SJ, et al, editors. Hematology, basic principles and practice. 4th edition. Philadelphia (PA): Elsevier Churchill Livingstone; 2005. p. 2197–224.

43. Zawadzki C, Gaveriaux V, Trillot N, et al. Homozygous G20210A transition in the prothrombin gene associated with severe venous thrombotic disease: two cases in a French family. Thromb Haemost 1998;80(6):1027–8.

44. Kosch A, Junker R, Wermes C, et al. Recurrent pulmonary embolism in a 13-year-old homozygous for the prothrombin G20210A mutation combined with protein S deficiency and increased lipoprotein (a). Thromb Res 2002;105(1):49–53.

45. Kraaijenhagen RA, in't Anker PS, Koopman MM, et al. High plasma concentration of factor VIIIc is

a major risk factor for venous thromboembolism. Thromb Haemost 2000;83(1):5—9.

46. Meijers JC, Tekelenburg WL, Bouma BN, et al. High levels of coagulation factor XI as a risk factor for venous thrombosis. N Engl J Med 2000;342(10): 696—701.

47. van Hylckama Vlieg A, van der Linden IK, Bertina RM, et al. High levels of factor IX increase the risk of venous thrombosis. Blood 2000;95(12): 3678—82.

48. Lim W, Crowther MA, Eikelboom JW. Management of antiphospholipid antibody syndrome. JAMA 2006;295(9):1050—7.

49. Rai RS, Clifford K, Cohe H, et al. High prospective fetal loss rate in untreated pregnancies of women with recurrent miscarriage and antiphospholipid antibodies. Humanit Rep 1995;10(12):3301—4.

50. Brandt JT, Barna LK, Triplett DA. Laboratory identification of lupus anticoagulants: results of the Second International Workshop for Identification of Lupus Anticoagulants. Thromb Haemost 1995; 74(6):1597—603.

51. Harris EN, Gharavi AE, Boey ML, et al. Anticardiolipin antibodies: detection by radioimmunoassay and association with thrombosis in systemic lupus erythematosus. Lancet 1983;2(8361):1211—4.

52. Long A, Ginsberg JS, Brill-Edwards P. The relationship of antiphospholipid antibodies to thromboembolic disease in systemic lupus erythematosus: a cross-sectional study. Thromb Haemost 1991; 66(5):520—4.

53. Brey RL, Chapman J, Levine SR. Stroke and the antiphospholipid syndrome: consensus meeting Taormina 2002. Lupus 2003;12(7):508—13.

54. Brey RL, Escalante A. Neurological manifestations of antiphospholipid antibody syndrome. Lupus 1998;7(Suppl 2):S67—74.

55. Carhuapoma JR, Mitsias P, Levine SR. Cerebral venous thrombosis and anticardiolipin antibodies. Stroke 1997;28(12):2363—9.

56. Warkentin TE. Heparin-induced thrombocytopenia. In: Colman RW, Marder VJ, Clowes AW, et al, editors. Hemostasis and thrombosis basic principles and clinical practice. 5th edition. Philadelphia: Lippincott, Williams and Wilkins; 2006. p. 1649—61.

57. Warkentin TE. Heparin-induced thrombocytopenia: pathogenesis and management. Br J Haematol 2003;121(4):535—55.

58. Warkentin TE, Kelton JG. Delayed-onset heparin-induced thrombocytopenia and thrombosis. Ann Intern Med 2001;135(7):502—6.

59. Warkentin TE, Roberts RS, Hirsh J. An improved definition of immune heparin-induced thrombocytopenia in postoperative orthopedic patients. Arch Intern Med 2003;163(20):2518—24.

60. Lee DH, Warkentin TE. Frequency of heparin-induced thrombocytopenia. In: Warkentin TE,

Greinacher A, editors. Heparin induced thrombocytopenia. 3rd edition. New York: Marcel Dekker Inc; 2004. p. 107—48.

61. Sheridan D, Carter C, Kelton JG. A diagnostic test for heparin-induced thrombocytopenia. Blood 1986;67(1):27—30.

62. Greinacher A, Amiral J, Dummel V, et al. Laboratory diagnosis of heparin-associated thrombocytopenia and comparison of platelet aggregation test, heparin-induced platelet activation test, and platelet factor 4/heparin enzyme-linked immunosorbent assay. Transfusion 1994;34(5):381—5.

63. Lee AY, Levine MN. Venous thromboembolism and cancer: risks and outcomes. Circulation 2003; 107(23 Suppl 1):I17—121.

64. Lee AY. Management of thrombosis in cancer: primary prevention and secondary prophylaxis. Br J Haematol 2006;128:291—302.

65. Ruf W. Molecular regulation of blood clotting in tumor biology. Haemostasis 2001;31(Suppl 1):5—7.

66. Gale AJ, Gordon SG. Update on tumor cell procoagulant factors. Acta Haematol 2001;106(1—2):25—32.

67. Bertomeu MC, Gallo S, Lauri D, et al. Chemotherapy enhances endothelial cell reactivity to platelets. Clin Exp Metastasis 1990;8(6):511—8.

68. Pritchard KI, Paterson AH, Paul NA, et al. Increased thromboembolic complications with concurrent tamoxifen and chemotherapy in a randomized trial of adjuvant therapy for women with breast cancer. J Clin Oncol 1996;14(10):2731—7.

69. Levine MN, Lee AY, Kakkar AK. Cancer and thrombosis. In: Colman RW, Marder VJ, Clowes AW, et al, editors. Hemostasis and thrombosis. basic principles and clinical practice. 5th edition. Philadelphia: Lippincott, Williams and Wilkins; 2006. p. 1251—62.

70. Greer IA. Thrombosis in pregnancy: maternal and fetal issues. Lancet 1999;353(9160):1258—65.

71. McColl MD, Ramsay JE, Tait RC, et al. Risk factors for pregnancy associated venous thromboembolism. Thromb Haemost 1997;78(4):1183—8.

72. Cockett FB, Thomas ML. The iliac compression syndrome. Br J Surg 1965;52(10):816—21.

73. Ginsberg JS, Brill-Edwards P, Burrows RF, et al. Venous thrombosis during pregnancy: leg and trimester of presentation. Thromb Haemost 1992; 67(5):519—20.

74. Clark P. Changes of hemostasis variables during pregnancy. Semin Vasc Med 2003;3(1):13—24.

75. Bremme K. Haemostatic changes in pregnancy. Best Pract Res Clin Haematol 2003;16(2):153—68.

76. Comp P, Thurnau GR, Welsh J, et al. Functional and immunologic protein S levels are decreased during pregnancy. Blood 1986;68(4):881—5.

77. Clark P, Brennand J, Conkie JA, et al. Activated protein C sensitivity, protein C, protein S and coagulation in normal pregnancy. Thromb Haemost 1998;79(6):1166—70.

78. Stirling Y, Woolf L, North WR, et al. Haemostasis in normal pregnancy. Thromb Haemost 1984;52: 176–82.

79. Eichinger S, Weltermann A, Philipp K, et al. Prospective evaluation of hemostatic system activation and thrombin potential in healthy pregnant women with and without factor V Leiden. Thromb Haemost 1999;82(4):1232–6.

80. Martinelli I, Legnani C, Bucciarelli P. Risk of pregnancy-related venous thrombosis in carriers of severe inherited thrombophilia. Thromb Haemost 2001;86(3):800–3.

81. Greer IA. Inherited thrombophilia and venous thromboembolism. Best Pract Res Clin Obstet Gynaecol 2003;17(3):413–25.

82. Gerhardt A, Scharf R, Beckmann M, et al. Prothrombin and factor V mutations in women with a history of thrombosis during pregnancy and the puerperium. N Engl J Med 2000;342(6):374–80.

83. Friederich PW, Sanson BJ, Simioni P, et al. Frequency of pregnancy-related venous thromboembolism in anticoagulant factor-deficient women: implications for prophylaxis. Ann Intern Med 1996;125(12):955–60.

84. Bates SM, Greer IA, Hirsh J, et al. Use of antithrombotic agents during pregnancy: the Seventh ACCP Conference on antithrombotic and thrombolytic therapy. Chest 2006;126(Suppl 3):627S.

85. Vandenbroucke JP, Rosing J, Bloemenkamp KW, et al. Oral contraceptives and the risk of venous thrombosis. N Engl J Med 2001;344(20):1527–35.

86. Daly E, Vessey MP, Hawkins MM, et al. Risk of venous thromboembolism in users of hormone replacement therapy. Lancet 1996;348(9033):977–80.

87. Martinelli I. Risk factors in venous thromboembolism. Thromb Haemost 2001;86(1):395–403.

88. Rosendaal FR. Oral contraceptives and screening for factor V Leiden. Thromb Haemost 1996;75(3): 524–5.

89. Prandoni P, Lensing AW, Cogo A, et al. The long-term clinical course of acute deep venous thrombosis. Ann Intern Med 1996;125(1):1–7.

90. Heit JA, Silverstein MD, Mohr DN, et al. Risk factors for deep vein thrombosis and pulmonary embolism: a population-based case-control study. Arch Intern Med 2000;160(6):809–15.

91. Kearon C, Gent M, Hirsh J, et al. A comparison of three months of anticoagulation with extended anticoagulation for a first episode of idiopathic venous thromboembolism. N Engl J Med 1999;340(12): 901–7.

92. Cattaneo M. Hyperhomocysteinemia, atherosclerosis and thrombosis. Thromb Haemost 1999;81 (2):165–76.

93. Ray J. Meta-analysis of hyperhomocysteinemia as a risk factor for venous thromboembolic disease. Arch Intern Med 1998;158(19):2101–6.

94. Finkelstein JD. Methionine metabolism in mammals. J Nutr Biochem 1990;1(5):228–37.

95. Kluijtmans LA, van den Huevel LP, Boers GH, et al. Molecular genetic analysis in mild hyperhomocysteinemia: a common mutation in the methylenetetrahydrofolate reductase gene is a genetic risk factor for cardiovascular disease. Am J Hum Genet 1996;58(1):35–41.

96. Jacques PF, Selhub J, Bostom AG, et al. The effect of folic acid fortification on plasma folate and total homocysteine concentrations. N Engl J Med 1999;340(19):1449–54.

97. Molloy AM, Scott JM. Folates and prevention of disease. Public Health Nutr 2001;4(2B):601–9.

98. Homocysteine Lowering Trialists' Collaboration. Lowering blood homocysteine with folic acid based supplements: meta-analysis of randomised trials. BMJ 1998;316:894–8.

99. Lonn E, Yusuf S, Arnold MJ, et al. Homocysteine lowering with folic acid and B vitamins in vascular disease. N Engl J Med 2006;354(15):1567–77.

100. Dreyfus M, Magny JF, Bridey F, et al. Treatment of homozygous protein C deficiency and neonatal purpura fulminans with a purified protein C concentrate. N Engl J Med 1991;325(22):1565–8.

101. Monagle P, Chan A, Massicotte P, et al. Antithrombotic therapy in children: the Seventh ACCP Conference on Antithrombotic and Thrombolytic Therapy. Chest 2004;126(3):645–87.

102. Lechner K, Kyrle P. Antithrombin III concentrates—are they clinically useful? Thromb Haemost 1995;73(3):340–8.

103. Crowther MA, Ginsberg JS, Julian J, et al. A comparison of two intensities of warfarin for the prevention of recurrent thrombosis in patients with the antiphospholipid antibody syndrome. N Engl J Med 2003;349(7):631–9.

104. Finazzi G, Marchioli R, Brancaccio V. A randomised clinical trial of high-intensity warfarin versus conventional antithrombotic therapy for the prevention of recurrent thrombosis in patients with the antiphospholipid antibody syndrome. J Thromb Haemost 2005;3(5):848–53.

105. Lee AYY, Levine MN, Baker RI, et al. Low-molecular-weight heparin versus a coumarin for the prevention of recurrent venous thromboembolism in patients with cancer. N Engl J Med 2003;349(2):146–53.

106. Marchetti M, Pistorio A, Barone M, et al. Low-molecular-weight heparin versus warfarin for secondary prophylaxis of venous thromboembolism: a cost-effectiveness analysis. Am J Med 2001;111(2):130–9.

107. Levine MN, Hirsh J, Gent M, et al. Optimal duration of oral anticoagulant therapy: a randomized trial comparing four weeks with three months of warfarin in patients with proximal deep venous thrombosis. Thromb Haemost 1995;74(2):606–11.

108. Agnelli G, Prandoni P, Santamaria MG, et al. Three months versus one year of oral anticoagulant therapy for idiopathic deep vein thrombosis. N Engl J Med 2001;345(3):165—9.

109. Buller HR, Agnelli G, Hull RD, et al. Antithrombotic therapy for venous thromboembolic disease: the Seventh ACCP Conference on Antithrombotic and Thrombolytic Therapy. Chest 2004;126(3):401S—28S.

110. Ridker PM, Goldhaber SZ, Danielson E, et al. Long-term, low-intensity warfarin therapy for the prevention of recurrent venous thromboembolism. N Engl J Med 2003;348(15):1425—34.

111. Gallus AS. Management options for thrombophilias. Semin Thromb Hemost 2005;31(1):118—26.

112. Mazzolai L, Hohlfeld P, Spertini F, et al. Fondaparinux is a safe alternative in case of heparin intolerance during pregnancy. Blood 2006;108(5):1569—70.

113. McKenna R, Cole ER, Vasan U. Is warfarin sodium contraindicated in lactating mothers? J Pediatr 1983;103(2):325—7.

114. Brill-Edwards P, Ginsberg JA, Gent M, et al. Safety of withholding heparin in pregnant women with a history of venous thromboembolism. N Engl J Med 2000;343(20):1439—44.

115. Greaves M, Baglin T. Laboratory testing for heritable thrombophilia; impact on clinical management of thrombotic disease. Br J Haematol 2000;109(4):699—703.

116. Mannucci PM. Genetic hypercoagulability: prevention suggests testing family members. Blood 2001;98(1):21—2.

117. Heron E, Lozinguez O, Alhenc-Gelas M, et al. Hypercoagulable states in primary upper-extremity deep vein thrombosis. Arch Intern Med 2000;160(3):382—6.

Deep Vein Thrombosis Prophylaxis in Hospitalized Medical Patients: Current Recommendations, General Rates of Implementation, and Initiatives for Improvement

Scott M. Stevens, MD[a,b,*],
James D. Douketis, MD, FRCP(C), FCCP[c]

KEYWORDS

- Venous thromboembolism • Deep vein thrombosis
- Pulmonary embolism • Prophylaxis

Venous thromboembolism (VTE), which encompasses deep vein thrombosis (DVT) and pulmonary embolism (PE), is a leading cause of preventable morbidity and mortality following hospitalization.[1] In the last decade, investigators have used randomized controlled trials (RCTs) to assess the efficacy and safety of various methods of VTE prevention for more than 20,000 medical patients.[2] Identifying medical patients at risk for VTE and providing effective prophylaxis is now an important health care priority to reduce the burden of this morbid and sometimes fatal disease.

SCOPE OF THE PROBLEM: THE IMPORTANCE OF VENOUS THROMBOEMBOLISM IN THE MEDICAL PATIENT

As many as one-third of all cases of VTE occur in the 3 months following hospitalization[3,4] and VTE accounts for approximately 10% of all in-hospital mortality.[5] Of all patients diagnosed with hospital-associated VTE, half to three-quarters are medical patients without antecedent trauma or lower extremity injury[6,7] and 70% to 80% of inpatient deaths due to PE occur in medical patients.[8] An analysis of data from the 2003 United States Healthcare Cost and Use Project estimated that more than 8 million hospitalized patients are at risk for VTE annually, that almost 200,000 experience hospital-associated VTE, and that appropriate prophylaxis would have averted more than 110,000 of these events.[9]

The absolute risk for symptomatic VTE occurring within 3 months of medical hospitalization, according to linked administrative databases, is 1.7%[10]; however, this estimate includes all hospital discharges, regardless of patient VTE risk. When prospective studies have evaluated medical patients with one or more recognized VTE risk factors, the incidence of venographically detected VTE rises to 10% to 15%[11,12] with even higher rates in critically ill patients.[13] In the

[a] Department of Medicine, Intermountain Medical Center, 5169 South Cottonwood Street, Suite 300, Murray, UT 84107, USA
[b] University of Utah, Salt Lake City, UT, USA
[c] Department of Medicine, McMaster University, 1280 Main Street West, Hamilton, ON L8S4L8, Canada
* Corresponding author. Department of Medicine, Intermountain Medical Center, 5169 South Cottonwood Street, Suite 300, Murray, UT 84107.
E-mail address: Scott.StevensMD@imail.org

Clin Chest Med 31 (2010) 675–689
doi:10.1016/j.ccm.2010.07.005
0272-5231/10/$ – see front matter

absence of prophylaxis, the rate of symptomatic proximal DVT (which is more likely to result in PE or the post-thrombotic syndrome) in medical patients with risk factors for VTE is approximately 5%[14]; PE has been reported in 0.5% of patients.[15]

Hospital-associated VTE carries substantial cost, similar to that incurred by stroke or myocardial infarction.[16] Post-thrombotic syndrome occurs in approximately one-third of patients with symptomatic DVT, and is a source of additional medical cost and long-term morbidity.[17]

These findings highlight the significant association between medical hospitalization and VTE, and the importance of effective strategies to mitigate this risk and reduce associated patient morbidity and mortality. PE is considered the most common preventable cause of hospital mortality,[13] and its prevention has been given the highest priority among 79 interventions detailed in a report by the Agency for Health Research and Quality (AHRQ).[18] Use of VTE prophylaxis in medical patients is cost effective, and results in net health savings that may extend for as long as 2 years following hospitalization.[19]

PROPHYLAXIS OF VTE: IMPORTANCE TO PATIENTS AND BARRIERS TO IMPLEMENTATION

Over 3 decades, a large number of RCTs and prospective cohort studies have validated the effectiveness of various prophylactic strategies to reduce the incidence of DVT, PE, and even fatal PE that is associated with hospitalization.[13] Studies have validated that VTE prophylaxis is safe and results in only a small excess risk for bleeding.[12,20,21] Furthermore, implementation of an effective prophylaxis strategy results in net cost savings.[22]

Despite the significance of these benefits, the rate of implementation of VTE prevention strategies in medical inpatients is disappointing. Multiple registries and queries of administrative data reveal rates of VTE prophylaxis in medical patients ranging from 15% to 49%.[9,23,24] This rate is markedly lower than that reported in similar analyses of surgical patients, which have reported rates of VTE prophylaxis of as high as 90%.[25,26]

Several reasons may explain the lower rate of implementation of VTE prophylaxis in medical patients. Prophylaxis decisions in surgical patients are often driven by the surgical procedure, whereas medical inpatients are a more diverse and heterogeneous population. Risk assessment for VTE in medical patients is complex, with many recognized risk factors noted in assessment tools, and a lack of precision regarding indications and contraindications for prophylaxis. In addition, concerns regarding bleeding risk and lack of clinician time have been cited as barriers to implementing prophylaxis in all patients.[27]

IDENTIFYING PATIENTS FOR PROPHYLAXIS: VTE RISK FACTORS

Although a large majority of medical inpatients are considered at risk for VTE,[13] pharmacologic prophylaxis incurs expense and a small increased risk for bleeding. Therefore, most practitioners select patients for prophylaxis on the basis of a sufficiently high perceived risk of VTE. Unfortunately, the list of putative risk factors for VTE in medical patients is extensive (Table 1), and there is limited validation of methods to stratify the relative contribution of individual factors or assess the additive risk when multiple factors coexist.

These limitations impede implementing an individual-based system for prophylaxis decisions, whereby a practitioner determines a patient's individual risk for hospital-associated VTE and responds with a targeted prophylaxis decision based on this risk estimate. When assessing a medical patient for VTE risk, admission illness, activity level, and patient history may all contribute to the VTE risk profile. Admitting diagnoses of heart failure, acute stroke, chronic obstructive pulmonary disease (COPD), respiratory infection, and cancer are considered to confer a higher risk for VTE. Presence of vascular devices and location of admission (medical ward vs intensive care unit [ICU]) also influences the risk for VTE.

Heart failure has long been recognized as an admitting diagnosis associated with an increased risk for VTE. Some of the earliest studies of pharmacologic prophylaxis focused on this patient group.[20,28] The risk appears to be amplified by the severity of symptoms, with higher risk observed in patients with New York Heart Association class III or IV symptoms. Other cardiovascular diseases, including myocardial infarction, have also been associated with VTE risk; however, this risk may be mitigated in many patients by the use of anticoagulant medications for treatment of acute coronary artery disease.

Respiratory disease, particularly respiratory failure, carries a strong association with increased VTE risk. COPD and severe respiratory infection have been among the inclusion criteria for several studies of pharmacologic prophylaxis.[29,30] In addition to COPD and respiratory infection, acute respiratory distress syndrome, parenchymal lung disease, and pulmonary hypertension have also been associated with increased VTE risk.

Table 1
Recognized risk factors for VTE in hospitalized inpatients

Risk Factor	Comments
Age	Age >60–65 has been used to define risk groups in controlled trials. Age >40 is often used as a threshold after which the addition of other risk factors confers significant risk
Obesity	No threshold body mass index has clearly been defined at which significant VTE risk begins
Immobility	No standard definition. Bed rest or bed rest with ambulation only to bathroom has been used in prophylaxis trials to define immobility
Previous VTE	Major risk factor for hospital-associated VTE
Ischemic stroke	Risk particularly high in those with paralysis or paresis of a lower limb
Heart failure	Defining risk condition in many prophylaxis trials. Hospitalization with heart failure usually implies severe functional impairment
Severe respiratory disease	Defining risk condition in many prophylaxis trials. Hospitalization for respiratory disease usually implies severe functional impairment
Severe inflammatory disease	Examples include rheumatologic conditions such as systemic lupus erythematosis; flares of inflammatory bowel disease
Active cancer	Includes cancer under palliative care; cancer with any form of active treatment (radiation, chemotherapy, or biologic therapy), or cancer with completion of treatment in the preceding 6 months
Severe infectious disease	Includes pneumonia, sepsis syndromes, meningitis
Hypercoagulability and thrombophilia	Includes acquired and hereditary thrombophilias, as well as myeloproliferative syndromes, nephrotic syndrome, and protein-losing enteropathy
Recent surgery	Generally defined as surgery under general or regional anesthesia in the preceding 3 months

Cancer is a common diagnosis or comorbidity in hospitalized medical patients. Cancer patients are as much as 6 times more likely to develop VTE than patients without cancer[15,31]; moreover, VTE is one of the most common complications of malignancy[31–34] and results in decreased survival.[35–37] Several mechanisms contribute to this increase in risk. Many tumors have been associated with hypercoagulability through a variety of biochemical mechanisms, and this risk varies by type of malignancy.[31,38] Adenocarcinomas of the abdominal and pelvic viscera and brain tumors confer a particularly strong association with VTE.[38,39] In addition, certain tumors may cause venous thrombosis through mechanical compression of veins. Cancer therapy, including chemotherapy agents, radiation therapy, hormonal therapies, and use of indwelling venous catheters, also contributes to this risk. Despite these factors, cancer patients have been reported to have lower rates of VTE prophylaxis than other patient groups.[23]

Bed rest or limited ambulation, increased patient age, and a history of prior VTE are patient-specific factors that confer higher risk.[11,40,41] A derivation-validation of a simplified risk-assessment tool, which analyzed 18 potential risk factors in approximately 120,000 medical hospitalizations against the outcome of VTE diagnosed within 3 months of discharge, found that patient age, prior VTE, and cancer are dominant risk factors in predicting development of VTE (Woller SC and colleagues, in preparation; data obtained by personal communication, July, 2010).

The presence of a peripherally inserted central venous catheter (PICC), typically inserted in the brachial veins, is also associated with an increased risk for upper extremity VTE. A risk prediction model, derived from analysis of in-hospital DVT rates following 2014 PICC placements, revealed that a history of prior VTE (odds ratio [OR] 9.92) and increasing catheter diameter and number of lumens (OR 7.54 for 5F double-lumen; 19.50 for 6F triple-lumen) were most predictive of PICC-associated DVT (Evans RS, Sharp, JH, Linford LH and colleagues, Chest, in press data obtained by personal communication, July, 2010).

Reported rates of VTE in critically ill patients in an ICU have varied widely[42] but with upper-range estimates far in excess of the rates reported in medical ward patients (**Table 2**). ICU patients

Table 2
Rates of VTE in various groups of hospitalized patients without prophylaxis

Patient Group	Rate of VTE
General medical ward	10%–20%
ICU	10%–80%
Stroke patients	20%–50%
with paralysis	40%–60%

Abbreviation: ICU, intensive care unit.

are likely to have multiple risk factors for VTE (see **Table 1**) and the ICU environment may contribute to VTE risk, in that patients are more likely to be immobilized, may be mechanically ventilated, may be medically sedated and/or paralyzed, and may be more likely to have central venous catheters.[13]

Several studies have attempted to develop formal risk assessment models (RAMs), containing individual risk factors, usually in combination with the patient's admission diagnosis.[40,41,43,44] None of these tools are used commonly; their implementation has likely been hampered by complexity. Furthermore, validation of these RAMs has been limited outside of the original study populations.[13]

INITIATIVES FOR IMPROVEMENT: STRATEGIES TO INCREASE RATES OF PROPHYLAXIS

Initiatives to improve the uptake of VTE prophylaxis in medical patients can be separated into general and specific strategies.

General Strategies to Improve VTE Prophylaxis

General strategies to improve the use of VTE prophylaxis include (a) identification of easily identified and targeted patient groups who are likely to benefit from prophylaxis, or (b) broad application of a prophylaxis strategy to encompass all patients, except those in whom anticoagulants are contraindicated or in whom therapeutic-dose anticoagulation is being administered for other clinical indications.

With the first approach, one can target 5 large patient groups, to include congestive heart failure, respiratory disease, ischemic stroke, serious infection, and advanced cancer.[13] With the second approach, all medical patients would be candidates for anticoagulant VTE prophylaxis unless they had a contraindication, such as active bleeding, or were already receiving anticoagulant therapy. The first approach has the merit that

these patient groups were the dominant patient groups studied in RCTs of pharmacologic VTE prophylaxis.[20,28–45] A limitation of this approach is that it may overlook some patients at increased risk for VTE. The second approach has the merit of being more inclusive and not predicating prophylaxis on the basis of admission diagnosis—a more simplified approach that may optimize anticoagulant prophylaxis. Its drawbacks include possible administration of anticoagulant prophylaxis, with its inherent risks, to patients who may derive little if any benefit. The authors suggest that the approach used should depend on patient demographics at each institution. Thus, hospitals that have a high volume of less acute, less ill patients may opt for the disease-specific approach, targeting anticoagulant prophylaxis to selected higher-risk medical patients. Other hospitals, such as tertiary care facilities, which typically have a high volume of acutely ill patients, may opt for the more inclusive approach, as one would anticipate few patients who are considered "low risk." Whichever general approach is taken, the American College of Chest Physicians (ACCP) consensus guideline recommends (Level 1A) that every hospital have an institution-wide policy for VTE prophylaxis that, ideally, should reflect patient demographics.[13]

Specific Strategies to Improve VTE Prophylaxis

A variety of more specific strategies has been studied to attempt to overcome the barriers to successful implementation of VTE prophylaxis and increase rates of appropriate implementation. Strategies may be categorized as active (performance audit and feedback, reminder systems, preprinted orders) or passive (distribution of guidelines and educational sessions). Several active strategies have been shown to increase rates of prophylaxis[46–50] and decrease rates of VTE diagnosed following hospitalization.[51] The method of intervention chosen influences the rate of success. Kucher and colleagues[51] implemented a computerized system that identified inpatients at high risk for VTE not receiving prophylaxis. The system then randomly assigned a group of providers to receive computerized alerts. The group of patients whose providers received the alert were more likely to receive VTE prophylaxis and less likely to experience VTE within 90 days of hospital discharge. However, such a system is highly dependent on the capabilities of the electronic medical record at the institution, limiting widespread use of the intervention. A second study used the same risk assessment system but provided the prophylaxis reminder in the form of a phone call from study personnel. The intervention group again received higher rates of prophylaxis, but did not attain a statistically significant reduction in the rate of VTE at 90 days post hospitalization.[52] While this system does not rely on an electronic medical information system, the human resources needed to perform the risk assessment and reminder calls may be a barrier to broad implementation. All reminder-based interventions have the possible benefit of diffusion (providers who do not receive a reminder may still improve their rates of prophylaxis based on knowledge of the system's existence) and the possible drawback of alert fatigue (a decrease in the rate of response to the reminder over time).[53]

Simpler active strategies have also been implemented and have demonstrated increases in prophylaxis rates and VTE outcome. In a group of medical and surgical patients, Maynard and colleagues[44] studied the effect of an embedded set of electronic orders that included a menu of VTE prophylaxis options. Over 3 years, the rate of prophylaxis increased from 58% to 98% and the rate of hospital-associated VTE detected by imaging review decreased by 30%. Although this intervention did not require an information system capable of automatic risk assessment and targeted alerting, it still required an electronic physician orders system that may not be widely available. Audit and feedback was also used, which requires additional resources. Paper-based systems, such as preprinted orders, have also been used. While arguably the simplest and most generalizable of the active interventions, the degree of effectiveness of such systems is more variable.[50,54,55] These systems are also subject to fatigue and likely require active upkeep by personnel tasked to maintain such a system.[55] Preprinted orders carry a lower level of recommendation in published guidelines.[13] Features shown to predict an effective prophylaxis program include use of a multifaceted approach and a system of audit and feedback.[50]

By contrast, passive interventions, while much easier to implement, appear to be ineffective at changing the rate of appropriate prophylaxis. Grand rounds or lectures, distribution of published guidelines, and dedicated education programs do not appreciably change prophylaxis practices.[46–56] However, such activities are often used in the creation of a program of active intervention to help increase acceptance of the active strategy, and may improve the success of implementation.[57,58] Several published guidelines make recommendations to hospitals regarding the type of prophylaxis programs that should be implemented (see "Prophylaxis Recommendations: Published Guidelines and Regulatory Statements").

PROPHYLAXIS INTERVENTIONS: OPTIONS AND EVIDENCE FOR EFFECTIVENESS
Nonpharmacologic and Mechanical Strategies

Nonpharmacologic strategies to reduce the risk of VTE include promoting patient activity through ambulation, graduated compression stockings (GCS), venous foot pumps (VFPs), and intermittent pneumatic compression devices (IPCs). These interventions are thought to prevent DVT through several mechanisms: they reduce stasis of blood in the veins through intermittent application of pressure, and enhance both local and systemic fibrinolysis, as has been shown by decreases in euglobin clot lysis time.[59–62] Many investigators have suggested that tPA-activity increases despite decreases in tPA-antigen, and that PAI-1 Ag and activity drop.[60,61] Others have shown decreases in Factor VIIa activity.[63] Enhancement of fibrinolysis likely explains the observation that patients with a device applied to one extremity experience a reduction in DVT rate in extremities without a device.[62,64] The attractiveness of these methods is that they are unlikely to increase the risk for bleeding.

Early and frequent ambulation is a simple intervention, but no studies have been performed to quantify its effectiveness as a sole method of VTE prophylaxis. The observation that most hospital-associated VTE events occur in patients who are ambulatory[13] argues against the effectiveness of ambulation as a solitary intervention for VTE prophylaxis. In addition, many hospitalized patients are unable to ambulate, particularly in ICU settings.

Mechanical methods of prophylaxis, while conferring a low risk for bleeding, also have limitations. Such devices are only effective when worn by the patient, and in the case of IPCs and VFPs, when the devices are activated and functioning properly. Observational studies show substantial noncompliance with mechanical devices,[65] with the highest rates of compliance in the ICU. The presence of devices also may be a barrier to patient ambulation. There are several different devices available, many of which have not been assessed in clinical trials but have achieved regulatory approval based on similarity to preexisting devices. Size, fit, pressure settings, and for IPCs, timing and mode of compression, have not been well standardized. Very obese patients may have leg circumferences that preclude being fit with any device. Furthermore, GCS can cause skin breakdown or ulceration, especially in the elderly or other patients with compromised skin integrity.[66] Finally,

IPCs can cause ecchymoses or other soft tissue injury when not properly fitted or if used excessively. Actual contraindications to mechanical prophylaxis include open skin lesions and preexisting DVT in the limb prior to application.

Studies in surgical populations have noted reduction in the risk of VTE when mechanical methods are the sole prophylaxis method employed,[67,68] but similar studies have not been performed in medical inpatients. One study suggested that VFPs were ineffective in surgical patients when compared with full-length IPCs.[68] It is also noteworthy that a large randomized trial reported no therapeutic benefit when mechanical antithrombotic devices were added to anticoagulant prophylaxis. Even in surgical populations, no study has affirmed a beneficial effect of mechanical prophylaxis as a sole intervention on rates of symptomatic PE or survival.[66] Existing studies of mechanical prophylaxis tend to be less methodologically rigorous than studies of pharmacologic prophylaxis, in part due to the difficulty inherent in blinding the intervention.

Given these limitations, mechanical methods of prophylaxis should not be considered a "benign" method of prophylaxis that should be widely used, but should be reserved for medical inpatients with contraindications to pharmacologic prophylaxis, such as active bleeding, hemorrhagic stroke, or a bleeding diathesis. Even then, patients assigned to a mechanical VTE prophylaxis should be frequently reevaluated and provided with pharmacologic prophylaxis when the contraindication abates.

Pharmacologic Prophylaxis

Prophylaxis using pharmacologic agents is the most effective means of VTE prevention in medical inpatients. A meta-analysis of studies totaling more than 20,000 medical inpatients showed that pharmacologic prophylaxis reduced symptomatic DVT by 53%, symptomatic PE by 58%, and fatal PE by 64%, although there was no improvement in all-cause mortality.[14]

Several medications have been approved by the United States Food and Drug Administration (FDA) for prevention of VTE in medical inpatients (**Table 3**). All presently approved medications are anticoagulants; antiplatelet agents are not approved for this purpose. Several studies have shown limited

Table 3
FDA-approved medications for VTE prophylaxis in medical patients

Medication	Dose	Dose if ClCr ≤30 mL/min	Comments
Unfractionated heparin	5000 units SC, BID, or TID	Same	The BID and TID doses have never been directly compared in an RCT. Meta-analyses have suggested greater efficacy but greater risk of bleeding with the TID dose. Current guidelines conclude that there is insufficient evidence to recommend one dosing strategy over the other
Low Molecular Weight Heparins			
Enoxaparin	40 mg SC daily	30 mg SC daily	The 30-mg SC daily dose is not FDA-approved for patients on hemodialysis. Dosing of all LMWHs is less certain for severely obese patients with a BMI ≥35. Experts have advocated use of enoxaparin 30 mg SC twice daily for patients with a BMI ≥35
Dalteparin	5000 units SC daily	No specifically approved dose	The 5000 units SC daily dose has been studied in ICU patients with severe renal failure, but is not specifically FDA-approved in this patient group
Pentasaccharides			
Fondaparinux	2.5 mg SC daily	No approved dose	Not labeled for patients <50 kg. Labeled "use with caution" when ClCr 30–50 mL/kg. Very unlikely to cause HIT

Abbreviations: BID, twice daily; ClCr, creatinine clearance; HIT, heparin-induced thrombocytopenia; LMWH, low molecular weight heparin; SC, subcutaneous; TID, 3 times daily.

beneficial effect of acetylsalicylic acid (ASA) in the prevention of VTE, largely in surgical populations,[69–71] but the effect is less than that of anticoagulant medications. Additional studies have shown no beneficial effect from ASA in orthopedic surgery patients.[72–74] There is no evidence that ASA is safer than anticoagulants presently employed for VTE prophylaxis in medical inpatients.[69,70]

The anticoagulant medications presently approved for VTE prophylaxis are effective, reducing the rate of symptomatic VTE by nearly two-thirds when compared in large randomized trials, and confer a minimal increased risk for major bleeding[13] While more beneficial than nonpharmacologic strategies, pharmacologic prophylaxis has limitations. All agents presently available are administered by subcutaneous injection, which carries minor inconvenience to patients and adds a burden to hospital staff. All agents are associated with a risk for heparin-induced thrombocytopenia (HIT), although this risk is low with low molecular weight heparins (LMWHs), estimated at less than 0.1%, and has occurred with fondaparinux in only one reported case.[75–77] Contraindications include active bleeding or elevated risk of bleeding, history of HIT (particularly with persistent elevation of antiplatelet factor 4 IgG antibodies),[76] and medication allergy. LMWHs and fondaparinux are primarily cleared by renal excretion, and renal dysfunction requires dose adjustment or use of unfractionated heparin (see "Low Molecular Weight Heparins" and "Fondaparinux").[13]

Unfractionated Heparin

Unfractionated heparin (UFH) is the agent with the longest history of use for VTE prophylaxis in medical inpatients, and was first studied against placebo as a method of VTE prophylaxis more than 25 years ago.[20] In addition to being compared with placebo, UFH prophylaxis has served as the comparator group for several studies of newer anticoagulant medications.[29,78–80]

The dosing of UFH (see **Table 3**) has varied in trials of medical prophylaxis, with 5000 units subcutaneously dosed either twice daily[81] or 3 times daily.[20,28] Controversy has existed over which dosing strategy is preferred. These 2 doses have never been directly compared, but the twice-daily regimen was shown to be similarly effective to enoxaparin, 20 mg subcutaneously once daily, in an RCT,[78] whereas the same dose of enoxaparin was no better than placebo in a second trial.[11] A meta-analysis of nearly 8000 patients showed a statistically significant increase in the rate of bleeding with the thrice-daily dose, and a nonsignificant

trend toward greater VTE with the twice-daily dose.[82] A meta-analysis of 36 trials concluded that the thrice-daily dose of UFH was more effective than the twice-daily dose for VTE prevention (relative risk, 0.27 vs 0.52).[83] Current guidelines conclude that there is insufficient evidence to recommend one dosing strategy over the other.[13]

UFH is a commonly used anticoagulant for VTE prophylaxis in medical inpatients. As other available agents are cleared predominantly by renal excretion, UFH may be the preferred agent in patients with severe renal dysfunction, although some LMWH preparations have been assessed in this patient group as well (see "Low Molecular Weight Heparins"). UFH is contraindicated in patients with a history of HIT, especially in those in whom persistent heparin-associated platelet factor 4 antibodies exist.[76] In 2008, a defect in the manufacturing process resulted in the distribution of UFH contaminated with oversulfated chondroitin sulfate, leading to cases of severe anaphylactoid reaction.[84] The FDA in the United States implemented a program to detect contaminated UFH and remove it from the United States drug supply. Recently, an update to the US Pharmacopeia (USP) heparin monograph, effective October 1, 2009, resulted in an approximate 10% reduction in heparin potency in the United States, bringing units of UFH in line with international standards. This potency change in UFH is unlikely to have any effect on UFH dosing for VTE prophylaxis, whereas higher doses may need to be administered to patients receiving therapeutic-dose UFH that is adjusted by monitoring of the activated partial thromboplastin time. Although the drug acquisition cost of UFH is less than that for other agents in the United States, the inherent expense of more frequent administration offsets this cost benefit.[19] In addition, a cost-effectiveness study, conducted with pharmaceutical industry funding at a tertiary center, concluded that LMWH has superior cost effectiveness to UFH due to the lower rate of HIT and avoidance of related costs of HIT management.[85] Fondaparinux has had favorable cost effectiveness when compared with enoxaparin in orthopedic patients,[86] but cost-effectiveness data are not available for prophylaxis in medical patients.

The evidence for the effectiveness of UFH is substantial, with several studies showing benefit compared with placebo[20,28,81,87,88] and effectiveness similar to that of LMWH[29,78–80,89–91] including efficacy results from a pooled analysis of more than 4500 patients, which examined symptomatic and asymptomatic DVT, clinically overt PE, and death.[92] Specific patient populations in which UFH has been studied and found to be beneficial include patients with stroke,[87,88] medical patients 65 years and older,[78] patients with heart failure and/or severe respiratory disease,[20,28,29] and general medical inpatients with one or more VTE risk factors.[11,80,93,90] ICU patients have had similar risk reduction in several studies,[94–96] but a study of the twice-daily regimen of UFH in ICU patients showed it to be no better than placebo for prevention of VTE using ultrasound-detected DVT as the clinical end point.[97] The effect of UFH on all-cause mortality in medical patients has been the subject of two adequately powered studies.[98,99] In one study, all-cause mortality was reduced from 10.9% to 7.8%[98] but the second, larger study showed no effect on mortality.[99] The majority of studies have not had sufficient power to assess mortality.[13] UFH prophylaxis is associated with a low overall rate of major bleeding, although a meta-analysis of more than 4500 patients found the incidence of bleeding was higher with UFH than LMWH prophylaxis (1.2% vs 0.4%, $P = .049$).[92]

Low Molecular Weight Heparin

Several preparations of LMWH are available for VTE prophylaxis in medical patients. LMWHs have less tendency to bind to plasma proteins and macrophages, and have a longer plasma half-life than UFH; this has led to the adoption of once-daily dose regimens for medical prophylaxis.[13,100] Three LMWHs have been assessed in randomized trials for VTE prophylaxis in medical patients: enoxaparin,[11,21,29,78,80] dalteparin,[101] and nadroparin.[79] Enoxaparin and dalteparin are approved by the FDA for this indication.

All LMWH preparations are dosed once daily for medical prophylaxis, with dosing varying by agent (see **Table 3**). Different LMWHs have not been directly compared in randomized trials, but the effectiveness appears to be similar between available agents. In patients with severe renal insufficiency, defined as estimated creatinine clearance (CrCl) less than 30 mL/min, enoxaparin has an FDA-approved adjusted dose of 30 mg subcutaneously once daily, although to the authors' knowledge this dose regimen has not been formally studied in clinical trials involving patients with severe renal insufficiency. This dose is not approved for dialysis-dependent patients. Dalteparin's labeling indicates it should be used with caution in patients with severe renal insufficiency. However, a single-arm study of dalteparin, 5000 units subcutaneously once daily, was performed in ICU patients with severe renal insufficiency (CrCl <30 mL/min), and detected no evidence of excess anticoagulation from bioaccumulation, determined by anti-factor Xa level monitoring,[102]

after a mean of 7 days of treatment. This study, therefore, suggests that dalteparin 5000 units once daily is an option for DVT prophylaxis in patients with renal insufficiency. An ongoing randomized trial (PROTECT) is comparing this regimen against UFH 5000 units twice daily for VTE prophylaxis in critically ill patients, including those with severe renal insufficiency (NCT00182364).

Dosing of all LMWHs is less certain for severely obese patients with a body mass index (BMI) of 35 or greater. Open-label studies using monitored, high doses of enoxaparin (40–60 mg subcutaneously twice daily) have been performed in bariatric surgery populations[103]; but studies of medical patients with similar degrees of obesity are lacking. Experts have advocated use of enoxaparin, 30 mg subcutaneously twice daily, for patients with a BMI of 35 or greater, which corresponds to a dose administered in high-risk surgical patients.[2]

RCTs against placebo and against UFH have validated the effectiveness of LMWHs for prevention of VTE in medically ill inpatients. Three doses of enoxaparin have been tested against placebo. In a study of medical inpatients aged 65 years or older, enoxaparin 60 mg daily provided a relative risk reduction for VTE of two-thirds as measured by mandatory fibrinogen uptake scan.[21] A second study of medical inpatients aged at least 40 with at least one VTE risk factor tested enoxaparin 20 mg daily and 40 mg daily against placebo.[11] The 40-mg dose conferred a relative risk reduction of approximately 60% whereas the 20-mg daily dose did not differ from placebo. Outcomes were measured by mandatory venography or venous ultrasound.

Dalteparin was tested against placebo in one randomized trial, enrolling acutely ill medical patients at least 40 years old. Clinically important VTE (PE, symptomatic DVT, asymptomatic proximal DVT on duplex ultrasound, sudden death) was reduced by almost 50%.[30]

Enoxaparin has been tested against UFH in 3 randomized trials. A 20-mg daily dose was tested against UFH dosed twice daily in a study of medical patients 65 years and older at bed rest. There was no significant difference in VTE event rates between the 2 groups as measured by fibrinogen uptake scan.[104] The 40-mg daily dose of enoxaparin has been compared with thrice-daily dosed UFH in 2 randomized trials of medical patients. The first enrolled patients at bed rest for at least 7 days with at least one additional VTE risk factor. The second enrolled patients with an admission diagnosis of heart failure or severe respiratory disease.[29,80] In both studies there was no significant difference in the rate of VTE between the LMWH and UFH groups, although a subgroup of patients with heart failure in the second trial[29] derived more benefit from LMWH (rate of VTE 3.6% vs 1.5%, P<.05).

Nadroparin was similarly effective to thrice-daily dosing of UFH in a randomized trial.[79] This medication is not available in the United States.

As noted earlier, a large meta-analysis has suggested a decrease in the rate of major bleeding for LMWH when compared with UFH, although the absolute rate of major bleeding for both strategies is very small.[92] An additional meta-analysis of 36 studies suggested greater reduction in VTE with LMWH (relative risk vs UFH 0.68; 95% confidence interval 0.52–0.88).[83]

Fondaparinux

The most recent agent to gain FDA approval for VTE prophylaxis in medical patients is fondaparinux, an injectable pentasaccharide. Fondaparinux consists of a moiety of 5 saccharides, analogous to the minimum fragment of a heparin molecule capable of binding to antithrombin.[105] The anticoagulant effect of fondaparinux is achieved through inhibition of activated factor X, and unlike UFH and LMWH it does not inhibit the effect of factor II.

Dosing of fondaparinux is similar to that of LMWH, and consists of once-daily subcutaneous injection of 2.5 mg. It has a longer pharmacologic half-life than any of the LMWH products presently available, and is cleared by renal excretion. Drug labeling suggests use with caution in patients with estimated creatinine clearance of 30 to 50 mL/min, and this drug is contraindicated in patients with a creatinine clearance of less than 30 mL/min. There is also no labeled dosing for medical prophylaxis for patients weighing less than 50 kg.

Indications for use of fondaparinux are similar to those of LMWH. There are no studies of fondaparinux in patients with severe renal insufficiency. As already noted, fondaparinux is extremely unlikely to cause HIT,[76] and is the pharmacologic agent of choice in medical inpatients with a history of this condition.

A randomized trial of fondaparinux versus placebo has been conducted in acutely ill medical patients aged at least 60 years. Mandatory venography was performed to assess outcome between study days 6 and 15. Fondaparinux reduced the rate of VTE by almost 50% in this population.[45] Major bleeding occurred in 1 patient (0.2%) in each study arm.

Future Pharmacologic Agents

Several classes of new anticoagulant medications are in ongoing trials. New oral anticoagulants, including anti-Xa inhibitors (rivaroxaban, apixaban), are being assessed in clinical trials of VTE prophylaxis in medical inpatients (NCT00571649, NCT00457002). If effective and approved by the FDA, such agents offer the benefit of more convenient oral dosing.

DURATION OF VTE PROPHYLAXIS

VTE prophylaxis is generally provided for the duration of hospitalization; however, the ideal duration of thromboprophylaxis in medical patients is unknown. Randomized trials have frequently assessed VTE outcomes following 7 to 14 days of pharmacologic prophylaxis. However, patients may be hospitalized for much longer than this and may be discharged to settings such as nursing facilities, in which they may have ongoing risk of VTE. Most VTE events diagnosed in association with hospitalization occur in the outpatient setting following discharge.[4] Whereas orthopedic and cancer surgery patients have been extensively studied with regard to extended prophylaxis (continued prophylaxis past the date of hospital discharge),[13] only limited study of this issue has occurred in medical patients. Hull and colleagues[106] assigned 2975 patients with acute medical illness who were receiving inpatient pharmacoprophylaxis to a program of extended prophylaxis with enoxaparin, 40 mg daily for 28 ± 4 days. The comparator group of 2988 patients received placebo in the outpatient setting (initial duration of pharmacoprophylaxis was 10 ± 4 days). VTE was reduced by 40% (from 4.0% to 2.5%) and symptomatic VTE by 73% (from 1.1% to 0.3%) in the extended prophylaxis group. The major safety outcome was any bleeding, occurring in 6.3% of the extended prophylaxis group and 3.9% of the placebo group (P = .007). Major bleeding also increased from 0.3% to 0.8% absolute risk difference, 0.51% (95% CI, 0.12% to 0.89%). The protocol was modified during the trial due to lower than expected VTE events, and authors concluded that extended prophylaxis benefits only certain higher risk subgroups of patients.

Piazza and colleagues are presently engaged in a multicenter quality improvement study (NCT00853463) testing the effect of a reminder to consider extended-duration thromboprophylaxis in medical patients when hospital discharge is planned. Results of this study are not yet available.

PROPHYLAXIS RECOMMENDATIONS: PUBLISHED GUIDELINES AND REGULATORY STATEMENTS

Over the past 25 years, more than 20 clinical practice guidelines regarding VTE prophylaxis in medical and surgical patients have been published by various groups. Recent guidelines of VTE prophylaxis in medical patients have been published by the ACCP in 2008.[13] Six North American and European entities have issued guidelines regarding prevention and management of VTE in patients with cancer, and have published a joint consensus statement in 2009.[107] A review of specific recommendations was also published by the American Heart Association in 2004.[108]

In addition to scientific guidelines, entities involved in health care regulation and accreditation have issued policy statements regarding VTE prophylaxis. The US Joint Commission and the

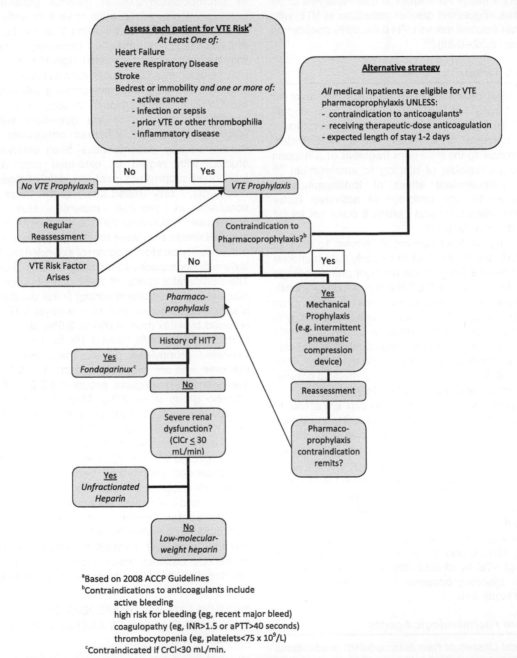

Assess each patient for VTE Risk[a]
At Least One of:
Heart Failure
Severe Respiratory Disease
Stroke
Bedrest or immobility *and one or more of:*
 - active cancer
 - infection or sepsis
 - prior VTE or other thrombophilia
 - inflammatory disease

Alternative strategy

All medical inpatients are eligible for VTE pharmacoprophylaxis UNLESS:
- contraindication to anticoagulants[b]
- receiving therapeutic-dose anticoagulation
- expected length of stay 1-2 days

No | Yes

No VTE Prophylaxis | VTE Prophylaxis

Regular Reassessment

Contraindication to Pharmacoprophylaxis?[b]

VTE Risk Factor Arises

No | Yes

Pharmaco-prophylaxis

<u>Yes</u> Mechanical Prophylaxis (e.g. intermittent pneumatic compression device)

History of HIT?

<u>Yes</u> *Fondaparinux[c]*

Reassessment

<u>No</u>

Severe renal dysfunction? (ClCr $\leq$ 30 mL/min)

Pharmaco-prophylaxis contraindication remits?

<u>Yes</u> *Unfractionated Heparin*

<u>No</u> *Low-molecular-weight heparin*

[a]Based on 2008 ACCP Guidelines
[b]Contraindications to anticoagulants include
    active bleeding
    high risk for bleeding (eg, recent major bleed)
    coagulopathy (eg, INR>1.5 or aPTT>40 seconds)
    thrombocytopenia (eg, platelets<75 x 10^9/L)
[c]Contraindicated if CrCl<30 mL/min.

Fig. 1. Suggested algorithm for VTE prophylaxis of medical inpatients. aPTT, activated partial thromboplastin time; CrCl, creatinine clearance; INR, international normalized ratio.

National Quality Forum (NQF) have endorsed standardized prophylaxis practices, and in May 2008 implemented a set of 6 VTE measurements as a core measure set for the ORYX program. Hospitals in the United States must select 4 such core measure sets as a component of accreditation as of May 1, 2009.[109]

As mentioned earlier, the AHRQ has given VTE prevention the highest priority among 79 patient safety practices.[18] In addition, the AHRQ and NQF together endorsed a practice guideline stating that all patients should have VTE risk assessed at admission and regularly thereafter, and have clinically appropriate methods of VTE prevention applied.[110] The US Surgeon General issued a call to action for the prevention of VTE in a 2008 statement.[111]

SUMMARY

A rational approach to assessing and implementing VTE prophylaxis in the medical patient, given the evidence and recommendations discussed, is summarized in **Fig. 1.**

VTE is a common and preventable complication of hospitalization in medical patients. All patients should be assessed for VTE risk at admission, and reassessed frequently during hospitalization. Most hospitalized medical patients are at sufficient risk of VTE to merit prophylaxis. Patient membership in certain groups, including ICU patients, the elderly, and those admitted with heart failure or severe respiratory disease, is adequate to confer high VTE risk. In other patients, the presence of individual risk factors defines sufficient risk to merit prophylaxis.

Pharmacologic prophylaxis is the mainstay of VTE prevention. It is effective, safe, and cost effective. LMWH can be considered the initial choice for prophylaxis based on its efficacy, safety, cost effectiveness, and easy-to-administer once-daily dose regimens. UFH is a reasonable alternative agent and should be initially considered in patients with severe renal insufficiency. Fondaparinux should be the initial choice in patients with a history of HIT. Mechanical prophylaxis should be used in patients in whom pharmacologic prophylaxis is contraindicated, although these devices should be used with care. The contraindication should be frequently reassessed, and pharmacologic prophylaxis should be initiated if the contraindication remits. There have been no studies to assess the use of inferior vena cava filter placement as a method of VTE prophylaxis in the medical inpatient.

Multiple scientific guidelines support VTE prophylaxis in medical patients. Regulatory and accreditation agencies have mandated that hospitals use formalized systems to assess VTE risk and provide clinically appropriate prophylaxis measures to patients at risk.

Additional research is needed to determine the optimal duration of VTE prophylaxis and to determine which patients would benefit from prophylaxis extended beyond hospital discharge.

REFERENCES

1. Zhan C, Miller MR. Excess length of stay, charges, and mortality attributable to medical injuries during hospitalization. JAMA 2003;290(14):1868–74.
2. Douketis JD. Prevention of venous thromboembolism in hospitalized medical patients: addressing some practical questions. Curr Opin Pulm Med 2008;14(5):381–8.
3. Heit JA, O'Fallon WM, Petterson TM, et al. Relative impact of risk factors for deep vein thrombosis and pulmonary embolism: a population-based study. Arch Intern Med 2002;162(11):1245–8.
4. Spencer FA, Lessard D, Emery C, et al. Venous thromboembolism in the outpatient setting. Arch Intern Med 2007;167(14):1471–5.
5. Hirsh J, Hoak J. Management of deep vein thrombosis and pulmonary embolism. A statement for healthcare professionals. Council on Thrombosis (in consultation with the Council on Cardiovascular Radiology), American Heart Association. Circulation 1996;93(12):2212–45.
6. Anderson FA Jr, Wheeler HB, Goldberg RJ, et al. A population-based perspective of the hospital incidence and case-fatality rates of deep vein thrombosis and pulmonary embolism. The Worcester DVT study. Arch Intern Med 1991;151(5):933–8.
7. Goldhaber SZ, Tapson VF. A prospective registry of 5,451 patients with ultrasound-confirmed deep vein thrombosis. Am J Cardiol 2004;93(2):259–62.
8. Lindblad B, Eriksson A, Bergqvist D. Autopsy-verified pulmonary embolism in a surgical department: analysis of the period from 1951 to 1988. Br J Surg 1991;78(7):849–52.
9. Piazza G, Fanikos J, Zayaruzny M, et al. Venous thromboembolic events in hospitalised medical patients. Thromb Haemost 2009;102(3):505–10.
10. Edelsberg J, Hagiwara M, Taneja C, et al. Risk of venous thromboembolism among hospitalized medically ill patients. Am J Health Syst Pharm 2006;63(20 Suppl 6):S16–22.
11. Samama MM, Cohen AT, Darmon JY, et al. A comparison of enoxaparin with placebo for the prevention of venous thromboembolism in acutely ill medical patients. Prophylaxis in medical patients with enoxaparin study group. N Engl J Med 1999;341(11):793–800.

12. Lloyd NS, Douketis JD, Moinuddin I, et al. Anticoagulant prophylaxis to prevent asymptomatic deep vein thrombosis in hospitalized medical patients: a systematic review and meta-analysis. J Thromb Haemost 2008;6(3):405–14.

13. Geerts WH, Bergqvist D, Pineo GF, et al. Prevention of venous thromboembolism: American College of Chest Physicians evidence-based clinical practice guidelines (8th edition). Chest 2008;133(Suppl 6): 381S–453S.

14. Dentali F, Douketis JD, Gianni M, et al. Meta-analysis: anticoagulant prophylaxis to prevent symptomatic venous thromboembolism in hospitalized medical patients. Ann Intern Med 2007;146(4): 278–88.

15. Heit JA, Silverstein MD, Mohr DN, et al. Risk factors for deep vein thrombosis and pulmonary embolism: a population-based case-control study. Arch Intern Med 2000;160(6):809–15.

16. Bergqvist D, Jendteg S, Johansen L, et al. Cost of long-term complications of deep venous thrombosis of the lower extremities: an analysis of a defined patient population in Sweden. Ann Intern Med 1997;126(6):454–7.

17. Kahn SR. Post-thrombotic syndrome after deep venous thrombosis: risk factors, prevention, and therapeutic options. Clin Adv Hematol Oncol 2009;7(7):433–5.

18. Shojania KG, Duncan BW, McDonald KM, et al. Making health care safer: a critical analysis of patient safety practices. Evid Rep Technol Assess (Summ) 2001;43:i–x, 1–668.

19. Deitelzweig SB, Becker R, Lin J, et al. Comparison of the two-year outcomes and costs of prophylaxis in medical patients at risk of venous thromboembolism. Thromb Haemost 2008;100(5):810–20.

20. Gallus AS, Hirsh J, Tutle RJ, et al. Small subcutaneous doses of heparin in prevention of venous thrombosis. N Engl J Med 1973;288(11):545–51.

21. Dahan R, Houlbert D, Caulin C, et al. Prevention of deep vein thrombosis in elderly medical in-patients by a low molecular weight heparin: a randomized double-blind trial. Haemostasis 1986;16(2): 159–64.

22. Avorn J, Winkelmayer WC. Comparing the costs, risks, and benefits of competing strategies for the primary prevention of venous thromboembolism. Circulation 2004;110(24 Suppl 1):IV25–32.

23. Kahn SR, Panju A, Geerts W, et al. Multicenter evaluation of the use of venous thromboembolism prophylaxis in acutely ill medical patients in Canada. Thromb Res 2007;119(2):145–55.

24. Cohen AT, Tapson VF, Bergmann JF, et al. Venous thromboembolism risk and prophylaxis in the acute hospital care setting (ENDORSE study): a multinational cross-sectional study. Lancet 2008;371(9610):387–94.

25. Stratton MA, Anderson FA, Bussey HI, et al. Prevention of venous thromboembolism: adherence to the 1995 American College of Chest Physicians consensus guidelines for surgical patients. Arch Intern Med 2000;160(3):334–40.

26. Caprini JA, Arcelus J, Sehgal LR, et al. The use of low molecular weight heparins for the prevention of postoperative venous thromboembolism in general surgery. A survey of practice in the United States. Int Angiol 2002;21(1):78–85.

27. Lloyd N HR, Haynes RB, Pai M. Barriers to and potential solutions towards optimal prophylaxis against deep vein thrombosis for hospitalized medical patients: a survey of healthcare professionals. Paper presented at: XXII Congress of the International Society of Thrombosis and Haemostasis. Boston, 16 July 2009.

28. Belch JJ, Lowe GD, Ward AG, et al. Prevention of deep vein thrombosis in medical patients by low-dose heparin. Scott Med J 1981;26(2):115–7.

29. Kleber FX, Witt C, Vogel G, et al. Randomized comparison of enoxaparin with unfractionated heparin for the prevention of venous thromboembolism in medical patients with heart failure or severe respiratory disease. Am Heart J 2003;145(4):614–21.

30. Leizorovicz A, Cohen AT, Turpie AG, et al. Randomized, placebo-controlled trial of dalteparin for the prevention of venous thromboembolism in acutely ill medical patients. Circulation 2004;110(7):874–9.

31. Blom JW, Doggen CJ, Osanto S, et al. Malignancies, prothrombotic mutations, and the risk of venous thrombosis. JAMA 2005;293(6):715–22.

32. Arkel YS. Thrombosis and cancer. Semin Oncol 2000;27(3):362–74.

33. Elting LS, Escalante CP, Cooksley C, et al. Outcomes and cost of deep venous thrombosis among patients with cancer. Arch Intern Med 2004;164(15):1653–61.

34. Blom JW, Vanderschoot JP, Oostindier MJ, et al. Incidence of venous thrombosis in a large cohort of 66,329 cancer patients: results of a record linkage study. J Thromb Haemost 2006;4(3): 529–35.

35. Sorensen HT, Mellemkjaer L, Olsen JH, et al. Prognosis of cancers associated with venous thromboembolism. N Engl J Med 2000;343(25):1846–50.

36. Alcalay A, Wun T, Khatri V, et al. Venous thromboembolism in patients with colorectal cancer: incidence and effect on survival. J Clin Oncol 2006; 24(7):1112–8.

37. Chew HK, Wun T, Harvey D, et al. Incidence of venous thromboembolism and its effect on survival among patients with common cancers. Arch Intern Med 2006;166(4):458–64.

38. Thodiyil PA, Kakkar AK. Variation in relative risk of venous thromboembolism in different cancers. Thromb Haemost 2002;87(6):1076–7.

39. Sallah S, Wan JY, Nguyen NP. Venous thrombosis in patients with solid tumors: determination of frequency and characteristics. Thromb Haemost 2002;87(4):575–9.

40. Cohen AT, Alikhan R, Arcelus JI, et al. Assessment of venous thromboembolism risk and the benefits of thromboprophylaxis in medical patients. Thromb Haemost 2005;94(4):750–9.

41. Zakai NA, Wright J, Cushman M. Risk factors for venous thrombosis in medical inpatients: validation of a thrombosis risk score. J Thromb Haemost 2004;2(12):2156–61.

42. Cook D, Crowther M, Meade M, et al. Deep venous thrombosis in medical-surgical critically ill patients: prevalence, incidence, and risk factors. Crit Care Med 2005;33(7):1565–71.

43. Chopard P, Dorffler-Melly J, Hess U, et al. Venous thromboembolism prophylaxis in acutely ill medical patients: definite need for improvement. J Intern Med 2005;257(4):352–7.

44. Maynard GA, Morris TA, Jenkins IH, et al. Optimizing prevention of hospital-acquired (HA) venous thromboembolism (VTE): prospective validation of a VTE risk assessment model (RAM). J Hosp Med 2009;5(1):10–8.

45. Cohen AT, Davidson BL, Gallus AS, et al. Efficacy and safety of fondaparinux for the prevention of venous thromboembolism in older acute medical patients: randomised placebo controlled trial. BMJ 2006;332(7537):325–9.

46. Tooher R, Middleton P, Pham C, et al. A systematic review of strategies to improve prophylaxis for venous thromboembolism in hospitals. Ann Surg 2005;241(3):397–415.

47. McMullin J, Cook D, Griffith L, et al. Minimizing errors of omission: behavioural reinforcement of heparin to avert venous emboli: the BEHAVE study. Crit Care Med 2006;34(3):694–9.

48. Timmons S, O'Callaghan C, O'Connor M, et al. Audit-guided action can improve the compliance with thromboembolic prophylaxis prescribing to hospitalized, acutely ill older adults. J Thromb Haemost 2005;3(9):2112–3.

49. Mosen D, Elliott CG, Egger MJ, et al. The effect of a computerized reminder system on the prevention of postoperative venous thromboembolism. Chest 2004;125(5):1635–41.

50. Michota FA. Bridging the gap between evidence and practice in venous thromboembolism prophylaxis: the quality improvement process. J Gen Intern Med 2007;22(12):1762–70.

51. Kucher N, Koo S, Quiroz R, et al. Electronic alerts to prevent venous thromboembolism among hospitalized patients. N Engl J Med 2005;352(10):969–77.

52. Piazza G, Rosenbaum EJ, Pendergast W, et al. Physician alerts to prevent symptomatic venous thromboembolism in hospitalized patients. Circulation 2009;119(16):2196–201.

53. Kucher N, Puck M, Blaser J, et al. Physician compliance with advanced electronic alerts for preventing venous thromboembolism among hospitalized medical patients. J Thromb Haemost 2009;7(8):1291–6.

54. Oghoetuoma J, Shahid N, Nuttall ID. Audit on the use of thromboprophylaxis during caesarean section. J Obstet Gynaecol 2001;21(2):138–40.

55. McCarthy MJ, Byrne G, Silverman SH. The setting up and implementation of a venous thromboembolism prophylaxis policy in clinical hospital practice. J Eval Clin Pract 1998;4(2):113–7.

56. Rashid ST, Thursz MR, Razvi NA, et al. Venous thromboprophylaxis in UK medical inpatients. J R Soc Med 2005;98(11):507–12.

57. Peterson GM, Drake CI, Jupe DM, et al. Educational campaign to improve the prevention of postoperative venous thromboembolism. J Clin Pharm Ther 1999;24(4):279–87.

58. McEleny P, Bowie P, Robins JB, et al. Getting a validated guideline into local practice: implementation and audit of the SIGN guideline on the prevention of deep vein thrombosis in a district general hospital. Scott Med J 1998;43(1):23–5.

59. Allenby F, Boardman L, Pflug JJ, et al. Effects of external pneumatic intermittent compression on fibrinolysis in man. Lancet 1973;2(7843):1412–4.

60. Comerota AJ, Chouhan V, Harada RN, et al. The fibrinolytic effects of intermittent pneumatic compression: mechanism of enhanced fibrinolysis. Ann Surg 1997;226(3):306–13 [discussion: 313–4].

61. Jacobs DG, Piotrowski JJ, Hoppensteadt DA, et al. Hemodynamic and fibrinolytic consequences of intermittent pneumatic compression: preliminary results. J Trauma 1996;40(5):710–6 [discussion: 716–7].

62. Tarnay TJ, Rohr PR, Davidson AG, et al. Pneumatic calf compression, fibrinolysis, and the prevention of deep venous thrombosis. Surgery 1980;88(4):489–96.

63. Chouhan VD, Comerota AJ, Sun L, et al. Inhibition of tissue factor pathway during intermittent pneumatic compression: a possible mechanism for antithrombotic effect. Arterioscler Thromb Vasc Biol 1999;19(11):2812–7.

64. Caprini JA. Mechanical methods for thrombosis prophylaxis. Clin Appl Thromb Hemost Oct 22 2009. [Epub ahead of print].

65. Bockheim HM, McAllen KJ, Baker R, et al. Mechanical prophylaxis to prevent venous thromboembolism in surgical patients: a prospective trial evaluating compliance. J Crit Care 2009;24(2):192–6.

66. Cohen AT, Skinner JA, Warwick D, et al. The use of graduated compression stockings in association

with fondaparinux in surgery of the hip. a multi-centre, multinational, randomised, open-label, parallel-group comparative study. J Bone Joint Surg Br 2007;89(7):887–92.

67. Geerts WH, Pineo GF, Heit JA, et al. Prevention of venous thromboembolism: the seventh ACCP conference on antithrombotic and thrombolytic therapy. Chest 2004;126(Suppl 3):338S–400S.

68. Elliott CG, Dudney TM, Egger M, et al. Calf-thigh sequential pneumatic compression compared with plantar venous pneumatic compression to prevent deep-vein thrombosis after non-lower extremity trauma. J Trauma 1999;47(1):25–32.

69. Collaborative overview of randomised trials of anti-platelet therapy—III: reduction in venous thrombosis and pulmonary embolism by antiplatelet prophylaxis among surgical and medical patients. Antiplatelet trialists' collaboration. BMJ 1994;308 (6923):235–46.

70. Prevention of pulmonary embolism and deep vein thrombosis with low dose aspirin: Pulmonary Embolism Prevention (PEP) trial. Lancet 2000;355 (9212):1295–302.

71. Hovens MM, Snoep JD, Tamsma JT, et al. Aspirin in the prevention and treatment of venous thrombo-embolism. J Thromb Haemost 2006;4(7):1470–5.

72. McKenna R, Galante J, Bachmann F, et al. Preven-tion of venous thromboembolism after total knee replacement by high-dose aspirin or intermittent calf and thigh compression. Br Med J 1980;280 (6213):514–7.

73. Powers PJ, Gent M, Jay RM, et al. A randomized trial of less intense postoperative warfarin or aspirin therapy in the prevention of venous thromboembo-lism after surgery for fractured hip. Arch Intern Med 1989;149(4):771–4.

74. Westrich GH, Sculco TP. Prophylaxis against deep venous thrombosis after total knee arthroplasty. Pneumatic plantar compression and aspirin compared with aspirin alone. J Bone Joint Surg Am 1996;78(6):826–34.

75. Girolami B, Prandoni P, Stefani PM, et al. The inci-dence of heparin-induced thrombocytopenia in hospitalized medical patients treated with subcuta-neous unfractionated heparin: a prospective cohort study. Blood 2003;101(8):2955–9.

76. Warkentin TE, Greinacher A, Koster A, et al. Treat-ment and prevention of heparin-induced thrombo-cytopenia: American College of Chest Physicians evidence-based clinical practice guidelines (8th edition). Chest 2008;133(Suppl 6):340S–80S.

77. Warkentin TE, Maurer BT, Aster RH. Heparin-induced thrombocytopenia associated with fonda-parinux. N Engl J Med 2007;356(25):2653–5 [discussion: 2653–5].

78. Bergmann JF, Neuhart E. A multicenter randomized double-blind study of enoxaparin compared with unfractionated heparin in the prevention of venous thromboembolic disease in elderly in-patients bedridden for an acute medical illness. The enoxa-parin in medicine study group. Thromb Haemost 1996;76(4):529–34.

79. Harenberg J, Roebruck P, Heene DL. Subcuta-neous low-molecular-weight heparin versus standard heparin and the prevention of thrombo-embolism in medical inpatients. The heparin study in internal medicine group. Haemostasis 1996;26 (3):127–39.

80. Lechler E, Schramm W, Flosbach CW. The venous thrombotic risk in non-surgical patients: epidemio-logical data and efficacy/safety profile of a low-molecular-weight heparin (enoxaparin). The prime study group. Haemostasis 1996;26(Suppl 2):49–56.

81. Cade JF. High risk of the critically ill for venous throm-boembolism. Crit Care Med 1982;10(7):448–50.

82. King CS, Holley AB, Jackson JL, et al. Twice vs three times daily heparin dosing for thromboembo-lism prophylaxis in the general medical population: a metaanalysis. Chest 2007;131(2):507–16.

83. Wein L, Wein S, Haas SJ, et al. Pharmacological venous thromboembolism prophylaxis in hospital-ized medical patients: a meta-analysis of random-ized controlled trials. Arch Intern Med 2007;167 (14):1476–86.

84. Kishimoto TK, Viswanathan K, Ganguly T, et al. Contaminated heparin associated with adverse clinical events and activation of the contact system. N Engl J Med 2008;358(23):2457–67.

85. Creekmore FM, Oderda GM, Pendleton RC, et al. Incidence and economic implications of heparin-induced thrombocytopenia in medical patients receiving prophylaxis for venous thromboembo-lism. Pharmacotherapy 2006;26(10):1438–45.

86. Gordois A, Posnett J, Borris L, et al. The cost-effectiveness of fondaparinux compared with enox-aparin as prophylaxis against thromboembolism following major orthopedic surgery. J Thromb Hae-most 2003;1(10):2167–74.

87. McCarthy ST, Turner JJ, Robertson D, et al. Low-dose heparin as a prophylaxis against deep-vein thrombosis after acute stroke. Lancet 1977;2 (8042):800–1.

88. McCarthy ST, Turner J. Low-dose subcutaneous heparin in the prevention of deep-vein thrombosis and pulmonary emboli following acute stroke. Age Ageing 1986;15(2):84–8.

89. Kleber FX, Witt C, Flosbach CW, et al. Study to compare the efficacy and safety of the LMWH enoxaparin and standard heparin in the prevention of thromboembolic events in medical patients with cardiopulmonary diseases [abstract]. Ann Hematol 1998;76(Suppl 1):A93.

90. Harenberg J, Schomaker U, Flosback CW, et al. Enoxaparin is superior to unfractionated heparin

in the prevention of thromboembolic events in medical patients at increased thromboembolic risk [abstract]. Blood 1999;94(Suppl 1):399a.

91. Hillbom M, Erila T, Sotaniemi CW, et al. Comparison of the efficacy and safety of the low-molecular-weight heparin enoxaparin with unfractionated heparin in the prevention of deep venous thrombosis in patients with acute ischemic stroke [abstract]. Blood 1999;94(Suppl 1):183a.

92. Mismetti P, Laporte-Simitsidis S, Tardy B, et al. Prevention of venous thromboembolism in internal medicine with unfractionated or low-molecular-weight heparins: a meta-analysis of randomised clinical trials. Thromb Haemost 2000;83(1):14−9.

93. Harenberg J, Kallenbach B, Martin U, et al. Randomized controlled study of heparin and low molecular weight heparin for prevention of deep-vein thrombosis in medical patients. Thromb Res 1990;59(3):639−50.

94. Ibarra-Perez K, Sandsest P. A double-blind and randomized placebo-controlled trial of low dose heparin in the intensive care unit. Semin Thromb Haemost 1988;11:25−33.

95. Marik PE, Andrews L, Maini B. The incidence of deep venous thrombosis in ICU patients. Chest 1997;111(3):661−4.

96. Kupfer Y, Anwar J, Seneviratne C, et al. Prophylaxis with subcutaneous heparin significantly reduces the incidence of deep venous thrombophlebitis in the critically ill [abstract]. Am J Respir Crit Care Med 1999;159(Suppl):A519.

97. Hirsch DR, Ingenito EP, Goldhaber SZ. Prevalence of deep venous thrombosis among patients in medical intensive care. JAMA 1995; 274(4):335−7.

98. Halkin H, Goldberg J, Modan M, et al. Reduction of mortality in general medical in-patients by low-dose heparin prophylaxis. Ann Intern Med 1982; 96(5):561−5.

99. Gardlund B. Randomised, controlled trial of low-dose heparin for prevention of fatal pulmonary embolism in patients with infectious diseases. The heparin prophylaxis study group. Lancet 1996; 347(9012):1357−61.

100. Parenteral anticoagulants: American College of Chest Physicians evidence-based clinical practice guidelines (8th edition). Addendum. Chest 2008; 134(2):474.

101. Alikhan R, Cohen AT. A safety analysis of thromboprophylaxis in acute medical illness. Thromb Haemost 2003;89(3):590−1.

102. Douketis J, Cook D, Meade M, et al. Prophylaxis against deep vein thrombosis in critically ill patients with severe renal insufficiency with the low-molecular-weight heparin dalteparin: an assessment of safety and pharmacodynamics: the DIRECT study. Arch Intern Med 2008;168(16):1805−12.

103. Borkgren-Okonek MJ, Hart RW, Pantano JE, et al. Enoxaparin thromboprophylaxis in gastric bypass patients: extended duration, dose stratification, and antifactor Xa activity. Surg Obes Relat Dis 2008;4(5):625−31.

104. Bergmann JF, Caulin C. Heparin prophylaxis in bedridden patients. Lancet 1996;348(9021):205−6.

105. Hirsh J, Bauer KA, Donati MB, et al. Parenteral anticoagulants: American College of Chest Physicians evidence-based clinical practice guidelines (8th edition). Chest 2008;133(Suppl 6):141S−59S.

106. Hull R, Schellong S, Tapson V, et al. Extended-duration venous thromboembolism prophylaxis in acutely Ill medical patients with recently reduced mobility. Ann Intern Med 2010;153(1):8−18.

107. Khorana AA, Streiff MB, Farge D, et al. Venous thromboembolism prophylaxis and treatment in cancer: a consensus statement of major guidelines panels and call to action. J Clin Oncol 2009;27(29): 4919−26.

108. Leizorovicz A, Mismetti P. Preventing venous thromboembolism in medical patients. Circulation 2004;110(24 Suppl 1):IV13−9.

109. Available at: http://www.jointcommission.org/PerformanceMeasurement/PerformanceMeasurement/VTE.htm. Accessed August 10, 2010.

110. Available at: http://www.ahrq.gov/qual/30safe.pdf. Accessed August 10, 2010.

111. Wakefield TW, McLafferty RB, Lohr JM, et al. Call to action to prevent venous thromboembolism. J Vasc Surg 2009;49(6):1620−3.

Established Venous Thromboembolism Therapies: Heparin, Low Molecular Weight Heparins, and Vitamin K Antagonists, with a Discussion of Heparin-Induced Thrombocytopenia

Robert C. Pendleton, MD[a],*,
George M. Rodgers, MD, PhD[b,c],
Russell D. Hull, MBBS, MSc, FRCPC[d]

KEYWORDS

- Venous thromboembolism • Heparin
- Low molecular weight heparin • Vitamin K antagonist
- Warfarin • Heparin-induced thrombocytopenia

Venous thromboembolism (VTE), encompassing both deep vein thrombosis (DVT) and pulmonary embolism (PE), is a common disease that carries a substantial risk of morbidity and mortality, is associated with high health care costs, and has become a national health priority in the United States.[1] Optimal treatment for patients with VTE continues to evolve. In 1960 Barritt and Jordan[2] first demonstrated the benefits of anticoagulant therapy in a randomized clinical trial of 35 patients with acute PE, wherein the combination of intravenous heparin and an oral vitamin K antagonist (VKA) substantially reduced death and recurrence. It is remarkable that with the exception of the low molecular weight heparins (LMWHs), few additional anticoagulants have gained regulatory approval over the past half-century for the treatment of venous thromboembolism. Rather, a standardized anticoagulant approach for a majority of patients with VTE has developed from numerous pivotal clinical trials completed over the past 3 decades (**Fig. 1**).

For most patients with VTE, treatment is straightforward and necessitates the immediate

[a] Department of Medicine, University Healthcare Thrombosis Service, University of Utah, 50 North Medical Drive, Room 4B120, Salt Lake City, UT 84132, USA
[b] Hemostasis and Thrombosis Laboratory, ARUP Laboratories, 500 Chipeta Way, Salt Lake City, UT 84108, USA
[c] Department of Medicine, University of Utah, 50 North Medical Drive, Salt Lake City, UT 84132, USA
[d] Department of Medicine, Thrombosis Research Unit, University of Calgary, 601 South Tower, Foothills Hospital, 1403 29th Street, NW, Calgary, Alberta T2N 2T9, Canada
* Corresponding author.
E-mail address: Robert.pendleton@hsc.utah.edu

Clin Chest Med 31 (2010) 691–706
doi:10.1016/j.ccm.2010.07.003
0272-5231/10/$ – see front matter © 2010 Elsevier Inc. All rights reserved.

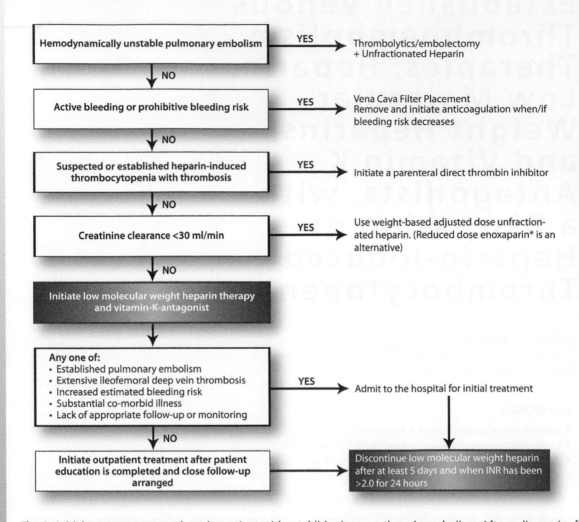

Fig. 1. Initial treatment approach to the patient with established venous thromboembolism. After a diagnosis of venous thromboembolism is established, the initial treatment is routine for a majority of patients. However, clinical scenarios that alter this routine management approach such as hemodynamic instability, active bleeding, heparin-induced thrombocytopenia, and renal impairment must be recognized. (*The Food and Drug Administration has approved a reduced dose of enoxaparin, specifically 1 mg/kg subcutaneous once daily, in patients with a creatinine clearance <30 mL/min.) INR, international normalized ratio.

initiation of a therapeutically dosed parenteral anticoagulant (eg, heparin or LMWH), simultaneous initiation of long-term therapy (eg, vitamin K antagonist), and discontinuation of the parenteral anticoagulant after at least 5 days, assuming that the VKA effect is therapeutic.[3–5] Yet, ongoing advances in standardized VTE treatment continue to evolve and include issues related to the selection and dosing of parenteral anticoagulants (eg, relative efficacy and dosing in obese patients, patients with impaired renal function, or pregnant patients), optimal location of initial care delivery, use of dosing initiation nomograms for vitamin K antagonists with the potential of gene-based dosing, and demonstration that long-term LMWH therapy may be optimal for some patient populations (eg, those with active cancer). Detailed discussion on duration of therapy for VTE, long-term warfarin monitoring, and issues related to periprocedural anticoagulant management are presented in this article.

ACUTE PARENTERAL ANTICOAGULANT USE: HEPARIN AND LOW MOLECULAR WEIGHT HEPARINS
The Need for a Parenteral Anticoagulant

The effectiveness of vitamin K antagonist therapy in impeding in vivo hemostasis is dependent on numerous variables, including the natural metabolism of circulating clotting factors present at the time of VKA initiation.[6] As such, VKAs have a delayed onset of action, which was demonstrated in a rabbit model of jugular vein thrombosis by Wessler and colleagues in 1959.[7] The necessity of instituting a rapid-onset parenteral anticoagulant (eg, heparin) during VKA initiation was subsequently highlighted by Brandjes and colleagues[8] in their pivotal trial of 120 patients with acute proximal DVT. In this study, patients were randomized to continuous intravenous heparin plus VKA or VKA alone. The study was stopped early because symptomatic recurrent VTE events occurred in 12 of 60 patients (20%) in the VKA versus 4 of 60 patients (6.7%) in the heparin plus VKA group ($P = .058$).[8] For years, patients with acute VTE were treated with approximately 10 days of initial heparin therapy. However, 2 different randomized studies directly compared shorter course heparin therapy (approximately 5 days) plus VKA started simultaneously with a longer course of heparin therapy (approximately 10 days) plus delayed VKA initiation.[9,10] In both studies, patients in the shorter course heparin group had no greater VTE recurrence, but had significantly shorter hospitalization.[9,10] For most patients with acute VTE, these studies provide the basis for contemporary recommendations to institute a parenteral anticoagulant and VKA simultaneously at the time of diagnosis and to continue the parenteral anticoagulant for a period of at least 5 days, at which time it can be discontinued if VKA therapy has been therapeutic for 24 hours.[5]

Parenteral Anticoagulants

Heparin and low molecular weight heparins
Heparin was discovered in the early 1900s at Johns Hopkins University in part through the efforts of Jay McLean, a second-year medical student, working in the laboratory of the physiologist Dr William Howell.[11] Initially isolated from canine liver, heparin was subsequently manufactured and commercialized from bovine lung through the efforts of Charles Best.[11] Unfractionated heparin (UFH) is now understood to be an indirect anticoagulant, which potentiates antithrombin activity and is most commonly isolated from porcine small intestine mucosa.[12] Heparin is a glycosaminoglycan that has a relatively large and heterogeneous molecular weight, is highly sulfated, and carries strong negative ionic charge.[12] These characteristics lead to inherent limitations of heparin; specifically, a rapid clearance phase through nonspecific binding to heparin-binding proteins, relatively low and variable bioavailability, a short elimination half-life,

and the common practice of monitoring and adjusting the dose based on the activated partial thromboplastin time (APTT).[12] Further, there have been 2 recent patient safety issues related to UFH: oversulfated chondroitin sulfate (OSCS) contaminants and a reduction in potency of available heparin in the United States. In late 2007, the Food and Drug Administration (FDA) recognized increased reporting of heparin-related deaths, leading to the release of a public health advisory.[13] A series of elegant observations led to the rapid discovery that these heparin-related deaths were due to activation of the plasma kallikrein system caused by the presence of OSCS contaminants in heparin products originating from a single manufacturing plant in Changzhou, China.[14,15,16] In response, heparin lots are now analyzed for the presence of OSCS contaminants through improved testing methods, which include harmonization of the United States Pharmacopeia (USP) unit dose potency with that of the World Health Organization. The clinical consequence of this revised testing process is an approximate 10% reduction in the potency of heparin now marketed in the United States.[17] With this, the FDA recommends clinicians to use clinical judgment in determining the dosing of heparin stating that: "heparin dosing is always individualized to the patient-specific situation. The FDA-approved labeling for heparin has not changed, including the recommended doses. Individualization of heparin dosing has long been the standard for clinical use of the drug and FDA reiterates the importance of clinical judgment in heparin dosing."[17]

Unfractionated heparin for VTE treatment
Administration of heparin either subcutaneously or as an intravenous infusion is acceptable.[5,18] Yet, adjusted-dose continuous intravenous heparin infusion has evolved as a common treatment approach for patients with acute VTE. When using intravenous heparin, the use of established nomogram-guided therapy is preferred.[19,20] In a clinical trial by Raschke and colleagues,[21] the initial dosing of a heparin bolus and subsequent infusion with a weight-based nomogram was shown to be superior to usual care dosing, wherein 60 of 62 patients (97%) in the weight-based group exceeded the therapeutic threshold (defined as an APTT >1.5 times the control) within 24 hours, compared with 37 of 48 (77%) in the standard care group ($P<.002$). Further, patients in the standard dosing group had a fivefold increase in recurrent thromboembolism (relative risk [RR] 5.0, 95% confidence interval [CI] 1.1–21.9).[21] Despite these

suggestive results and the widespread adoption of weight-based heparin dosing targeting an APTT greater than 1.5 times control, there has been controversy about the importance of APTT response in reducing recurrent thromboembolism as long as the patient's initial heparin dose is greater than 30,000 U/d.[22–25] However, the Galilei Study in 2004[26] confirmed the importance of achieving a therapeutic APTT within 24 hours, supporting the findings by Hull and colleagues.[24] Further, the dogma that therapeutic heparin therapy must be monitored and dose-adjusted has been challenged in a recent clinical trial. The FIxed-DOse (FIDO) heparin study randomized 708 patients with acute VTE to either unmonitored fixed-dose subcutaneous heparin (n = 345) (initial dose 333 U/kg followed by 250 U/kg every 12 hours) or LMWH (n = 352).[27] At 3 months recurrent VTE was similar, occurring in 3.8% in the heparin group and 3.4% in the LMWH group (absolute difference −0.4%, 95% CI −2.6%–3.3%) and without a difference in major bleeding.[27]

These studies collectively support the recommendation that when heparin is used for the treatment of VTE, administration as monitored subcutaneous adjusted-dose, intravenous infusion, or unmonitored subcutaneous fixed-dose are all acceptable treatment options.[5]

Low molecular weight heparins for VTE treatment

The LMWHs (eg, dalteparin, enoxaparin, and tinzaparin) are manufactured through the chemical or enzymatic depolymerization of UFH, leading to smaller and more uniform molecular weight and less resultant negative ionic charge.[28] These chemical differences are associated with less nonspecific protein binding, more predictable anticoagulant response, and a longer elimination half-life, which allows for once or twice-daily subcutaneous administration without requisite laboratory monitoring.[12,28] Primarily because of dose predictability and ease of use, the introduction of LMWH therapy as a treatment option for VTE has revolutionized patient management. In 1992, 2 separate groups of investigators demonstrated that fixed-dose LMWH therapy was at least as safe and effective as adjusted-dose intravenous heparin in patients with proximal vein thrombosis.[29,30] Subsequently, numerous other comparative trials have been performed, and in a meta-analysis of 13 comparative trials Dolovich and colleagues[31] demonstrated the LMWHs to be favorable compared with heparin for the initial treatment of VTE with regard to recurrence (RR 0.85, 95% CI 0.65–1.12), major bleeding (RR 0.63, 95% CI 0.37–1.05), and total mortality

(RR 0.76, 95% CI 0.59–0.98). Similarly, in a subsequent meta-analysis of 2110 patients who presented with acute symptomatic PE, LMWH were found to be at least as effective (odds ratio [OR] for recurrence 0.68, 95% CI 0.42–1.09) and safe (OR for major bleeding 0.67, 95% CI 0.36–1.27) as heparin.[32] Of note, the mortality benefit of initial LMWH therapy compared with heparin is primarily realized in patients with VTE in the setting of cancer. In these patients, meta-analysis of 11 studies showed a significant reduction in mortality if LMWHs are used rather than heparin (RR 0.71, 95% CI 0.52–0.98).[33] Because of their favorable profile and ease of administration, LMWHs are the preferred initial anticoagulant as recommended by current practice guidelines.[5]

Special dosing considerations of low molecular weight heparins

The widespread adoption of LMWH therapy has simplified parenteral anticoagulant dosing and administration for many patients. However, clinical questions of the differences between once- versus twice-daily dosing regimens and dosing in obese patients, patients with impaired renal function, and pregnant patients are encountered commonly.

Once- versus twice-daily LMWH dosing Clinical trials of the commonly prescribed LMWHs have used either once- or twice-daily dosing regimens, and an indirect comparative analysis suggests no differences between dosing regimens.[31] More recently, a Cochrane Systematic Review of 5 trials directly comparing once- versus twice-daily dosing regimens showed statistically nonsignificant differences favoring once-daily administration in recurrent venous thromboembolism (OR 0.82, 95% CI 0.49–1.39) and major bleeding events (OR 0.77, 95% CI 0.40–1.45). Further, mortality was not significantly higher with once-daily administration (OR 1.14, 95% CI 0.62–2.08)[34] Similarly, in a 3-arm comparative study of intravenous heparin, once-daily enoxaparin (1.5 mg/kg every 24 hours), and twice-daily enoxaparin (1 mg/kg every 12 hours), there were no overall differences in outcomes, but subgroup analysis suggested higher recurrent event rates with once-daily dosing in those patients with cancer or ileofemoral DVT.[35] Caution should be used when using once-daily enoxaparin in those patients. For most patients, however, once-daily administration may lead to greater convenience without compromising outcomes.

Dosing of LMWH in patients with obesity and those with impaired renal function Obese patients are underrepresented in VTE treatment trials, which has led to uncertainty about optimal LMWH dosing in these patients.[36,37] Studies evaluating drug (eg, dalteparin, enoxaparin, tinzaparin) activity with the use of anti-Xa activity levels, suggest the pharmacodynamics of LMWHs in obese patients (weighing up to 190 kg) are similar to those in nonobese patients.[38–40] Further, in a meta-analysis of LMWH dosing in patients with acute coronary syndrome, there was no increased bleeding in obese compared with nonobese patients when LMWH was dosed using total body weight (TBW) without dose capping.[41] Consequently, weight-based dosing (using TBW) in obese patients without dose capping and without anti-Xa monitoring seems appropriate.[12,36] However, due to limited published experience, anti-Xa monitoring with subsequent dose adjustment should be considered in patients at extreme weights, that is, those patients weighing more than 190 kg.[36]

The concomitant presence of renal insufficiency (creatinine clearance [CrCl] <30 mL/min) is associated with worse outcomes, including fatal bleeding, in patients with VTE.[42] Although inconsistent, the LMWHs have a significant degree of renal clearance with anti-Xa activity levels strongly correlating with CrCl, and drug accumulation occurring in those patients with a CrCl less than 30 mL/min.[12] Unadjusted LMWH therapy is associated clinically with greater bleeding complications (OR 2.25, 95% CI 1.19–4.27) in patients with CrCl less than 30 mL/min compared with those without renal impairment.[43] Because of potentially worse outcomes with LMWHs in patients with significant renal impairment, weight-based adjusted-dose UFH is recommended over LMWH for VTE treatment.[12,36,37] If LMWHs are used, enoxaparin adjusted to 1 mg/kg subcutaneous once daily has been approved by the FDA for patients with a CrCl of less than 30 mL/min.[44]

Dosing of LMWH in pregnant patients The LMWHs are the preferred anticoagulant for VTE treatment in most pregnant women, and standard weight-adjusted dosing has been recommended.[45] As pregnancy progresses, the volume of distribution of LMWHs may change, and clearance may become more efficient as glomerular filtration rate increases. However, the clinical consequence of these pregnancy-associated physiologic changes is uncertain. Recommendations include adjusting the dose of LMWH as weight increases or assessing periodic peak (4–6 hours postinjection) anti-Xa levels and adjusting the dose to keep levels in therapeutic range (eg, 0.6–1.0 IU/mL for twice-daily dosing regimens).[45] Although there is inadequate clinical trials experience to establish a preferred

management approach, the American College of Chest Physicians (ACCP) evidence-based guidelines (2008) recommend the monitoring of anti-Xa levels.[12]

Is treatment at home safe for patients with acute VTE?

The initial treatment of VTE used to be confined to the inpatient setting; however, 2 clinical trials demonstrated that outpatient LMWH treatment for carefully selected patients with acute DVT is safe and effective, and can lead to substantial cost savings.[46–48] Assuming an appropriate care delivery system is in place, outpatient DVT treatment has become appropriate for a majority of DVT patients, except perhaps those with massive ileofemoral DVT, a high bleeding risk, or substantial comorbid illness that otherwise necessitates hospitalization.[49]

Appropriate initial site of care for patients who present with acute PE is more controversial. Unlike patients with acute DVT, patients with acute PE represent a very heterogeneous risk group, with 3-month mortality rates ranging from 1.4% to 17.4%.[50,51] Clinical severity assessments such as the pulmonary embolism severity index (PESI), cardiac biomarkers such as troponin and B-type natriuretic peptide, and imaging results such as right ventricular enlargement on computed tomographic pulmonary angiogram or right ventricular dysfunction on echocardiogram, have all been demonstrated to have prognostic value in patients with acute PE.[52–56] Two recent systematic reviews suggest outpatient treatment of low-risk pulmonary embolism to be safe, but recognize that this conclusion is based on several small cohort studies with few randomized data to support the practice.[57,58] In fact, a recent small randomized clinical trial was stopped early due to an unexpectedly high short-term mortality rate (2.8%, 95% CI 0.8%–9.6%) in presumed low-risk PE patients randomized to outpatient therapy.[59] The lack of supportive clinical trial data for outpatient PE therapy is discordant with clinical practice. In a recent analysis from the National Hospital Discharge Survey from 1979 to 2005, there has been a 59% reduction in length of stay (LOS) in patients with PE, and in 2005, 13% of PE patients were discharged after a 1- to 2-day hospitalization and an additional 30% were discharged within 3 to 4 days.[60] In a separate study, adjusted postdischarge mortality was found to be significantly higher in patients with PE who had a LOS of 4 days or less (OR 1.55, 95% CI 1.21–2.00).[61] Although inferential, the increased mortality in patients with acute PE and short LOS may be due to inadequate provider assessment of patient risk or inadequate length of parenteral anticoagulant therapy. If providers choose to manage patients with an acute PE as outpatients, careful risk assessment should be performed, an adequate system of monitoring should be in place, and patients should receive at least 5 days of parenteral anticoagulant with discontinuation only after the International Normalized Ratio (INR) is in the range of 2.0 to 3.0 for 24 hours. Without randomized clinical trials, however, the safety of this approach remains uncertain.

INITIATION OF LONG-TERM THERAPY: VITAMIN K ANTAGONISTS

Rationale for Long-term Therapy in Patients with VTE

The need for therapeutic long-term antithrombotic use in patients with acute VTE is well established. In 1979 Hull and colleagues[62] randomized 68 patients with acute proximal DVT to low-dose subcutaneous heparin (LDUH) or VKA after initial heparin infusion. Recurrent VTE occurred in 25.7% of those treated with LDUH compared with none of the VKA-treated patients. A separate trial demonstrated a 20% rate of symptomatic recurrence/extension rate in patients with calf-vein DVT who were not treated with long-term therapy.[63] Due to their oral administration and low cost, VKA have emerged as the primary long-term anticoagulant for patients with VTE who have received an initial parenteral agent.

Vitamin K Antagonists

Mechanism and monitoring

The oral anticoagulant warfarin was discovered in the early 1900s by Dr Karl Link after identifying a coumarin from spoiled sweet clover that had been responsible for a hemorrhagic disorder of cattle in the United States.[11] This discovery led to the synthesis and commercialization of warfarin, which was approved for medical use in the 1950s.[11] Warfarin exerts its anticoagulant effect through inhibition of vitamin K–dependent clotting factors. The enzyme γ-carboxylase is responsible for the activation of clotting factors II, VII, IX, and X through the γ-carboxylation of glutamate residues. This enzymatic reaction relies on the reduced form of vitamin K as a critical cofactor. The VKAs such as warfarin exhibit their anticoagulant properties through the inhibition of vitamin-K-epoxide reductase (VKOR), leading to less available reduced vitamin K and in turn incomplete synthesis of the clotting factors II, VII, IX, and X (Fig. 2).[6] A measurable anticoagulant effect occurs within the first few days of VKA therapy and primarily reflects reduction of clotting factor VII, due to its short half-life

of approximately 6 hours.[6] However, it requires approximately 5 to 6 days of VKA therapy to exert an antithrombotic effect because of the critical importance of prothrombin (factor II) with its relatively long half-life of 60 to 72 hours. Consequently, a measurable anticoagulant effect in the first 4 to 5 days of VKA primarily reflects reduced levels of Factor VII and may not correlate with an in vivo antithrombotic effect.[6,64] This in part forms the basis of the recommendation to ensure that patients with acute VTE receive at least 5 days of overlap therapy with a rapidly acting anticoagulant while warfarin therapy is being initiated.[5]

Intensity of initial warfarin dosing

In early clinical trials, warfarin was dosed to achieve a prothrombin time of 1.5 to 2.0 times control. Although effective, this was associated with a high risk of bleeding, especially in trials conducted in North America.[62] To reduce the risk of bleeding without compromising efficacy, improved methods and standardization of prothrombin time reporting were necessary. Through a series of elegant clinical observations and experiments, the INR was introduced.[65] An important prior study (using prothrombin time) compared moderate-intensity VKA therapy (an INR range of approximately 2.0–3.0) with more intense therapy (an INR range of approximately 3.0–4.5) and demonstrated that moderate intensity is as effective as higher intensity in reducing recurrent VTE with a significantly lower risk of bleeding.[66] Moderate-intensity warfarin therapy, targeting an INR of 2.0 to 3.0, is the recommended standard initial treatment approach for patients with VTE.[5]

Dosing initiation of VKA therapy in patients with VTE

Efficient initial dosing of VKA therapy in patients with VTE minimizes excessive duration (ie, beyond 5–7 days) of potentially costly parenteral anticoagulants and may allow for shorter hospitalization. The use of standardized warfarin initiation dosing nomograms has been shown to be efficient and safe.[67–69] In 2 separate studies of predominantly inpatients, dosing nomograms using a 5-mg (milligram) initial dose was compared with 10 mg and shown to be effective in achieving a therapeutic INR within 5 days, with less risk of excessive anticoagulation.[67,68] More recently, Kovacs and colleagues[69] compared a 5-mg nomogram and 10-mg nomogram in 210 patients being treated as outpatients for VTE. The 10-mg nomogram group had a greater percentage of patients achieving a therapeutic INR by day 5 of therapy (86% vs 45%, $P<.001$) with no difference in

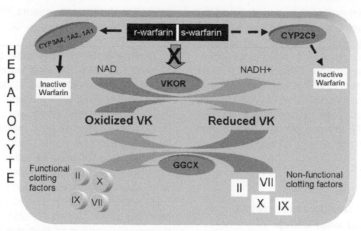

Fig. 2. Warfarin: mechanism of action. Warfarin inhibits vitamin-K-epoxide reductase (VKOR) from reducing vitamin K, a necessary cofactor in the γ-carboxylation of clotting factors II, VII, IX, and X. In turn, fewer functional clotting factors are formed and an anticoagulant effect is achieved. Recent advancements have identified common polymorphisms in the genes encoding VKOR and CYP2C9, which affect maintenance warfarin dose requirements. VK, vitamin K; NAD, nicotinamide adenine dinucleotide; GGCX, γ-carboxylase.

excessive anticoagulation or adverse events. Of note, the 10-mg dosing group only required INR assessment on days 3 and 5 in the first week of therapy. These data collectively suggest that flexibility is necessary in initiating warfarin therapy. Lower initial doses (eg, 5 mg or less) may be most appropriate for those patients who are elderly, have low body weight, are on interacting medications, or have poor nutrition, whereas a higher dose (eg, 10 mg) may be acceptable for others.

The emerging role of genetic-based VKA dosing

There are wide interindividual dosing requirements of warfarin that make dosing initiation problematic. Although clinical features such as age, body mass, nutrition, and concomitant medications are important variables, common genetic polymorphisms are now known to explain a significant percentage of warfarin dosing variability, both in the kinetics of warfarin metabolism and its pharmacodynamic effect.[6] Warfarin is metabolized by the cytochrome P450 system with the more potent *S*-enantiomer being metabolized by the cytochrome enzyme CYP2C9. Identifiable polymorphisms (ie, the common, non–wild-type alleles defined as *2 and *3) in the gene that encode CYP2C9 occur in approximately 20% of Caucasian individuals, and lead to a longer elimination half-life and lower dose requirements.[70] Similarly, common haplotypes of the gene (VKORC1) encoding VKOR have been identified and are strongly associated with warfarin dose requirements.[71] Together, these commonly identifiable polymorphisms have been integrated with clinical variables into several

different dosing prediction algorithms that account for more than 70% of the dosing variability of warfarin.[72] This application of gene-based warfarin dosing to clinical care has the potential to lead to more efficient and stable anticoagulation initiation and to improve patient outcomes.[73] Yet to date, limited prospective data suggest the possibility of improved anticoagulation control but no convincing benefit in patient outcomes.[74,75] Further, the cost effectiveness of gene-based warfarin dosing remains uncertain.[76] The role of gene-based warfarin dosing will be clarified in ongoing clinical trials, and until then standard, non–gene-based dosing approaches are recommended.[6,77]

LONG-TERM THERAPY: THE ROLE OF THE LOW MOLECULAR WEIGHT HEPARINS

Due to the cost and inconvenience of daily injections, most patients with VTE are transitioned from initial LMWH or heparin therapy to a VKA. However, VKA therapy is not without its well-documented limitations such as variable dose response and dietary and drug interactions, which necessitate frequent INR monitoring. Alternative treatment options to VKA would be beneficial. It has been suggested that long-term LMWH therapy may be an option for some patients such as those with the antiphospholipid antibody syndrome and warfarin resistance (defined as warfarin dose requirements >105 mg/wk), and those who have had recurrent VTE despite adequate VKA therapy.[78–80] For those with recurrent VTE despite adequate VKA therapy, management options include placement of a vena cava filter, increasing the intensity of VKA therapy, stopping VKA and implementing long-term LMWH therapy, or a combination of approaches.[37] Without prospective study, it is uncertain which of these approaches (or combination of approaches) is optimal, although institution of long-term LMWH has been recommended.[37,79] Further, long-term LMWH therapy has evolved as the preferred treatment strategy for patients with VTE in the setting of cancer, and may have an emerging role in a broader number of patients.

The Role of Extended-Duration LMWH Therapy in Patients with Cancer

The management, efficacy, and safety of VKA are particularly problematic in cancer patients with VTE.[81] Both recurrent VTE and major bleeding events are significantly more common in patients with cancer than in those without cancer in the first month of therapy, and are not explained by anticoagulant intensity outside the target range.[82] Due to the limitations of VKA in this population, long-term LMWH therapy has been evaluated as an alternative to LMWH followed by VKA in cancer patients with VTE. In the pivotal 2003 CLOT trial, Lee and colleagues[83] randomized 672 patients with acute proximal DVT, PE, or both to either 6 months of dalteparin (200 IU/kg body weight once daily for 1 month followed by 150 IU/kg once daily for 5 months) to 5 to 7 days of dalteparin followed by 6 months of VKA, with a target INR of 2.5. During the 6-month study period, recurrent VTE was significantly less common in the long-term LMWH group (hazard ratio [HR] 0.48, 95% CI 0.30–0.77) without a difference in bleeding events or mortality. In a separate randomized open-label clinical trial comparing usual care to long-term tinzaparin in patients with a proximal DVT in the setting of cancer (n = 200), Hull and colleagues[84] demonstrated long-term tinzaparin to be associated with fewer recurrent VTE events, 16% versus 7% (absolute risk difference −9%, 95% CI −21.7% to −0.7%). Most recently, a Cochrane meta-analysis of 6 randomized trials showed that long-term LMWH compared with usual therapy provided a reduction in VTE (HR 0.47, 95% CI 0.32–0.71), with no statistically significant survival benefit (HR 0.96, 95% CI 0.81–1.14) or difference in bleeding outcomes (RR 0.91, 95% CI 0.64–1.31).[85] From a patient perspective, long-term LMWH therapy is deemed acceptable and is preferable to VKA.[86] Based on favorable outcomes, long-term LMWH therapy for cancer patients is currently endorsed by numerous practice guidelines as the preferred therapeutic approach in these patients.[5,87–89] A treatment approach is outlined in **Fig. 3**.

Is There a Role for Extended-Duration LMWH Therapy Beyond Patients with Cancer?

LMWH has been studied as a long-term management option in a broad range of patients with VTE. In 2002, a Cochrane Review of 7 published studies (3 of which were of high methodological quality) found that compared with usual care (ie, a parenteral anticoagulant for at least 5 days followed by VKA therapy), long-term LMWH therapy was associated with a nonsignificant reduction in recurrent VTE (OR 0.70, 95% CI 0.42–1.16) and caused significantly less bleeding (OR 0.38, 95% CI 0.15–0.94).[90] When only studies of high methodological quality were analyzed, differences in bleeding were no longer significant but still favored LMWH (OR 0.80, 95% CI 0.21–3.00).[90] Subsequently, in a large multicenter trial, Hull and colleagues[91] randomized 737 patients with proximal DVT to receive either intravenous heparin followed by VKA or long-term tinzaparin (175 IU/kg once daily). At 3 months, recurrent VTE occurred in 4.9% of the LMWH patients compared with 5.7% of those in the usual care group (absolute difference −0.8%; 95% CI, −4.1–2.4), and bleeding was less common in those treated with tinzaparin, 13% versus 19.8% (absolute difference −6.8%; 95% CI, −12.4 to −1.5).[91] In composite, these data suggest that long-term LMWH therapy is an acceptable alternative to usual care with outcomes that are at least as good, and that this approach may be cost effective for high-risk patients.[92]

More recently, other potential advantages of long-term LMWH therapy have been demonstrated. The Home-LITE trial was designed to determine if there are benefits of long-term once-daily LMWH in patients with acute proximal DVT treated at home as compared with usual therapy, and if this treatment approach is associated with improved quality of life.[93] In this multicenter trial, 480 patients were randomized to receive either initial tinzaparin (175 IU/kg once daily) followed by VKA or long-term tinzaparin at the same dose.[93] At 3 months, the rates of recurrent VTE (3.3% vs 3.3%), bleeding (9.2% vs 9.2%), and death (3.8% vs 3.8%) were the same, but patients treated in the long-term LMWH group expressed significantly greater overall treatment satisfaction as assessed by the Medical Outcome Study Short Form-20 (P = .0024). It is remarkable that patients in the tinzaparin group were also less likely to report signs/symptoms of the post-thrombotic syndrome (PTS) (overall OR 0.77, P = .001) and had fewer leg ulcers at 12 weeks (0.5%

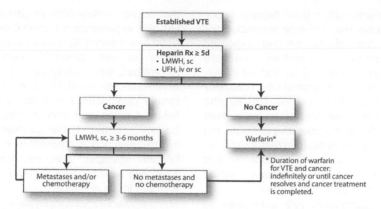

Fig. 3. Treatment approach in patients with cancer-associated venous thromboembolism. Patients with venous thromboembolism (VTE) associated with cancer have a lower risk of VTE recurrence with long-term low molecular weight heparin (LMWH) therapy as opposed to warfarin, and patients with metastatic disease or those undergoing chemotherapy derive the greatest benefit from ongoing LMWH treatment. Consensus groups like the American College of Chest Physicians evidence-based guidelines and the National Comprehensive Cancer Network recommend LMWH as the preferred long-term therapy. UFH, unfractionated heparin; sc, subcutaneous; iv, intravenous. (*Data from* Kearon C, Kahn SR, Agnelli G, et al. Antithrombotic therapy for venous thromboembolic disease: American College of Chest Physicians evidence-based clinical practice guidelines (8th edition). Chest 2008;133 (Suppl 6):454–545S; National Comprehensive Cancer Network. NCCN clinical practice guidelines in oncology. Venous thromboembolic disease, V.2.2009. Available at: http://www.nccn.org. Accessed January 25, 2010.)

vs 4.1%, P = .02).[93] The findings in the Home-LITE trial of a lower risk of PTS risk with long-term LMWH treatment compared with usual therapy are plausible. A recent randomized open-label trial (n = 241) comparing long-term tinzaparin with usual care in patients with proximal DVT showed significantly greater vein recanalization at 6 months (73% vs 47.5%) and at 1 year (91.5% vs 69.2%) in the tinzaparin group.[94] Other studies have also demonstrated greater thrombus resolution and less venous reflux in patients with acute proximal DVT who are treated with long-term LMWH as compared with usual care.[95,96] Of importance is that lack of recanalization of proximal DVT in the first 6 months of treatment is an important predictor of PTS.[97] Given the association of inflammation and PTS, it is plausible that additional features of LMWHs such as their anti-inflammatory properties may also be beneficial in reducing the risk of PTS.[98] As PTS is a common, morbid, and costly complication of patients with proximal DVT, treatment strategies that prevent its occurrence would be welcome.[99] Further confirmatory study of the role of long-term LMWH in this regard is urgently needed.

HEPARIN-INDUCED THROMBOCYTOPENIA

Although bleeding is the most common adverse event associated with heparin and LMWH therapy,

heparin-induced thrombocytopenia/thrombosis (HIT) is increasingly recognized as a serious, albeit paradoxic, complication of heparin therapy. HIT is a "clinical-pathologic" syndrome, meaning that the diagnosis is optimally based on compatible clinical features as well as laboratory assay results positive for heparin-dependent antibodies.

Mechanism of HIT

Platelet activation occurs in vivo in normal people; this results in release of platelet factor 4 (PF4), a tetrameric platelet α-granule constituent, into blood where it may also bind to the external platelet surface. Negatively charged heparin can bind to positively charged PF4 tetramers, resulting in heparin-PF4 complex formation that is immunogenic under certain circumstances.[100] Binding of IgG to the heparin-PF4 complex forms an immune complex that triggers cross-linking of the platelet Fcγlla receptor, an event that leads to platelet activation and formation of thrombogenic microparticles.[101] The end result is development of thrombocytopenia in the setting of a profound hypercoagulable state.

Clinical Features of HIT

In sensitive patients who receive heparin (in any form, route, or dose, including heparin-coated catheters), thrombocytopenia typically begins 5 to 10 days following initial exposure.[102]

Alternatively, patients with a prior heparin exposure within 30 days may develop thrombocytopenia within 1 day of the second exposure (anamnestic response). Nadir platelet counts are typically in the range of 60,000/μL and the development of severe thrombocytopenia (<20,000/μL) is rarely seen in HIT.[102] In some patients who develop reactive thrombocytosis (elevated platelet count), for example, in postoperative patients, the diagnosis of HIT may be difficult. In these patients, recognition of a 50% decrease in the platelet count from baseline after exposure to heparin should prompt consideration of an HIT diagnosis.

UFH induces pathogenic HIT antibodies to a greater extent than LMWH (~5% vs ~1%, respectively, in orthopedic patients).[103] The clinical setting also influences the frequency of HIT; patients undergoing cardiac surgery who receive UFH have a higher incidence of pathogenic HIT antibodies (2.5%) than medical (<1%) or obstetric (<0.1%) patients.[103]

The feared complication of HIT is thrombosis. Despite development of significant thrombocytopenia, bleeding rarely occurs in HIT, even in postoperative patients. Studies have demonstrated that approximately 50% of patients who develop HIT will experience an arterial or venous thrombotic event within 30 days if alternative anticoagulation is not given.[104] Historically, arterial thrombosis was initially described as the thrombotic association with HIT, but subsequent studies clearly demonstrate that venous thromboembolism is 4 times more common than arterial thrombosis.[102] Other HIT-associated complications include injection site reactions (for subcutaneous heparin therapy), skin necrosis, venous limb gangrene (which occurs when HIT is treated with warfarin in the absence of an adequate alternative anticoagulant), and anaphylaxis (which may occur with intravenous bolus heparin).[102]

A clinical scoring system for HIT

Limitations of laboratory assays for HIT (discussed below) have led to development of a scoring system to determine the pretest probability of HIT, in an attempt to more rapidly identify patients with the likely diagnosis. Analogous to the Wells criteria used to formulate a pretest probability of DVT, the "4Ts" scoring system (**Table 1**) uses easily available clinical information (nadir platelet

Table 1
The 4T's scoring system for HIT

4T's Parameter	2 Points	1 Point	0 Point
Thrombocytopenia	Platelet count decrease >50% with nadir >20 K	Platelet count decrease 30%–50% or nadir 10–19 K	Platelet count decrease <30% or nadir <10 K
Timing	Onset between days 5 and 10 or ≤1 day (prior heparin exposure within 30 days)	Consistent with platelet count decrease between days 5 and 10, but missing data; onset after 10 days; decrease ≤1 day with prior heparin exposure 30–100 days ago	Platelet count decrease <4 days without recent exposure
Thrombosis or other complications	New thrombosis (confirmed); skin necrosis; systemic reaction after IV heparin bolus	Progressive or recurrent thrombosis; erythematous skin lesions; suspected (nonproven) thrombosis	—
Other causes for thrombocytopenia	None apparent	Possible	Definite

Patients suspected as having HIT are clinically evaluated with the 4T's parameters in the table. Points are assessed as described. Patients who score 6–8 points are classified as high-probability; those with 4–5 points are classified as intermediate-probability; and those with ≤3 points are classified as low-probability.
Data from Lo GK, Juhl D, Warkentin TE, et al. Evaluation of pretest clinical score (4 T's) for the diagnosis of heparin-induced thrombocytopenia in two clinical settings. J Thromb Haemost 2006;4:759–65.

count, timing of thrombocytopenia, presence or absence of thrombosis, and alternative explanations for thrombocytopenia) to classify patients into high (score of 6–8), intermediate (score of 4–5), or low (score of ≤3) probability of HIT.[105] Study results indicate that this scoring system has a high negative predictive value. Consequently, a low pretest score may be useful in ruling out an HIT diagnosis.[105]

Laboratory assays for HIT

In general, there are 2 types of assays used to diagnose HIT: immunoassays and functional assays. Immunoassays detect antibodies to the heparin-PF4 complex either by enzyme-linked immunosorbent assay (ELISA) or by particle immunofiltration methods.[106] Functional assays measure the ability of heparin-PF4 antibodies to activate platelets, and include methods such as the serotonin release assay (SRA), heparin-induced platelet aggregation (HIPA) assay, and flow cytometry.[106]

Immunoassays

HIT ELISAs have high sensitivity, but poor specificity for the diagnosis.[106] Most will detect IgG, IgM, and IgA antibodies, but only IgG antibodies are thought to be pathogenic in the disorder. In addition, not all antibodies to the heparin-PF4 complex will induce platelet activation.[106] Recent data indicate that the optimum immunoassay uses ELISA methodology to detect only IgG antibodies.[107] The particle immunofiltration assay may yield false-negative results in patients with likely HIT, and cannot be recommended at this time. The reliability of an IgG ELISA in diagnosing HIT can be further improved by considering the "positivity" of the result. ELISA optical density results near the upper limit of the normal range (usually ~0.4 OD units) are less likely to be associated with clinical HIT than a much higher positive result (≥1.0 OD units).[108] Most hospital laboratories should provide HIT ELISA results within 48 hours.

Functional assays

The SRA is considered to be the "gold standard" test for HIT because this test measures only clinically relevant, pathogenic antibodies to the heparin-PF4 complex.[106] However, few laboratories offer the SRA because it is technically demanding to perform. Results may take up to a week or more to be reported, so the SRA is usually ordered as a confirmation test for patients with intermediate probability of having HIT. Other functional assays (HIPA, flow cytometry) have fewer data supporting their use.[106]

Diagnosing HIT

One approach to diagnosing HIT is shown in **Fig. 4**. Patients should be assessed clinically (**Table 1**) to determine their likelihood of having HIT while awaiting immunoassay results. Those patients having a low pretest likelihood for HIT probably need no further testing or alternative anticoagulation. Patients with a high pretest probability for HIT should receive alternative anticoagulation, and for any positive immunoassay result, no further testing is indicated. Patients with a high pretest probability but who have negative immunoassay results should be tested with the SRA to confirm or refute a diagnosis of HIT. Patients with an intermediate likelihood of HIT should receive an alternative anticoagulant while awaiting immunoassay results. If the result is strongly positive, no further testing may be

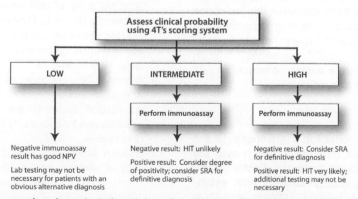

Fig. 4. Diagnostic approach to heparin-induced thrombocytopenia. This approach uses the 4T's scoring system to assess the pretest probability combined with results of an HIT immunoassay. The optimal immunoassay uses ELISA methodology to detect IgG antibodies to the heparin-platelet factor 4 complex. Clinical reassessment and repeat laboratory testing may be necessary for some patients. NPV, negative predictive value; SRA, serotonin release assay. (*Reprinted* with permission of AACC, Washington, DC, from Clinical Laboratory News 2009;35:8–10.)

necessary. If the result is negative or only weakly positive, the SRA should be performed to definitively diagnose or exclude HIT. Alternative anticoagulation should be continued while awaiting the SRA results.

Treatment of HIT

The initial treatment of HIT is to discontinue all exposure to heparin or LMWHs (including heparin-coated catheters) and immediately begin an alternative anticoagulant, usually a direct thrombin inhibitor (DTI) (such as argatroban, lepirudin, or bivalirudin).[109] Pharmacy-driven protocols are available to simplify the use of these drugs. DTI therapy is continued as monotherapy until normalization of the platelet count, at which time bridging therapy with warfarin is started. Both drugs are continued for at least 5 days, or until a therapeutic INR (2.0–3.0) is achieved on warfarin alone. Screening ultrasonography of the lower extremities is recommended in patients with apparent "isolated HIT" (no thrombosis).[109]

For isolated HIT, warfarin therapy duration of 6 to 8 weeks is suggested. For HIT patients with thrombosis, a longer period of warfarin therapy (ie, at least 12 weeks) is recommended. Fondaparinux has been used to treat HIT in small case series, but is not approved to treat HIT. Patients should be informed that they should never be exposed to heparin again, although protocols are available in which short-term exposure to heparin can be safely tolerated in patients who require heparin therapy.

Prevention of HIT

The cornerstone of preventing HIT is minimizing the use of UFH. Although some exposure to UFH may be unavoidable, the availability and use of LMWH and fondaparinux, which are approved for a large number of prophylactic and treatment indications, will substantially decrease the incidence of HIT. Platelet count monitoring recommendations in patients receiving heparin have been published in the recent ACCP guidelines.[109] Such monitoring may enable earlier detection of HIT and perhaps prevent complications.

SUMMARY

There have been remarkable advances in the treatment of venous thromboembolism over the past 30 years. Through numerous pivotal clinical trials and observations, treatments with established therapies (eg, heparin, LMWHs, and VKA) have become straightforward for a majority of patients. Further study to better define appropriate patient selection for outpatient PE treatment, the role of long-term LMWH in reducing PTS, and

the role of warfarin pharmacogenetics will continue to provide advances in these long-established treatments. In parallel, HIT has been identified as an important complication of parenteral anticoagulant use. Advances in our understanding of this disorder have allowed for more accurate diagnosis and improved treatment alongside preventive strategies.

REFERENCES

1. Galson SK, U.S. Department of Health & Human Services. The surgeon general's call to action to prevent deep vein thrombosis and pulmonary embolism 2008. Available at: http://www.surgeongeneral.gov/topics/deepvein/. Accessed January 25, 2010.
2. Barritt DW, Jordan SC. Anticoagulant drugs in the treatment of pulmonary embolism. A controlled trial. Lancet 1960;1(7138):1309–12.
3. Prevention and treatment of venous thromboembolism. International Consensus Statement (guidelines according to scientific evidence). Int Angiol 2006;25(2):101–61.
4. Snow V, Qaseem A, Barry P, et al. Management of venous thromboembolism: a clinical practice guideline from the American College of Physicians and the American Academy of Family Physicians. Ann Intern Med 2007;146(3):204–10.
5. Kearon C, Kahn SR, Agnelli G, et al. Antithrombotic therapy for venous thromboembolic disease: American College of Chest Physicians evidence-based clinical practice guidelines (8th edition). Chest 2008;133(Suppl 6):454S–545S.
6. Ansell J, Hirsh J, Hylek E, et al. Pharmacology and management of the vitamin K antagonists: American College of Chest Physicians evidence-based clinical practice guidelines (8th edition). Chest 2008;133(Suppl 6):160S–98S.
7. Wessler S, Reiner L, Freiman DG, et al. Serum-induced thrombosis. Studies of its induction, and evolution under controlled conditions in vivo. Circulation 1959;20:864–74.
8. Brandjes DP, Heijboer H, Buller HR, et al. Acenocoumarol and heparin compared with acenocoumarol alone in the initial treatment of proximal-vein thrombosis. N Engl J Med 1992;327(21):1485–9.
9. Gallus A, Jackaman J, Tillett J, et al. Safety and efficacy of warfarin started early after submassive venous thrombosis or pulmonary embolism. Lancet 1986;2(8519):1293–6.
10. Hull RD, Raskob GE, Rosenbloom D, et al. Heparin for 5 days as compared with 10 days in the initial treatment of proximal venous thrombosis. N Engl J Med 1990;322(18):1260–4.

11. Wardrop D, Keeling D. The story of the discovery of heparin and warfarin. Br J Haematol 2008;141(6): 757–63.

12. Hirsh J, Bauer KA, Donati MB, et al. Parenteral anticoagulants: American College of Chest Physicians evidence-based clinical practice guidelines (8th edition). Chest 2008;133(Suppl 6):141S–59S.

13. U.S. Food and Drug Administration. Public health advisory: important warnings and instructions for heparin sodium injection (Baxter). FDA Web site. Available at: http://www.fda.gov/Drugs/DrugSafety/PublicHealthAdvisories/ucm051133.html. Accessed February 17, 2010.

14. U.S. Food and Drug Administration. Update to healthcare facilities and healthcare professionals about heparin and heparin-containing medical products. FDA Web site. Available at: http://www.fda.gov/MedicalDevices/Safety/AlertsandNotices/ucm135355.htm. Accessed February 17, 2010.

15. Guerrini M, Beccati D, Shriver Z, et al. Oversulfated chondroitin sulfate is a contaminant in heparin associated with adverse clinical events. Nat Biotechnol 2008;26(6):669–75.

16. Kishimoto TK, Viswanathan K, Ganguly T, et al. Contaminated heparin associated with adverse clinical events and activation of the contact system. N Engl J Med 2008;358(23):2457–67.

17. U.S. Food and Drug Administration. FDA Public health alert: change in heparin USP monograph. FDA Web site. Available at: http://www.fda.gov/Drugs/DrugSafety/PostmarketDrugSafetyInformationforPatientsandProviders/ucm184502.htm. Accessed February 17, 2010.

18. Hommes DW, Bura A, Mazzolai L, et al. Subcutaneous heparin compared with continuous intravenous heparin administration in the initial treatment of deep vein thrombosis. A meta-analysis. Ann Intern Med 1992;116(4):279–84.

19. Cruickshank MK, Levine MN, Hirsh J, et al. A standard heparin nomogram for the management of heparin therapy. Arch Intern Med 1991; 151(2):333–7.

20. Raschke RA, Gollihare B, Peirce JC. The effectiveness of implementing the weight-based heparin nomogram as a practice guideline. Arch Intern Med 1996;156(15):1645–9.

21. Raschke RA, Reilly BM, Guidry JR, et al. The weight-based heparin dosing nomogram compared with a "standard care" nomogram. A randomized controlled trial. Ann Intern Med 1993; 119(9):874–81.

22. Anand S, Ginsberg JS, Kearon C, et al. The relation between the activated partial thromboplastin time response and recurrence in patients with venous thrombosis treated with continuous intravenous heparin. Arch Intern Med 1996;156(15): 1677–81.

23. Anand SS, Bates S, Ginsberg JS, et al. Recurrent venous thrombosis and heparin therapy: an evaluation of the importance of early activated partial thromboplastin times. Arch Intern Med 1999;159 (17):2029–32.

24. Hull RD, Raskob GE, Brant RF, et al. Relation between the time to achieve the lower limit of the APTT therapeutic range and recurrent venous thromboembolism during heparin treatment for deep vein thrombosis. Arch Intern Med 1997;157 (22):2562–8.

25. Hull RD, Raskob GE, Hirsh J, et al. Continuous intravenous heparin compared with intermittent subcutaneous heparin in the initial treatment of proximal-vein thrombosis. N Engl J Med 1986;315 (18):1109–14.

26. Writing Committee for the Galilei Investigators. Subcutaneous adjusted-dose unfractionated heparin vs fixed-dose low-molecular-weight heparin in the initial treatment of venous thromboembolism. Arch Intern Med 2004;164(10):1077–83.

27. Kearon C, Ginsberg JS, Julian JA, et al. Comparison of fixed-dose weight-adjusted unfractionated heparin and low-molecular-weight heparin for acute treatment of venous thromboembolism. JAMA 2006;296(8):935–42.

28. Weitz JI. Low-molecular-weight heparins. N Engl J Med 1997;337(10):688–98.

29. Hull RD, Raskob GE, Pineo GF, et al. Subcutaneous low-molecular-weight heparin compared with continuous intravenous heparin in the treatment of proximal-vein thrombosis. N Engl J Med 1992;326 (15):975–82.

30. Prandoni P, Lensing AW, Buller HR, et al. Comparison of subcutaneous low-molecular-weight heparin with intravenous standard heparin in proximal deep-vein thrombosis. Lancet 1992;339 (8791):441–5.

31. Dolovich LR, Ginsberg JS, Douketis JD, et al. A meta-analysis comparing low-molecular-weight heparins with unfractionated heparin in the treatment of venous thromboembolism: examining some unanswered questions regarding location of treatment, product type, and dosing frequency. Arch Intern Med 2000;160(2):181–8.

32. Quinlan DJ, McQuillan A, Eikelboom JW. Low-molecular-weight heparin compared with intravenous unfractionated heparin for treatment of pulmonary embolism: a meta-analysis of randomized, controlled trials. Ann Intern Med 2004;140 (3):175–83.

33. Akl EA, Rohilla S, Barba M, et al. Anticoagulation for the initial treatment of venous thromboembolism in patients with cancer. Cochrane Database Syst Rev 2008;1:CD006649.

34. van Dongen CJ, MacGillavry MR, Prins MH. Once versus twice daily LMWH for the initial treatment

of venous thromboembolism. Cochrane Database Syst Rev 2005;1:CD003074.

35. Merli G, Spiro TE, Olsson CG, et al. Subcutaneous enoxaparin once or twice daily compared with intravenous unfractionated heparin for treatment of venous thromboembolic disease. Ann Intern Med 2001;134(3):191–202.

36. Nutescu EA, Spinler SA, Wittkowsky A, et al. Low-molecular-weight heparins in renal impairment and obesity: available evidence and clinical practice recommendations across medical and surgical settings. Ann Pharmacother 2009;43(6): 1064–83.

37. Rondina MT, Pendleton RC, Wheeler M, et al. The treatment of venous thromboembolism in special populations. Thromb Res 2007;119(4):391–402.

38. Bazinet A, Almanric K, Brunet C, et al. Dosage of enoxaparin among obese and renal impairment patients. Thromb Res 2005;116(1):41–50.

39. Hainer JW, Barrett JS, Assaid CA, et al. Dosing in heavy-weight/obese patients with the LMWH, tinzaparin: a pharmacodynamic study. Thromb Haemost 2002;87(5):817–23.

40. Wilson SJ, Wilbur K, Burton E, et al. Effect of patient weight on the anticoagulant response to adjusted therapeutic dosage of low-molecular-weight heparin for the treatment of venous thromboembolism. Haemostasis 2001;31(1):42–8.

41. Spinler SA, Inverso SM, Cohen M, et al. Safety and efficacy of unfractionated heparin versus enoxaparin in patients who are obese and patients with severe renal impairment: analysis from the ESSENCE and TIMI 11B studies. Am Heart J 2003;146(1):33–41.

42. Falga C, Capdevila JA, Soler S, et al. Clinical outcome of patients with venous thromboembolism and renal insufficiency. Findings from the RIETE registry. Thromb Haemost 2007;98(4):771–6.

43. Lim W, Dentali F, Eikelboom JW, et al. Meta-analysis: low-molecular-weight heparin and bleeding in patients with severe renal insufficiency. Ann Intern Med 2006;144(9):673–84.

44. Product Information. Lovenox (enoxaparin sodium injection). Bridgewater (NJ): Sanofi-aventis US LLC; 2009.

45. Bates SM, Greer IA, Pabinger I, et al. Venous thromboembolism, thrombophilia, antithrombotic therapy, and pregnancy: American College of Chest Physicians evidence-based clinical practice guidelines (8th edition). Chest 2008;133(Suppl 6): 844S–86S.

46. Koopman MM, Prandoni P, Piovella F, et al. Treatment of venous thrombosis with intravenous unfractionated heparin administered in the hospital as compared with subcutaneous low-molecular-weight heparin administered at home. The Tasman Study Group. N Engl J Med 1996;334(11):682–7.

47. Levine M, Gent M, Hirsh J, et al. A comparison of low-molecular-weight heparin administered primarily at home with unfractionated heparin administered in the hospital for proximal deep-vein thrombosis. N Engl J Med 1996;334(11):677–81.

48. O'Brien B, Levine M, Willan A, et al. Economic evaluation of outpatient treatment with low-molecular-weight heparin for proximal vein thrombosis. Arch Intern Med 1999;159(19):2298–304.

49. Douketis JD. Treatment of deep vein thrombosis: what factors determine appropriate treatment? Can Fam Physician 2005;51:217–23.

50. Douketis JD, Kearon C, Bates S, et al. Risk of fatal pulmonary embolism in patients with treated venous thromboembolism. JAMA 1998;279(6): 458–62.

51. Goldhaber SZ, Visani L, De Rosa M. Acute pulmonary embolism: clinical outcomes in the International Cooperative Pulmonary Embolism Registry (ICOPER). Lancet 1999;353(9162):1386–9.

52. Becattini C, Vedovati MC, Agnelli G. Prognostic value of troponins in acute pulmonary embolism: a meta-analysis. Circulation 2007;116(4):427–33.

53. Goldhaber SZ. Echocardiography in the management of pulmonary embolism. Ann Intern Med 2002;136(9):691–700.

54. Jimenez D, Yusen RD, Otero R, et al. Prognostic models for selecting patients with acute pulmonary embolism for initial outpatient therapy. Chest 2007; 132(1):24–30.

55. Klok FA, Mos IC, Huisman MV. Brain-type natriuretic peptide levels in the prediction of adverse outcome in patients with pulmonary embolism: a systematic review and meta-analysis. Am J Respir Crit Care Med 2008;178(4):425–30.

56. Schoepf UJ, Kucher N, Kipfmueller F, et al. Right ventricular enlargement on chest computed tomography: a predictor of early death in acute pulmonary embolism. Circulation 2004;110(20): 3276–80.

57. Janjua M, Badshah A, Matta F, et al. Treatment of acute pulmonary embolism as outpatients or following early discharge. A systematic review. Thromb Haemost 2008;100(5):756–61.

58. Squizzato A, Galli M, Dentali F, et al. Outpatient treatment and early discharge of symptomatic pulmonary embolism: a systematic review. Eur Respir J 2009;33(5):1148–55.

59. Otero R, Uresandi F, Jimenez D, et al. Home treatment in pulmonary embolism. Thromb Res 2010; 126(1):e1–5.

60. Stein PD, Hull RD, Matta F, et al. Early discharge of patients with venous thromboembolism: implications regarding therapy. Clin Appl Thromb Hemost 2010;16(2):141–5.

61. Aujesky D, Stone RA, Kim S, et al. Length of hospital stay and postdischarge mortality in

patients with pulmonary embolism: a statewide perspective. Arch Intern Med 2008;168(7):706–12.

62. Hull R, Delmore T, Genton E, et al. Warfarin sodium versus low-dose heparin in the long-term treatment of venous thrombosis. N Engl J Med 1979;301(16): 855–8.

63. Lagerstedt CI, Olsson CG, Fagher BO, et al. Need for long-term anticoagulant treatment in symptomatic calf-vein thrombosis. Lancet 1985;2(8454): 515–8.

64. Wessler S, Gitel SN. Warfarin. From bedside to bench. N Engl J Med 1984;311(10):645–52.

65. Hirsh J, Bates SM. Clinical trials that have influenced the treatment of venous thromboembolism: a historical perspective. Ann Intern Med 2001;134 (5):409–17.

66. Hull R, Hirsh J, Jay R, et al. Different intensities of oral anticoagulant therapy in the treatment of proximal-vein thrombosis. N Engl J Med 1982;307 (27):1676–81.

67. Crowther MA, Ginsberg JB, Kearon C, et al. A randomized trial comparing 5-mg and 10-mg warfarin loading doses. Arch Intern Med 1999; 159(1):46–8.

68. Harrison L, Johnston M, Massicotte MP, et al. Comparison of 5-mg and 10-mg loading doses in initiation of warfarin therapy. Ann Intern Med 1997;126(2):133–6.

69. Kovacs MJ, Rodger M, Anderson DR, et al. Comparison of 10-mg and 5-mg warfarin initiation nomograms together with low-molecular-weight heparin for outpatient treatment of acute venous thromboembolism. A randomized, double-blind, controlled trial. Ann Intern Med 2003;138(9):714–9.

70. Sanderson S, Emery J, Higgins J. CYP2C9 gene variants, drug dose, and bleeding risk in warfarin-treated patients: a HuGEnet systematic review and meta-analysis. Genet Med 2005;7(2):97–104.

71. Rieder MJ, Reiner AP, Gage BF, et al. Effect of VKORC1 haplotypes on transcriptional regulation and warfarin dose. N Engl J Med 2005;352(22): 2285–93.

72. Grice GR, Laramie D, Anderson DC Jr. Periprocedural anticoagulation management in orthopedic patients: overview and description of a program utilizing pharmacogenetics. J Clin Outcome Manag 2008;15(4):183–90.

73. McWilliam A, Lutter R, Nardinelli C. AEI-Brookings joint center regulatory studies report: health care savings from personalized medicine using genetic testing. Available at: http://www.aei-brookings.org/publications/abstract.php?pid=1127. Accessed January 25, 2010.

74. Anderson JL, Horne BD, Stevens SM, et al. Randomized trial of genotype-guided versus standard warfarin dosing in patients initiating oral anticoagulation. Circulation 2007;116(22):2563–70.

75. Caraco Y, Blotnick S, Muszkat M. CYP2C9 genotype-guided warfarin prescribing enhances the efficacy and safety of anticoagulation: a prospective randomized controlled study. Clin Pharmacol Ther 2008;83(3):460–70.

76. Eckman MH, Rosand J, Greenberg SM, et al. Cost-effectiveness of using pharmacogenetic information in warfarin dosing for patients with nonvalvular atrial fibrillation. Ann Intern Med 2009;150(2):73–83.

77. Rosove MH, Grody WW. Should we be applying warfarin pharmacogenetics to clinical practice? No, not now. Ann Intern Med 2009;151(4): 270–3, W295.

78. Dentali F, Manfredi E, Crowther M, et al. Long-duration therapy with low molecular weight heparin in patients with antiphospholipid antibody syndrome resistant to warfarin therapy. J Thromb Haemost 2005;3(9):2121–3.

79. Luk C, Wells PS, Anderson D, et al. Extended outpatient therapy with low molecular weight heparin for the treatment of recurrent venous thromboembolism despite warfarin therapy. Am J Med 2001;111(4):270–3.

80. Osinbowale O, Al Malki M, Schade A, et al. An algorithm for managing warfarin resistance. Cleve Clin J Med 2009;76(12):724–30.

81. Lee AY. Cancer and venous thromboembolism: prevention, treatment and survival. J Thromb Thrombolysis 2008;25(1):33–6.

82. Prandoni P, Lensing AW, Piccioli A, et al. Recurrent venous thromboembolism and bleeding complications during anticoagulant treatment in patients with cancer and venous thrombosis. Blood 2002; 100(10):3484–8.

83. Lee AY, Levine MN, Baker RI, et al. Low-molecular-weight heparin versus a coumarin for the prevention of recurrent venous thromboembolism in patients with cancer. N Engl J Med 2003;349(2): 146–53.

84. Hull RD, Pineo GF, Brant RF, et al. Long-term low-molecular-weight heparin versus usual care in proximal-vein thrombosis patients with cancer. Am J Med 2006;119(12):1062–72.

85. Akl EA, Barba M, Rohilla S, et al. Anticoagulation for the long term treatment of venous thromboembolism in patients with cancer. Cochrane Database Syst Rev 2008;2:CD006650.

86. Noble SI, Finlay IG. Is long-term low-molecular-weight heparin acceptable to palliative care patients in the treatment of cancer related venous thromboembolism? A qualitative study. Pa Med 2005;19(3):197–201.

87. National Comprehensive Cancer Network. NCCN Clinical practice guidelines in oncology. Venous thromboembolic disease, V.2.2009. Available at: www.nccn.org. Accessed January 25, 2010.

88. Lyman GH, Khorana AA, Falanga A, et al. American Society of Clinical Oncology guideline: recommendations for venous thromboembolism prophylaxis and treatment in patients with cancer. J Clin Oncol 2007;25(34):5490–505.

89. Mandala M, Falanga A, Roila F. Management of venous thromboembolism in cancer patients: ESMO clinical recommendations. Ann Oncol 2009;20(Suppl 4):182–4.

90. van der Heijden JF, Hutten BA, Buller HR, et al. Vitamin K antagonists or low-molecular-weight heparin for the long term treatment of symptomatic venous thromboembolism. Cochrane Database Syst Rev 2002;1:CD002001.

91. Hull RD, Pineo GF, Brant RF, et al. Self-managed long-term low-molecular-weight heparin therapy: the balance of benefits and harms. Am J Med 2007;120(1):72–82.

92. Marchetti M, Pistorio A, Barone M, et al. Low-molecular-weight heparin versus warfarin for secondary prophylaxis of venous thromboembolism: a cost-effectiveness analysis. Am J Med 2001;111(2):130–9.

93. Hull RD, Pineo GF, Brant R, et al. Home therapy of venous thrombosis with long-term LMWH versus usual care: patient satisfaction and post-thrombotic syndrome. Am J Med 2009;122(8): 762–9, e763.

94. Romera A, Cairols MA, Vila-Coll R, et al. A randomised open-label trial comparing long-term sub-cutaneous low-molecular-weight heparin compared with oral-anticoagulant therapy in the treatment of deep venous thrombosis. Eur J Vasc Endovasc Surg 2009;37(3):349–56.

95. Daskalopoulos ME, Daskalopoulou SS, Tzortzis E, et al. Long-term treatment of deep venous thrombosis with a low molecular weight heparin (tinzaparin): a prospective randomized trial. Eur J Vasc Endovasc Surg 2005;29(6):638–50.

96. Lopez-Beret P, Orgaz A, Fontcuberta J, et al. Low molecular weight heparin versus oral anticoagulants in the long-term treatment of deep venous thrombosis. J Vasc Surg 2001;33(1):77–90.

97. Prandoni P, Frulla M, Sartor D, et al. Vein abnormalities and the post-thrombotic syndrome. J Thromb Haemost 2005;3(2):401–2.

98. Shbaklo H, Holcroft CA, Kahn SR. Levels of inflammatory markers and the development of the post-thrombotic syndrome. Thromb Haemost 2009;101 (3):505–12.

99. Prandoni P, Kahn SR. Post-thrombotic syndrome: prevalence, prognostication and need for progress. Br J Haematol 2009;145(3):286–95.

100. Amiral J, Bridey F, Dreyfus M, et al. Platelet factor 4 complexed to heparin is the target for antibodies generated in heparin-induced thrombocytopenia. Thromb Haemost 1992;68(1):95–6.

101. Warkentin TE, Hayward CP, Boshkov LK, et al. Sera from patients with heparin-induced thrombocytopenia generate platelet-derived microparticles with procoagulant activity: an explanation for the thrombotic complications of heparin-induced thrombocytopenia. Blood 1994;84(11):3691–9.

102. Warkentin TE. Clinical picture of heparin-induced thrombocytopenia. In: Warkentin TE, Greinacher A, editors. Heparin-induced thrombocytopenia. 4th edition. New York: Informa Healthcare USA, Inc; 2008. p. 21–66.

103. Lee DH, Warkentin TE. Frequency of heparin-induced thrombocytopenia. In: Warkentin TE, Greinacher A, editors. Heparin-induced Thrombocytopenia. 4th edition. New York: Informa Healthcare USA, Inc; 2008. p. 67–116.

104. Warkentin TE, Kelton JG. A 14-year study of heparin-induced thrombocytopenia. Am J Med 1996;101(5):502–7.

105. Lo GK, Juhl D, Warkentin TE, et al. Evaluation of pretest clinical score (4 T's) for the diagnosis of heparin-induced thrombocytopenia in two clinical settings. J Thromb Haemost 2006;4(4): 759–65.

106. Warkentin TE. Laboratory testing for heparin-induced thrombocytopenia. In: Warkentin TE, Greinacher A, editors. Heparin-induced thrombocytopenia. 4th edition. New York: Informa Healthcare USA, Inc; 2008. p. 227–60.

107. Bakchoul T, Giptner A, Najaoui A, et al. Prospective evaluation of PF4/heparin immunoassays for the diagnosis of heparin-induced thrombocytopenia. J Thromb Haemost 2009;7(8):1260–5.

108. Zwicker JI, Uhl L, Huang WY, et al. Thrombosis and ELISA optical density values in hospitalized patients with heparin-induced thrombocytopenia. J Thromb Haemost 2004;2(12):2133–7.

109. Warkentin TE, Greinacher A, Koster A, et al. Treatment and prevention of heparin-induced thrombocytopenia: American College of Chest Physicians evidence-based clinical practice guidelines (8th edition). Chest 2008;133(Suppl 6):340S–80S.

New Synthetic Antithrombotic Agents for Venous Thromboembolism: Pentasaccharides, Direct Thrombin Inhibitors, Direct Xa Inhibitors

Timothy A. Morris, MD

KEYWORDS

- Anticoagulation • Pulmonary embolism
- Venous thromboembolism • Management

Although heparin and low molecular weight heparins are the most widely used anticoagulant medication for the acute treatment of thromboembolic disease, there are instances where their usefulness is limited. For example, one of the major complications of unfractionated and low molecular weight heparins is the development of immune-mediated heparin-induced thrombocytopenia.[1] Although the mechanisms involved in HIT are complex and incompletely understood,[2–6] the current evidence suggests that the pathogenic antibodies are specific for epitopes within Platelet Factor 4,[7,8] that are exposed after binding by unfractionated heparin or by low molecular weight heparin.[9] The immune reaction causing heparin-induced thrombocytopenia between the heparin class of drugs (unfractionated heparin or low molecular weight heparin) and Platelet Factor 4 depends on the amount of the (larger) molecules in either drug that bind Platelet Factor 4.[10] In one recent meta-analysis, the risk of immune-mediated heparin-induced thrombocytopenia appears equal between unfractionated heparin and low molecular weight heparin.[11] There is some controversy surrounding this, however, as other investigators have suggested a lower risk of heparin-induced thrombocytopenia with the low molecular weight heparins (see articles by Pendleton and colleagues and Anderson and colleagues elsewhere in this issue). If heparin-induced thrombocytopenia does occur, heparin and low molecular weight heparin must be immediately withdrawn and an alternative form of anticoagulation should be used.[12] In those situations the anticoagulant medications discussed in this article, which do not increase the formation and binding of the antibodies, may help avoid further thrombosis.[13,14]

SYNTHETIC PENTASACCHARIDES
Mechanism of Action

Synthetic pentasaccharides (fondaparinux and idraparinux) are analogues of the specific (5-sugar)

This work was supported by Grant No. HL095089 from the National Institutes of Health as well as a grant from the CHEST Foundation and the American College of Chest Physicians.
Division of Pulmonary and Critical Care Medicine, University of California, San Diego Medical Center, 200 West Arbor Drive, San Diego, CA 92103-8378, USA
E-mail address: t1morris@ucsd.edu

Clin Chest Med 31 (2010) 707–718
doi:10.1016/j.ccm.2010.06.006

sequence that must be present on unfractionated heparin or low molecular weight heparin molecules to catalyze the inhibitory action of antithrombin (also referred to as antithrombin III). Unfractionated heparins and low molecular weight heparins are heterogeneous mixtures of modified polysaccharides (glycosaminoglycans) derived from animal products, and only about 1 in 3 molecules in unfractionated heparin and an even smaller proportion of low molecular weight heparin molecules contain the specific pentasaccharide sequence.[15,16] Those that lack it have no significant potentiating effect on antithrombin.[17] In contrast, fondaparinux is a synthetic pentasaccharide, and its molecules uniformly have the antithrombin-binding sequence identical to the active sites of unfractionated heparin or low molecular weight heparin.[18] Idraparinux is similar to fondaparinux, but has been modified to have a higher affinity for antithrombin and exhibit a longer half-life in the blood after administration.[19]

A major portion of the clinical effects of unfractionated heparin and of low molecular weight heparin occurs through enhancement of the inhibitory action of antithrombin on factor IIa (thrombin) and factor Xa. The fundamental biologic difference between unfractionated heparin and low molecular weight heparin stems from the relative potency with which each drug accelerates the basal rate of antithrombin-mediated thrombin and/or factor Xa inactivation.[20] Unfractionated heparin preparations enhance inactivation of both thrombin and factor Xa while low molecular weight heparins catalyze factor Xa inactivation predominantly. The small size and relatively simple structure of fondaparinux and idraparinux make both drugs specific for enhancing antithrombin-mediated inhibition of factor Xa, rather than thrombin. Enhancement of thrombin inhibition by antithrombin requires larger, more negatively charged polysaccharides. The same characteristic of these 2 drugs makes them less likely to induce the conformational change in Platelet Factor 4 that has been implicated in heparin-induced thrombocytopenia.

The synthetic pentasaccharides have other notable differences with heparin, which contains larger, more negatively charged molecules. First, heparin tends to bind to several other plasma proteins, decreasing the bioavailability of at least a portion of the drug. Whether this property of heparin makes its pharmacokinetic profile after subcutaneous administration less predictable than low molecular weight heparins with regard to their mechanisms of action is controversial.[21] High-dose subcutaneous unfractionated heparin was as effective and as safe as high-dose low molecular weight heparin when they were compared in a clinical trial of venous thromboembolism (VTE) treatment.[22] Heparin has not been compared in this fashion with synthetic pentasaccharides. Second, because binding to plasma proteins is a major factor in the elimination of heparin, it is not dependent on normal hepatic or renal function for clearance. Like low molecular weight heparins, the synthetic pentasaccharides are eliminated largely by glomerular filtration and so are highly dependent on renal function for clearance. Finally, the anticoagulant effects of heparin can be largely reversed by administration of protamine, a negatively charged medication that can separate heparin:antithrombin complexes. For this reason, protamine can be used as an "antidote" to heparin if serious bleeding should occur following administration. However, protamine does not separate the pentasaccharides from antithrombin, and so does not reverse their anticoagulant activity. Treatment of bleeding after pentasaccharide administration is limited to more generic methods, such as factor VII administration and (of course) discontinuation of the drug itself.

Fondaparinux

Fondaparinux is approved by the Food and Drug Administration (FDA) for prophylaxis of deep venous thrombosis (DVT) in patients undergoing hip fracture surgery (including extended prophylaxis), hip replacement surgery, knee replacement surgery, or abdominal surgery. Fondaparinux is also approved for treatment of DVT or acute pulmonary embolism (PE) when administered in conjunction with warfarin.

Fondaparinux is administered subcutaneously once per day. It is completely absorbed by this route, reaching peak steady-state plasma levels within 3 hours of administration. The dosages for prophylaxis are lower than the doses for treatment. Unlike heparin, fondaparinux is eliminated renally as unchanged drug. These properties bestow a predictable pharmacokinetic profile in patients with normal renal function. However, as noted later, fondaparinux may be problematic if renal function is compromised.

Safety and efficacy for VTE prevention

Fondaparinux has been tested in several well-run randomized controlled clinical trials that have established its safety and efficacy for VTE prophylaxis in specific clinical situations (**Table 1**). The dose used for prophylaxis is typically 2.5 mg subcutaneously once per day. In a double-blind randomized controlled trial of patients undergoing major knee surgery, fondaparinux at this dose (beginning 4–8 hours postoperatively) resulted in a lower overall incidence of VTE (screened for by venography) in the first postoperative week than enoxaparin, 30 mg subcutaneously twice per day (beginning 12–24 hours postoperatively).[23] In that trial, however, fondaparinux was also associated with more episodes of major bleeding than enoxaparin, at least at the dosing regimens used in that trial. In a similar trial performed on patients undergoing surgical repair of hip fractures, the same prophylactic regimen of fondaparinux was also associated with a lower occurrence of VTE in the first postoperative week than enoxaparin, 40 mg given subcutaneously once per week (beginning 10–14 hours postoperatively).[24] Two similar trials were performed using the same prophylactic regimen of fondaparinux following hip replacement surgery. In one trial, fondaparinux was associated with the a lower incidence of VTE than enoxaparin, 40 mg given 12 hours preoperatively and continued daily.[25] However, in the other hip replacement trial, there was no difference in VTE incidences between patients who received fondaparinux and those who received enoxaparin, 30 mg twice daily, begun 12 hours postoperatively.[26] In the hip fracture surgery trial[24] and the 2 hip replacement surgery trials,[25,26] there were no differences in bleeding rates between the fondaparinux and enoxaparin groups. In none of these trials did the incidences of the secondary outcomes of symptomatic DVT, nonfatal PE, or fatal PE in the fondaparinux group differ from the enoxaparin groups.

A subsequent double-blind randomized controlled trial in hip fracture surgery patients compared extended prophylaxis with fondaparinux, 2.5 mg per day, to placebo.[27] Both treatments began after 6 to 8 days of postoperative prophylaxis with fondaparinux and continued for 19 to 23 days. In that trial, there were substantial and statistically significant reductions in VTE (screened for by venography), as well as symptomatic VTE in those who were treated with fondaparinux as compared with placebo. Although this trial did not evaluate the relative merits of fondaparinux as compared with other forms of extended prophylaxis, it does validate fondaparinux as a useful agent for this purpose.

Safety and efficacy for VTE treatment

The acute treatment of VTE with fondaparinux has also been well validated by double-blind randomized controlled trials (**Table 2**). The dosing regimen used in these trials was straightforward: 7.5 mg subcutaneously in patients who weighed from 50 to 100 kg (85% of cases). The dose was decreased to 5.0 mg patients weighing less than 50 kg and increased to 10.0 mg in those weighing

more than 100 kg. As is the case for unfractionated heparin and low molecular weight heparin, the treatment was continued for at least 5 days, during which time warfarin was administered. After 5 days, treatment with fondaparinux was stopped once warfarin was therapeutic. In a double-blind randomized trial for the treatment of acute proximal lower extremity DVT,[28] this regimen was as effective in preventing recurrent symptomatic VTE as enoxaparin, 1.0 mg/kg body weight twice per day. A randomized, open-label clinical trial compared the same fondaparinux treatment regimen to intravenous unfractionated heparin (using standard activated partial thromboplastin time–driven dosage adjustments) for the treatment of PE.[29] The outcomes of the 2 treatments appeared identical: the fondaparinux and "standard therapy" groups did not significantly differ with respect to the incidence of recurrent VTE, bleeding, overall mortality, or mortality due to PE.

Other advantages and disadvantages

Fondaparinux is highly bioavailable when given subcutaneously and is cleared renally, both of which contribute to its predictable pharmacokinetics in patients with normal renal function. However, its renal clearance raises the possibility of cumulative overdosage in patients with severe renal impairment. Clinical trials using fondaparinux typically excluded patients with creatinine levels above 2 mg per deciliter.[23,24,28,29] Despite this restriction, the incidence of major bleeding was more than sevenfold higher in DVT patients and in PE patients treated with fondaparinux whose creatinine clearance was less than 30 mL/min, compared with those with better renal function.[28,29] Although it may be feasible to adjust the dose downward for renal impairment, it is currently recommended that fondaparinux be avoided in patients with creatinine clearance rates below 30 mL/min, and that is be used with caution in patients with rates between 30 and 50 mL/min.[30]

Fondaparinux has a smaller size and less negative charge density than unfractionated heparin and low molecular weight heparin, which makes it less likely to induce the molecular changes associated with heparin-induced thrombocytopenia. However, it bears comment that the rates of thrombocytopenia were similar between fondaparinux and the comparator drugs during the prophylaxis and treatment trials described.[23,24,28,29] Furthermore, no cases of immune-mediated heparin-induced thrombocytopenia with thrombosis were observed in any of the experimental groups, including the trial comparing fondaparinux to intravenous heparin for the treatment of PE.[29] Although it is unusual, there have been isolated

Table 1
Randomized controlled trials of prophylaxis against VTE

Agent / Author,Ref. Year	Population	Intervention		VTE Outcome	VTE		Major Bleeding	
		Study Drug	Control		Study Drug	Control	Study Drug	Control
Fondaparinux								
Bauer et al,[23] 2001	Major knee surgery	Fondaparinux 2.5 mg SC qd, beginning 4–8 h postop, for 5–9 d	Enoxaparin 30 mg SC bid, beginning 12–24 h postop, for 5–9 d	Asymptomatic DVT (venography), symptomatic DVT, PE within 11 d	45/361 (12.5%)	101/363 (27.8%)	11/517 (2.1%)	1/517 (0.2%)
Eriksson et al,[24] 2001	Hip fracture surgery	Fondaparinux 2.5 mg SC qd, beginning 4–8 h postop, for 5–9 d	Enoxaparin 40 mg SC qd, beginning 10–14 h preop, for 5–9 d	Asymptomatic DVT (venography), symptomatic DVT, PE within 11 d	52/626 (8.3%)	119/624 (19.1%)	18/831 (2.2%)	19/842 (2.3%)
Lassen et al,[25] 2002	Hip arthroplasty	Fondaparinux 2.5 mg SC qd, beginning 4–8 h postop, for 5–9 d	Enoxaparin 40 mg SC qd, beginning 10–14 h preop, for 5–9 d	Asymptomatic DVT (venography), symptomatic DVT, PE within 11 d	37/908 (4.1%)	85/919 (9.2%)	47/1140 (4.1%)	32/1133 (2.8%)
Turpie et al,[26] 2002	Hip arthroplasty	Fondaparinux 2.5 mg SC qd, beginning 4–8 h postop, for 5–9 d	Enoxaparin 30 mg SC qd, beginning 10–14 h postop, for 5–9 d	Asymptomatic DVT (venography), symptomatic DVT, PE within 11 d	48/787 (6.1%)	66/797 (8.3%)	20/1128 (1.8%)	11/1129 (1.0)
Eriksson and Lassen[27] 2003	Hip fracture surgery	Fondaparinux 2.5 mg SC qd, beginning after fondaparinux for 6–8 d, extending for 19–23 d	Placebo, beginning after fondaparinux for 6–8 d, extending for 19–23 d	Asymptomatic DVT (venography), symptomatic DVT, PE within 32 d	3/208 (1.4%)	77/220 (35.0%)	8/327 (2.4%)	2/329 (0.6%)
Dabigatran								
Eriksson et al,[38] 2007	Hip arthroplasty	Dabigatran etexilate 220 mg PO qd, (half-dose 1–4 h postop) for 28–35 d. Dabigatran etexilate 150 mg PO qd (half-dose 1–4 h postop) for 28–35 d	Enoxaparin 40 mg SC qd, beginning the evening preop for 28–35 d	Asymptomatic DVT (venography), symptomatic DVT, PE or mortality during treatment	53/880 (6.0%) 75/874 (8.6%)	60/897 (6.7%)	23/1126 (2.0%) 15/1163 (1.3%)	18/1154 (1.6%)

Study	Procedure	Intervention	Comparator	Outcome				
Eriksson et al,[39] 2007	Knee arthroplasty	Dabigatran etexilate 220 mg PO qd, (half-dose 6–12 h postop) for 6–10 d	Enoxaparin 40 mg SC qd, beginning the evening preop for 6–10 d	Asymptomatic DVT (venography), symptomatic DVT, PE or mortality within 3 d of last dose	183/503 (36.4%)	193/512 (37.7%)	10/679 (1.5%)	9/694 (1.3%)
		Dabigatran etexilate 150 mg PO qd (half-dose 6–12 h postop) for 6–10 d			213/526 (40.5%)		9/703 (1.3%)	
Ginsberg et al,[40] 2009	Knee arthroplasty	Dabigatran etexilate 220 mg PO qd, (half-dose 6–12 h postop) for 12–15 d	Enoxaparin 30 mg SC bid, beginning 12–24 h postop for 12–15 d	Asymptomatic DVT (venography), symptomatic DVT, PE or mortality within 3 d of last dose	188/857 (31.1%)	163/868 (25.3%)	5/857 (0.6%)	12/868 (1.4%)
		Dabigatran etexilate 150 mg PO qd (half-dose 6–12 h postop) for 12–15 d			219/871 (33.7%)		5/871 (0.6%)	
Rivaroxaban								
Eriksson et al,[47] 2008	Hip arthroplasty	Rivaroxaban 10 mg PO qd. First dose 6–8 h postop for 31–39 d	Enoxaparin 40 mg SC qd, beginning 12 h preop, then 6–8 h postop for 31–39 d	Asymptomatic DVT (venography), symptomatic DVT, PE or mortality within 1 day of last dose	18/1595 (1.1%)	58/1558 (3.7%)	6/2209 (0.3%)	2/224 (0.1%)
Lassen et al,[49] 2008	Knee arthroplasty	Rivaroxaban 10 mg PO qd. First dose 6–8 h postop for 10–14 d	Enoxaparin 40 mg SC qd, beginning 12 h preop, then 6–8 h postop for 10–14 d	Asymptomatic DVT (venography), symptomatic DVT, PE or mortality within 3 d of last dose	79/824 (9.6%)	166/878 (18.9%)	7/1220 (0.6%)	6/1239 (0.5%)
Kakkar et al,[48] 2008	Hip arthroplasty	Rivaroxaban 10 mg PO qd. First dose 6–8 h postop for 31–39 d	Enoxaparin 40 mg SC qd, beginning 12 h preop, then 6–8 h postop for 10–14 d	Asymptomatic DVT (venography), symptomatic DVT, PE or mortality within 30–42 d	17/864 (2.0%)	81/869 (9.3%)	81/1228 (6.6%)	68/1229 (5.5%)
Apixaban								
Lassen et al,[54] 2009	Knee arthroplasty	Apixaban 2.5 mg orally bid, beginning 12–24 h postop, for 10–14 d	Enoxaparin 30 mg SC bid beginning 12–24 h postop, for 10–14 d	Asymptomatic DVT (venography), symptomatic DVT, PE during treatment	104/1157 (9.0%)	100/1130 (8.8%)	11/1596 (0.7%)	22/1588 (1.4%)

Abbreviations: aPTT, activated partial thromboplastin time; bid, twice per day; DVT, deep venous thrombosis; PE, pulmonary embolism; PO, by mouth; postop, postoperatively; preop, preoperatively; qd, every day; SC, subcutaneous; VTE, venous thromboembolism.

Table 2
Phase III trials for the treatment of DVT, PE, or both

Agent / Author, Ref. Year	Population	Study Drug	Control	VTE Outcome	Recurrent VTE Study Drug	Recurrent VTE Control	Major Bleeding Study Drug	Major Bleeding Control	Mortality Study Drug	Mortality Control
Fondaparinux										
Buller et al,[28] 2004	Acute symptomatic proximal LE DVT	Fondaparinux, 7.5 mg (5.0 mg if <50 kg and 10.0 mg if >100 kg) SC qd	Enoxaparin, 1 mg/kg body weight, SC bid	Symptomatic recurrent DVT or PE within 3 mo	43/1098 (3.9%)	45/1107 (4.1%)	12/1091 (1.1%)	13/1101 (1.2%)	41/1098 (3.8%)	33/1107 (3.0%)
Buller et al,[29] 2003	Acute symptomatic PE	Fondaparinux, 7.5 mg (5.0 mg if <50 kg and 10.0 mg if >100 kg) qd	Unfractionated heparin IV, adjusted to aPTT	Symptomatic recurrent DVT or PE within 3 mo	42/1103 (3.8%)	56/1110 (5.0%)	14/1092 (1.3%)	12/1092 (1.1%)	57/1092 (5.2%)	48/1092 (4.4%)
Idraparinux										
Buller et al,[34] 2007	Acute symptomatic proximal LE DVT	Idraparinux 2.5 mg SC every week for 3–6 mo	Unfractionated heparin IV or LMWH SC for at least 5 d, followed by warfarin for 3–6 mo	Symptomatic recurrent DVT or PE within 3 mo	42/1452 (2.9%)	43/1452 (3.0%)	12/1452 (0.8%)	17/1452 (1.2%)	33/1452 (2.3%)	29/1452 (2.0%)
Buller et al,[34] 2007	Acute symptomatic PE	Idraparinux 2.5 mg SC every week for 3–6 mo	Unfractionated heparin IV or LMWH SC for at least 5 d, followed by warfarin for 3–6 mo	Symptomatic recurrent DVT or PE within 3 mo	37/1095 (3.4%)	18/1120 (1.6%)	12/1095 (1.1%)	24/1120 (2.1%)	56/1095 (5.1%)	32/1120 (2.9%)
Buller et al,[35] 2007	VTE previously treated for 6 mo	Idraparinux 2.5 mg SC every week for 6 mo	Placebo	Symptomatic recurrent DVT or PE within 6 mo	6/594 (1.0%)	23/621 (3.7%)	11/594 (1.9%)	0/616 (0%)	9/594 (1.5%)	4/616 (0.6%)
Dabigatran										
Schulman et al,[41] 2009	VTE previously treated with LMWH or UH for at least 5 d	Dabigatran 150 mg oral bid for 6 mo	Warfarin oral qd, adjusted to an INR of 2–3 for 6 mo	Symptomatic recurrent DVT or PE or death associated with VTE within 6 mo	30/1274 (2.4%)	27/1265 (2.1%)	20/1274 (1.6%)	24/1265 (1.9%)	21/1274 (1.6%)	21/1265 (1.7%)

Abbreviations: INR, international normalized ratio; IV, intravenous; LE, lower extremity; LMWH, low molecular weight heparin; UH, unfractionated heparin.

reports of thrombosis associated with thrombocytopenia in patients receiving fondaparinux.[31,32]

Idraparinux

Idraparinux is an analogue of the pentasaccharide sequence that makes up fondaparinux. The modifications to the synthesis of idraparinux confer on it a higher affinity to antithrombin, which make it a more potent anti-Xa anticoagulant. For this reason, it is typically given in much smaller doses than fondaparinux. Perhaps more importantly, idraparinux has a very long half-life,[19] which permits subcutaneous treatment once per week,[33] rather than once or more daily. Idraparinux is not approved for use by the FDA.

Safety and efficacy for VTE treatment
Two consecutive randomized open-label controlled trials were performed to evaluate the efficacy of idraparinux: one trial for the treatment of symptomatic acute DVT and the other for the treatment of symptomatic acute PE (see **Table 2**).[34] In both trials, idraparinux, 2.5 mg administered subcutaneously every week, was compared with standard treatment regimens that included heparin or low molecular weight heparin for the acute treatment, followed by an adjusted dose vitamin K antagonist such as warfarin. In patients treated for DVT, the outcomes of therapy did not significantly differ between idraparinux and standard therapy with regard to recurrent VTE, major bleeding, or death. However, in patients treated for PE, the idraparinux group had a significantly higher incidence of recurrent VTE and mortality, as well as a trend toward more deaths attributed to PE itself. Why the efficacy of idraparinux differed between the two groups is unknown, but the finding does call into question the wisdom of extrapolating the results of DVT treatment trials to the treatment of PE.

A follow-on substudy to the idraparinux trial randomized patients who had received 6 months of anticoagulant therapy (idraparinux or a vitamin K antagonist) to an additional 6 months of idraparinux versus placebo.[35] Although the idraparinux-treated group had a lower incidence of recurrent VTE, they also had a higher incidence of major bleeding episodes, more than one-fourth of which were fatal. It is possible the long half-life, without a specific antidote, contributed to the bleeding risk observed with idraparinux. The bleeding risk may be less with a modification of idraparinux that includes biotin. Because biotin binds to avidin with tremendous affinity, the anticoagulant effects of biotinylated idraparinux ("idrabiotaparinux") may be neutralized by administration of avidin.[36] Clinical trials are ongoing to determine if long-term treatment with idrabiotaparinux would have less bleeding risk than idraparinux.

SYNTHETIC DIRECT THROMBIN INHIBITORS
Dabigatran

Dabigatran is a novel synthetic anticoagulant, designed by molecular analysis of thrombin-thrombin inhibitor complexes.[37] Unlike heparin, low molecular weight heparin, and the pentasaccharides, dabigatran inhibits thrombin directly, without involvement of antithrombin. A theoretical advantage of dabigatran is that it can inhibit fibrin-bound thrombin, which is typically protected against the action of antithrombin. Dabigatran is cleared by renal excretion, with a relatively long half-life.[37] Dabigatran etexilate is an orally absorbed prodrug of dabigatran that has undergone clinical trials for VTE prevention and treatment.

Safety and efficacy for VTE prevention
A large randomized controlled trial in hip replacement surgery patients (see **Table 1**) compared the efficacy of 2 different dose regimens of oral dabigatran etexilate (220 mg or 150 mg once daily, starting with a half-dose 1–4 hours after surgery) to enoxaparin (40 mg subcutaneously per day, starting the evening before surgery).[38] The rates of symptomatic VTE and major bleeding were small, and the study was not powered to detect differences in these indices. However, the efficacy and safety of the 2 oral dabigatran etexilate regimens appeared similar to the enoxaparin regimen.

The data are less straightforward in patients undergoing total knee arthroplasty, who have a higher risk of VTE. In 2 randomized controlled trials that compared the efficacy of oral dabigatran etexilate to enoxaparin, the results were different. In the first trial, 2 dosage regimens of oral dabigatran etexilate (220 mg every day and 150 mg every day, initiated at half-dose 4–8 hours postoperatively) were compared with enoxaparin (40 mg subcutaneously every day, initiated the night before surgery).[39] This dosage regimen of enoxaparin is commonly used for knee arthroplasty in Europe, Australia, and South Africa. The efficacies of both dosages of oral dabigatran etexilate were noninferior to enoxaparin: they were associated with similar rates of postoperative VTE (venographically detected asymptomatic DVT and symptomatic VTE). The rates of symptomatic VTE and major bleeding were small, and similar among the treatment groups.

By contrast, a subsequent trial of VTE prophylaxis for knee replacement surgery compared the same 2 dosage regimens of oral dabigatran etexilate to a more aggressive enoxaparin regimen (30 mg subcutaneously twice per day), which is reflective of practice in North America.[40] In that trial, both dabigatran dosage regimens were inferior to enoxaparin for the prevention of VTE. Major bleeding was rare and tended to be less than in the enoxaparin group, suggesting that a higher (and possibly more effective) dosage of dabigatran might be tolerated in this patient population.

Safety and efficacy for VTE treatment
Dabigatran has been compared in a randomized controlled trial with warfarin for the follow-up treatment of VTE (see **Table 2**).[41] After acute treatment with heparin or low molecular weight heparin, patients were randomized to dabigatran, 150 mg orally twice per day without dosage adjustment, or warfarin, adjusted to an international normalized ratio (INR) of 2 to 3. The outcome of the 2 groups was similar with respect to symptomatic recurrent VTE and major bleeding. These results suggest that dabigatran would be an acceptable alternative to warfarin for the 6-month treatment of VTE following acute therapy with heparin or low molecular weight heparin. Dabigatran has the advantage of not requiring INR-guided dosage adjustment, which can be labor intensive for clinicians as well as patients.

Other advantages and disadvantages
The clinical trials performed to date suggest that dabigatran is a promising agent for prophylaxis against of VTE, and for the first 6 months of therapy following acute VTE treatment. (A study concerning treatment for longer than 6 months is ongoing at the time of writing.) The somewhat conflicting results of the VTE prophylaxis trials suggest that higher doses might be applicable for knee arthroplasty to achieve comparable outcomes to an aggressive enoxaparin regimen.

Dabigatran is well absorbed orally and has a pharmacokinetic profile in most patients that allows dosing for either prophylaxis or treatment of VTE without adjustment in most patients. The studies described here excluded patients with creatinine clearances less than 30 mL/min, and it is currently unknown whether dosage adjustment (and perhaps therapeutic monitoring) would be feasible or safe in patients with renal dysfunction. However, the simplicity of the dosing regimens suggests that dabigatran would be an attractive option for patients with normal renal function.

Unlike ximelagatran,[42] a previously tested direct thrombin inhibitor, there did not appear to be an excess of liver toxicity with dabigatran, compared with enoxaparin[38–40] or warfarin.[41] However, patients with severe hepatic enzyme elevations were excluded from these trials and it is unclear whether dabigatran would have adverse effects on patients with preexisting liver dysfunction.

SYNTHETIC DIRECT FACTOR XA INHIBITORS
Rivaroxaban
Rivaroxaban is a synthetic drug that selectively binds to and inhibits the active site of factor Xa reversibly.[43,44] Because it works without the requirement for the enzyme antithrombin, it is termed a "direct Xa inhibitor." Rivaroxiban is well absorbed orally and is cleared by both hepatic metabolism (two-thirds) and renal excretion (one-third).[45,46]

Safety and efficacy for VTE prevention
A randomized controlled trial in hip replacement surgery disclosed that rivaroxaban (10 mg orally every day) was associated with significantly fewer episodes of VTE than enoxaparin (40 mg subcutaneously every day) when both drugs were administered for 31 to 39 days (see **Table 1**).[47] Rivaroxaban was also significantly more effective in preventing "major VTE," defined as proximal DVT, PE, and death from VTE. There were no differences in postoperative bleeding.

Because a potential advantage of once-daily oral rivaroxaban is the ease of outpatient administration, extended (5-week) prophylaxis with rivaroxiban was also compared with short-term (2-week) prophylaxis with enoxaparin.[48] As expected, the incidence of VTE was substantially lower in the rivaroxaban-treated group. Major VTE (as defined above) and symptomatic VTE also occurred with significantly less frequency in the rivaroxaban group. Bleeding occurred with nearly the same frequency with either drug.

A randomized controlled study in knee replacement surgery also demonstrated superiority of rivaroxaban (10 mg orally every day) over enoxaparin (40 mg subcutaneously every day).[49] Patients who had been prophylaxed with rivaroxaban had a lower overall incidence of VTE and a lower incidence of major VTE than those treated with enoxaparin. Postoperative bleeding was rare, and occurred with nearly the same frequency in the 2 groups.

None of these prophylactic trials compared rivaroxiban to the "North American" prophylactic regimen of enoxaparin, 30 mg administered twice per day postoperatively, as had been done for dabigatran.[40]

Safety and efficacy for VTE treatment
Rivaroxiban has shown promising, albeit preliminary, results in phase 2 (dose-ranging) trials for the treatment of acute DVT. In the first

open-label trial, patients with DVT were randomized to 4 different dose regimens of rivaroxiban (10, 20, or 30 mg twice a day, or 40 mg every day) or standard therapy with enoxaparin followed by warfarin.[50] Treatment continued for 12 weeks. The surrogate end point of "clot burden" as assessed by compression ultrasonography was similar between the experimental and standard therapy groups. Minor trends toward increased bleeding in the rivaroxaban groups were not statistically significant.

A second phase 2 study tested 3 different once-daily dose regimens of rivaroxaban: (20, 30, or 40 mg every day) in an open-label comparison with locally determined standard therapy with heparin or low molecular weight heparin followed by a vitamin K antagonist such as warfarin or acenocoumarol.[51] All groups were treated for 84 days. The composite end point of symptomatic recurrent DVT, symptomatic fatal or nonfatal PE, and asymptomatic deterioration in thrombotic burden (assessed by compression ultrasound) occurred less often in the rivaroxaban groups than in the standard treatment groups. Bleeding was comparable among the groups.

The results of both phase 2 trials supported the performance of phase 3 trials, which are currently underway.

Other advantages and disadvantages

The high bioavailability and pharmacokinetic predictability of once- or twice-daily oral rivaroxaban[45,46] is advantageous for extended prophylaxis and for treatment. Rivaroxiban is cleared by both renal and hepatic routes, including cytochrome P450-mediated metabolism. In the trials listed here, patients with severe renal or hepatic dysfunction were excluded. There are also potential drug interactions with agents that inhibit cytochrome P450 3A4, such as azole compounds or human immunodeficiency virus–protease inhibitors.

Rivaroxiban does not appear to pose a particular risk of liver damage. Transaminase elevations were observed with similar frequency among rivaroxaban- and enoxaparin-treated groups in most trials,[47,49,51] whereas one treatment trial disclosed far fewer transaminase elevations with rivaroxaban than with enoxaparin.[50]

Apixaban

Like rivaroxaban, apixaban is a potent, reversible, and highly selective direct inhibitor of activated factor X.[52] Apixaban is well absorbed after oral administration and is cleared both renally and by multiple metabolic pathways.[53] These properties make it an attractive candidate as an antithrombotic agent.

Safety and efficacy for VTE prevention

A large phase 3 randomized controlled trial was performed that compared apixaban (2.5 mg orally twice per day) for prophylaxis after knee replacement surgery to the "North American" regimen of enoxaparin (30 mg subcutaneously twice per day) (see **Table 1**).[54] The trial was inconclusive because the incidence of the primary end point of asymptomatic and symptomatic VTE was unexpectedly low in both groups: 9.0% in those treated with apixaban and 8.8% in those treated with enoxaparin. Despite this close outcome, the study did not reach its prespecified criteria for noninferiority. The same result was observed for major VTE and symptomatic VTE, in which the groups differed by less than 0.5%. The maxim "absence of proof does not imply proof of absence" seems applicable in this case, where the outcome rates were so close between the groups. As it turns out, the rate of bleeding was significantly lower for those treated with apixaban: 0.7%, compared with 1.4% in the enoxaparin-treated group.

Safety and efficacy for VTE treatment

A phase 2, dose-ranging clinical trial compared 3 different oral apixaban potential treatment regimens (5 mg twice per day, 10 mg twice per day, and 20 mg once per day) to standard therapy with low molecular weight heparin followed by vitamin K antagonists.[55] The incidence of the composite outcome (symptomatic recurrent VTE and the surrogate marker of worsened compression ultrasound or perfusion lung scan findings) was similar between the experimental and standard care groups, as was the incidence of bleeding. These results prompted the performance of phase 3 studies, which are currently in progress.

Other advantages and disadvantages

Apixaban is well absorbed after oral administration, which makes it a promising agent for prolonged prophylaxis and treatment. Apixaban is cleared largely by the kidneys, but is also eliminated in the liver by multiple metabolic pathways other than the cytochrome P450 system. Thus it has some potential as an agent for patients with renal or hepatic impairment. However, this potential has yet to be validated in clinical trials, which excluded patients with low creatinine clearance or hepatic dysfunction.

Betrixaban

Betrixaban is an orally absorbed highly potent, selective inhibitor of factor Xa.[56] Like other direct Xa inhibitor drugs, it is highly selective for the active site of factor Xa, and does not require interaction with antithrombin. Betrixaban differs from the others in that its clearance is primarily by biliary excretion with very little urinary excretion. It therefore has potential in patients with renal dysfunction.

Safety and efficacy for VTE prevention
Betrixaban has been evaluated in a relatively small dose-ranging randomized trial for the prophylaxis of VTE after knee arthroplasty.[57] Two different dose regimens of oral betrixaban (15 mg twice a day or betrixaban 40 mg twice a day, beginning 6–8 hours postoperatively) were compared with subcutaneous enoxaparin (30 mg twice a day, beginning 12–24 hours postoperatively). Treatments were continued for 10 to 14 days and followed by mandatory venography. Although the study was not powered sufficiently to allow a useful statistical comparison of outcomes, the rates of VTE and bleeding appeared comparable among all 3 groups.

Other advantages and disadvantages
Betrixaban is undergoing preliminary clinical studies, and insufficient data exist to evaluate its relevant clinical characteristics at this time.

SUMMARY

Synthetic antithrombotic drugs are in various stages of clinical development. All of them offer at least theoretical advantages over heparin and low molecular weight heparins. Fondaparinux, an analogue of the antithrombin-binding site common to heparin and low molecular weight heparins, has undergone the most extensive testing. Clinical trials have demonstrated its usefulness for the prevention and treatment of VTE, and fondaparinux has been approved by the FDA for both purposes. Idraparinux, a long-acting analogue of fondaparinux, and its biotin-bound modification "idrabiotaparinux," are undergoing further study to identify their optimal role for VTE treatment. Specific enzyme inhibitors have been synthesized that do not require antithrombin and have the advantage of oral bioavailability. The direct thrombin inhibitor dabigatran has demonstrated efficacy and safety for the prevention and treatment of VTE in phase 3 clinical trials. There are several direct factor Xa inhibitors being developed for clinical use. Among them, rivaroxaban currently has the most clinical trial data supporting its use for VTE prophylaxis. Phase 3 trials are underway to study rivaroxaban for VTE treatment. Apixaban also has shown promise as a prophylactic and treatment drug for VTE, although further testing is necessary. Betrixaban has pharmacokinetic properties that may be advantageous in patients with renal and hepatic dysfunction, but is too early in its development for sound conclusions to be made about its safety and efficacy. All of these agents may prove to be beneficial, although clinical trials have not yet established their superiority to heparin and low molecular weight heparin with respect to efficacy and the avoidance of problems such as bleeding and immune-mediated thrombocytopenia/thrombosis.

REFERENCES

1. Chong BH. Heparin-induced thrombocytopenia. J Thromb Haemost 2003;1:1471–8.
2. Amiral J. Antigens involved in heparin-induced thrombocytopenia. Semin Hematol 1999;36:7–11.
3. Newman PM, Chong BH. Further characterization of antibody and antigen in heparin-induced thrombocytopenia. Br J Haematol 1999;107:303–9.
4. Amiral J, Pouplard C, Vissac AM, et al. Affinity purification of heparin-dependent antibodies to platelet factor 4 developed in heparin-induced thrombocytopenia: biological characteristics and effects on platelet activation. Br J Haematol 2000;109:336–41.
5. Horsewood P, Kelton JG. Investigation of a platelet factor 4 polymorphism on the immune response in patients with heparin-induced thrombocytopenia. Platelets 2000;11:23–7.
6. Ahmad S, Walenga JM, Jeske WP, et al. Functional heterogeneity of antiheparin-platelet factor 4 antibodies: implications in the pathogenesis of the HIT syndrome. Clin Appl Thromb Hemost 1999;5(Suppl 1):S32–7.
7. Ziporen L, Li ZQ, Park KS, et al. Defining an antigenic epitope on platelet factor 4 associated with heparin-induced thrombocytopenia. Blood 1998;92:3250–9.
8. Horsewood P, Warkentin TE, Hayward CP, et al. The epitope specificity of heparin-induced thrombocytopenia. Br J Haematol 1996;95:161–7.
9. Pouplard C, Amiral J, Borg JY, et al. Differences in specificity of heparin-dependent antibodies developed in heparin-induced thrombocytopenia and consequences on cross-reactivity with danaparoid sodium. Br J Haematol 1997;99:273–80.
10. Horne MK, Alkins BR. Platelet binding of IgG from patients with heparin-induced thrombocytopenia. [see comments]. J Lab Clin Med 1996;127:435–42.
11. Morris TA, Castrejon S, Devendra G, et al. No difference in risk for thrombocytopenia during treatment of pulmonary embolism and deep venous thrombosis with either low-molecular-weight heparin or unfractionated heparin: a meta-analysis. Chest 2007;132:1131–9.
12. Wallis DE, Workman DL, Lewis BE, et al. Failure of early heparin cessation as treatment for heparin-induced thrombocytopenia. Am J Med 1999;106:629–35.

13. Warkentin TE, Greinacher A, Koster A, et al. Treatment and prevention of heparin-induced thrombocytopenia: American College of Chest Physicians Evidence-Based Clinical Practice Guidelines (8th edition). Chest 2008;133:340S–80S.

14. Lewis BE, Wallis DE, Leya F, et al. Argatroban anticoagulation in patients with heparin-induced thrombocytopenia. Arch Intern Med 2003;163:1849–56.

15. Lam LH, Silbert JE, Rosenberg RD. The separation of active and inactive forms of heparin. Biochem Biophys Res Commun JID –0372516 1976;69:570–7.

16. Harenberg J. Pharmacology of low molecular weight heparins. Semin Thromb Hemost 1990;16(Suppl): 12–8.

17. Olson ST, Bjork I, Sheffer R, et al. Role of the antithrombin-binding pentasaccharide in heparin acceleration of antithrombin-proteinase reactions. Resolution of the antithrombin conformational change contribution to heparin rate enhancement. J Biol Chem JID –2985121R 1992;267:12528–38.

18. Beguin S, Choay J, Hemker HC. The action of a synthetic pentasaccharide on thrombin generation in whole plasma. Thromb Haemost 1989;61: 397–401.

19. Herbert JM, Herault JP, Bernat A, et al. Biochemical and pharmacological properties of SANORG 34006, a potent and long-acting synthetic pentasaccharide. Blood 1998;91:4197–205.

20. Hirsh J, Levine MN. Low molecular weight heparin. Blood 1992;79:1–17.

21. Morris TA, Jacobson A, Marsh JJ, et al. Pharmacokinetics of UH and LMWH are similar with respect to antithrombin activity. Thromb Res 2005;115:45–51.

22. Kearon C, Ginsberg JS, Julian JA, et al. Comparison of fixed-dose weight-adjusted unfractionated heparin and low-molecular-weight heparin for acute treatment of venous thromboembolism. JAMA 2006; 296:935–42.

23. Bauer KA, Eriksson BI, Lassen MR, et al. Fondaparinux compared with enoxaparin for the prevention of venous thromboembolism after elective major knee surgery. N Engl J Med JID –0255562 2001; 345:1305–10.

24. Eriksson BI, Bauer KA, Lassen MR, et al. Fondaparinux compared with enoxaparin for the prevention of venous thromboembolism after hip-fracture surgery. N Engl J Med 2001;345:1298–304.

25. Lassen MR, Bauer KA, Eriksson BI, et al. Postoperative fondaparinux versus preoperative enoxaparin for prevention of venous thromboembolism in elective hip-replacement surgery: a randomised double-blind comparison. Lancet JID –2985213R 2002;359:1715–20.

26. Turpie AG, Bauer KA, Eriksson BI, et al. Postoperative fondaparinux versus postoperative enoxaparin for prevention of venous thromboembolism after elective hip-replacement surgery: a randomised

double-blind trial. Lancet JID –2985213R 2002; 359:1721–6.

27. Eriksson BI, Lassen MR. Duration of prophylaxis against venous thromboembolism with fondaparinux after hip fracture surgery: a multicenter, randomized, placebo-controlled, double-blind study. Arch Intern Med 2003;163:1337–42.

28. Buller HR, Davidson BL, Decousus H, et al. Fondaparinux or enoxaparin for the initial treatment of symptomatic deep venous thrombosis: a randomized trial. Ann Intern Med 2004;140:867–73.

29. Buller HR, Davidson BL, Decousus H, et al. Subcutaneous fondaparinux versus intravenous unfractionated heparin in the initial treatment of pulmonary embolism. N Engl J Med 2003;349:1695–702.

30. Prescribing label for ARIXTRA, NDA no. 021345. Approved 12/23/2009, in Administration FaD (ed), 2009.

31. Warkentin TE, Maurer BT, Aster RH. Heparin-induced thrombocytopenia associated with fondaparinux. N Engl J Med 2007;356:2653–5 [discussion 2655].

32. Rota E, Bazzan M, Fantino G. Fondaparinux-related thrombocytopenia in a previous low-molecular-weight heparin (LMWH)-induced heparin-induced thrombocytopenia (HIT). Thromb Haemost 2008; 99:779–81.

33. Samama MM, Gerotziafas GT. Evaluation of the pharmacological properties and clinical results of the synthetic pentasaccharide (fondaparinux). Thromb Res 2003;109:1–11.

34. Buller HR, Cohen AT, Davidson B, et al. Idraparinux versus standard therapy for venous thromboembolic disease. N Engl J Med 2007;357: 1094–104.

35. Buller HR, Cohen AT, Davidson B, et al. Extended prophylaxis of venous thromboembolism with idraparinux. N Engl J Med 2007;357:1105–12.

36. Paty I, Trellu M, Destors JM, et al. Reversibility of the anti-FXa activity of idrabiotaparinux (biotinylated idraparinux) by intravenous avidin infusion. J Thromb Haemost 2010;8(4):722–9.

37. Hauel NH, Nar H, Priepke H, et al. Structure-based design of novel potent nonpeptide thrombin inhibitors. J Med Chem 2002;45:1757–66.

38. Eriksson BI, Dahl OE, Rosencher N, et al. Dabigatran etexilate versus enoxaparin for prevention of venous thromboembolism after total hip replacement: a randomised, double-blind, non-inferiority trial. Lancet 2007;370:949–56.

39. Eriksson BI, Dahl OE, Rosencher N, et al. Oral dabigatran etexilate vs. subcutaneous enoxaparin for the prevention of venous thromboembolism after total knee replacement: the RE-MODEL randomized trial. J Thromb Haemost 2007;5:2178–85.

40. Ginsberg JS, Davidson BL, Comp PC, et al. Oral thrombin inhibitor dabigatran etexilate vs North American enoxaparin regimen for prevention of

venous thromboembolism after knee arthroplasty surgery. J Arthroplasty 2009;24:1—9.

41. Schulman S, Kearon C, Kakkar AK, et al. Dabigatran versus warfarin in the treatment of acute venous thromboembolism. N Engl J Med 2009;361: 2342—52.

42. Schulman S, Wahlander K, Lundstrom T, et al. Secondary prevention of venous thromboembolism with the oral direct thrombin inhibitor ximelagatran. N Engl J Med 2003;349:1713—21.

43. Roehrig S, Straub A, Pohlmann J, et al. Discovery of the novel antithrombotic agent 5-chloro-N-({(5S)-2-oxo-3- [4-(3-oxomorpholin-4-yl)phenyl]-1,3-oxazolidin-5-yl}methyl)thiophene- 2-carboxamide (BAY 59-7939): an oral, direct factor Xa inhibitor. J Med Chem 2005;48:5900—8.

44. Perzborn E, Strassburger J, Wilmen A, et al. In vitro and in vivo studies of the novel antithrombotic agent BAY 59-7939—an oral, direct Factor Xa inhibitor. J Thromb Haemost 2005;3:514—21.

45. Mueck W, Borris LC, Dahl OE, et al. Population pharmacokinetics and pharmacodynamics of once- and twice-daily rivaroxaban for the prevention of venous thromboembolism in patients undergoing total hip replacement. Thromb Haemost 2008;100:453—61.

46. Mueck W, Eriksson BI, Bauer KA, et al. Population pharmacokinetics and pharmacodynamics of rivaroxaban—an oral, direct factor Xa inhibitor—in patients undergoing major orthopaedic surgery. Clin Pharmacokinet 2008;47:203—16.

47. Eriksson BI, Borris LC, Friedman RJ, et al. Rivaroxaban versus enoxaparin for thromboprophylaxis after hip arthroplasty. N Engl J Med 2008;358:2765—75.

48. Kakkar AK, Brenner B, Dahl OE, et al. Extended duration rivaroxaban versus short-term enoxaparin for the prevention of venous thromboembolism after total hip arthroplasty: a double-blind, randomised controlled trial. Lancet 2008;372:31—9.

49. Lassen MR, Ageno W, Borris LC, et al. Rivaroxaban versus enoxaparin for thromboprophylaxis after total knee arthroplasty. N Engl J Med 2008;358:2776—86.

50. Agnelli G, Gallus A, Goldhaber SZ, et al. Treatment of proximal deep-vein thrombosis with the oral direct factor Xa inhibitor rivaroxaban (BAY 59-7939): the ODIXa-DVT (Oral Direct Factor Xa Inhibitor BAY 59-7939 in Patients With Acute Symptomatic Deep-Vein Thrombosis) study. Circulation 2007;116:180—7.

51. Buller HR, Lensing AW, Prins MH, et al. A dose-ranging study evaluating once-daily oral administration of the factor Xa inhibitor rivaroxaban in the treatment of patients with acute symptomatic deep vein thrombosis: the Einstein-DVT Dose-Ranging Study. Blood 2008;112:2242—7.

52. Pinto DJ, Orwat MJ, Koch S, et al. Discovery of 1-(4-methoxyphenyl)-7-oxo-6-(4-(2-oxopiperidin-1-yl) phenyl)-4,5,6,7-tetrah ydro-1H-pyrazolo[3,4-c]pyridine-3-carboxamide (apixaban, BMS-562247), a highly potent, selective, efficacious, and orally bioavailable inhibitor of blood coagulation factor Xa. J Med Chem 2007;50:5339—56.

53. Raghavan N, Frost CE, Yu Z, et al. Apixaban metabolism and pharmacokinetics after oral administration to humans. Drug Metab Dispos 2009;37:74—81.

54. Lassen MR, Raskob GE, Gallus A, et al. Apixaban or enoxaparin for thromboprophylaxis after knee replacement. N Engl J Med 2009;361:594—604.

55. Buller H, Deitchman D, Prins M, et al. Efficacy and safety of the oral direct factor Xa inhibitor apixaban for symptomatic deep vein thrombosis. The Botticelli DVT dose-ranging study. J Thromb Haemost 2008;6: 1313—8.

56. Zhang P, Huang W, Wang L, et al. Discovery of betrixaban (PRT054021), N-(5-chloropyridin-2-yl)-2-(4-(N, N-dimethylcarbamimidoyl)benzamido)-5-meth oxybenzamide, a highly potent, selective, and orally efficacious factor Xa inhibitor. Bioorg Med Chem Lett 2009;19:2179—85.

57. Turpie AG, Bauer KA, Davidson BL, et al. A randomized evaluation of betrixaban, an oral factor Xa inhibitor, for prevention of thromboembolic events after total knee replacement (EXPERT). Thromb Haemost 2009;101:68—76.

Long-term Anticoagulation for Venous Thromboembolism: Duration of Treatment and Management of Warfarin Therapy

Clive Kearon, MB, MRCPI, FRCPC, PhD*

KEYWORDS

- Venous thromboembolism • Deep vein thrombosis
- Pulmonary embolism • Treatment • Warfarin
- Duration of therapy

Long-term anticoagulation for venous thromboembolism (VTE) refers to treatment that is continued after initial therapy, such as with heparin or thrombolytic agents, has been completed. Long-term treatment of VTE is usually with a vitamin K antagonist, which is almost always warfarin in North America, and less commonly with a low-molecular-weight heparin (mostly patients with active cancer). Long-term therapy has 2 goals that overlap in timing: (1) to complete treatment of the acute episode of VTE (first 3 months of therapy), and (2) to prevent new episodes of VTE that are not directly related to the acute event (after the first 3 months of therapy). This article focuses primarily on how long patients with VTE should be treated, and also considers how long-term warfarin therapy should be managed.

DURATION OF ANTICOAGULANT THERAPY

Anticoagulant therapy for VTE should be continued until: (1) its benefits (reduction of recurrent VTE) no longer clearly outweigh its risks (increase in bleeding), or (2) it is the patient's preference to stop treatment even if continuing treatment is expected to be of net benefit (eg, because of inconvenience, cost, or other personal dislike of being on warfarin). Therefore, in patients who are not at high risk for bleeding while on anticoagulant therapy, the decision to stop or continue therapy is dominated by the risk of recurrent VTE if treatment is stopped. Current evidence suggests that the risk of recurrence after stopping therapy is largely determined by 2 categories of factors: (1) whether the acute episode of VTE has been effectively treated, and (2) the patient's intrinsic risk of having a new episode of VTE (ie, not arising directly from the episode of thrombosis for which patients have been receiving treatment). If therapy is stopped before the acute episode of thrombosis is adequately treated, the risk of recurrent VTE is higher than if treatment was stopped after a longer course of anticoagulation. If patients still have a persistently high intrinsic risk for thrombosis after

Dr Kearon is a Career Investigator of the Heart and Stroke Foundation of Ontario and is supported by a Canadian Institutes of Health Research Team Grant in Venous Thromboembolism (FRN 79846).
Conflict of Interest: Dr Kearon is an advisor to Boehringer Ingelheim.
McMaster University, Hamilton, ON, Canada

* Henderson Division, Hamilton Health Sciences, Henderson General Hospital, 711 Concession Street, Hamilton, ON L8V 1C3, Canada.
E-mail address: kearonc@mcmaster.ca

Clin Chest Med 31 (2010) 719–730
doi:10.1016/j.ccm.2010.06.003

the acute episode of thrombosis has been effectively treated, indefinite therapy is likely to be indicated.

This article discusses risk factors for recurrence in individual patients and reviews studies that have compared different durations of vitamin K antagonist therapy in patients with VTE. Presence of the most important of these factors has also influenced the patients who have been enrolled in many of the trials that have compared 2 durations of therapy.

Patient-related Risk Factors for Recurrent VTE After Stopping Anticoagulant Therapy

Cancer

Cancer is associated with about a 3-fold increased risk of recurrent VTE both during[1-5] and after[4,6-8] anticoagulant therapy, and, among patients with cancer, the risk of recurrence is about 3-fold higher in those with metastatic disease.[5] The risk of recurrent VTE after stopping anticoagulant therapy is expected to be high (ie, 10%–20% in the first year) in patients with cancer, particularly if there is progressive or metastatic disease, poor mobility, or ongoing chemotherapy.[7-9] The risk of recurrence is uncertain, but is likely to be lower if the cancer has responded to therapy, or if the initial VTE was provoked by an additional reversible risk factor, such as surgery or chemotherapy (see later discussion). Because cancer is considered a strong risk factor for recurrent VTE, there is widespread agreement that most patients with VTE and active cancer require long-term anticoagulant therapy, and these patients have generally been excluded from the randomized trials that have compared different durations of anticoagulant therapy.[10]

Reversible provoking risk factor or unprovoked

Patients with VTE provoked by a major reversible risk factor, such as surgery, have a low risk of recurrence (about 2% in the first year and 6% in the first 5 years) if they stop treatment having completed 3 or more months of therapy, whereas this risk is high (about 10% in the first year and 30% in the first 5 years) in patients with an unprovoked VTE (also termed idiopathic; including those with and without nonmalignant chronic medical conditions).[8,9,11-17] If VTE was provoked by a minor reversible risk factor, such as leg trauma, estrogen therapy, or prolonged air travel (eg, a flight of more than 8 hours), there is an intermediate risk of recurrent VTE after stopping anticoagulant therapy (about 5% in the first year and 15% in the first 5 years).[7,16,18,19] Because patients with unprovoked VTE have a high risk of recurrence, such patients have often selectively been enrolled in studies that have compared longer durations of therapy for VTE.[17,20-25]

Isolated calf deep vein thrombosis versus proximal deep vein thrombosis

Patients with deep vein thrombosis (DVT) that is confined to the distal veins (often called isolated calf DVT) have about half the risk of recurrence as patients who have DVT that involves the proximal veins (ie, popliteal or more proximal veins).[13,15,26]

Second versus first episode of VTE

After a second or subsequent episode of VTE, the risk of recurrence seems to be about 1.5-fold higher than after a first episode.[17,27,28] If the second episode of VTE occurred soon after anticoagulant therapy was stopped (eg, within 1 or 2 years), this may suggest a higher subsequent risk of recurrence than if the 2 episodes were separated by many years.

Pulmonary embolism versus DVT

Patients who present with pulmonary embolism (PE) seem to have the same risk of recurrent VTE as those who present with proximal DVT.[7,13,27,29,30] However, after a PE, about 60% of recurrent episodes of VTE are also PE, whereas only about 20% of recurrent episodes of VTE are a PE after an initial DVT.[21,22,27,29,31,32] This pattern of recurrence, with about a 3-fold higher risk of PE after an initial PE than after an initial DVT, seems to persist long term.[27,31,32] About 10% of symptomatic PE are believed to be rapidly fatal,[33-35] and another 5% of patients whose PE is diagnosed and treated also die from PE.[27,31,36-39] Thus, after 3 or more months of treatment of DVT or PE, recurrent VTE that presents as PE probably has a case fatality of about 15%. The risk of dying from acute DVT, because of early PE or other complications (eg, bleeding, precipitation of myocardial infarction), seems to be 2% or less.[6,27,31-40] Based on these estimates, the case fatality associated with late recurrent VTE after a preceding PE is expected to be about 10%, whereas after a preceding DVT case fatality is expected to be about 5%. Consistent with the latter estimate, an overview of randomized trials calculated a 5.1% case fatality for recurrent VTE in patients with DVT who had completed 3 months of treatment.[29] Therefore, although the risk of a recurrence is the same after PE and proximal DVT, the case fatality for a recurrence is expected to be 2-fold higher after PE than after DVT.

Sex

Meta-analysis has estimated that the risk of recurrent VTE is higher in men than in women (relative risk 1.6, 95% confidence interval [CI] 1.2–2.0).[41] This difference seemed to be greater in cohort studies (relative risk 2.1, 95% CI 1.5–2.9) than in randomized trials (relative risk 1.3, 95% CI 1.0–1.8) A recent family study concluded that the lower risk of recurrence in women could be accounted for by many episodes of VTE in women being associated with estrogen therapy or pregnancy (reversible risk factors).[42] It is possible that this effect (ie, confounding between sex and presence of a reversible risk factor) may contribute to the overall lower risk of recurrence that has been reported in women, although this effect could not be detected in the previously noted meta-analysis.[41]

Hereditary thrombophilias

A recent meta-analysis estimated that the risk of recurrent VTE (odds ratio) with associated factor V Leiden was 1.6 (95% CI 1.1–2.1) when heterozygous (1.2, 95% CI 0.6–2.2, in the subset with unprovoked VTE), and 2.7 (95% CI 1.2–6.0) when homozygous, and for heterozygous prothrombin G20210A was 1.2 (95% CI 0.9–1.7).[43] In 5 large prospective studies that included a total of 2691 patients with a first episode of VTE (provoked and unprovoked), and of whom 117 (4.3%) had homozygous factor V Leiden, homozygous prothrombin gene G20210A, double heterozygous states for these 2 mutations, or deficiency of protein C, protein S, or antithrombin, the overall odds ratio for recurrent VTE associated with these major thrombophilias was 1.5 (95% CI 0.9–2.4).[16,44–47] Consequently, because thrombophilia does not appear to be a clinically important risk factor for recurrence, testing for thrombophilia has no clear role in guiding duration of treatment.

Antiphospholipid antibodies

Schulman and colleagues[48] found that an anticardiolipin antibody was associated with recurrent VTE in the first 4 years after a first VTE, but was no longer predictive of recurrence at the end of 10 years.[32] Kearon and colleagues[20] found that an anticardiolipin antibody or lupus anticoagulant was associated with recurrent VTE after an unprovoked VTE (hazard ratio 4.0, 95% CI 1.2–13), but not after a provoked VTE (hazard ratio 1.3, 95% CI 0.2–11).[49] Rodger and colleagues[30] found that an anticardiolipin antibody or lupus anticoagulant was not associated with recurrence in all patients after an unprovoked VTE (relative risk 1.1, 95% CI 0.7–1.7), but that the association did seem to be present in men (relative risk 1.8, 95% CI 1.1–3.0).

Residual DVT

An association between the presence of residual DVT on ultrasound and risk of recurrent VTE has been reported.[4,50–52] However, several other studies have not found that residual DVT is an independent predictor of recurrence,[20,22,30,49,53] and why residual DVT should be associated with recurrent DVT in the contralateral leg is unexplained.[50]

D-dimer level after withdrawal of treatment

A normal D-dimer level after a prolonged period of anticoagulant therapy, while still on treatment[30] but particularly about 1 month after withdrawal of warfarin,[19,24,44,54–60] has been shown to be associated with a substantially reduced risk of recurrent VTE (rate ratio [RR] by meta-analysis 0.5, 95% CI 0.3–0.6).[59]

Vena caval filter

In patients who have a vena caval filter inserted and then receive standard anticoagulant therapy there is a trend to a higher risk of a new episode of DVT (RR 1.3; 95% CI 0.9–1.8), a lower risk of PE (RR 0.4; 95% CI 0.2–0.9), and no difference in the risk of VTE (DVT and/or PE; RR 1.0, 95% CI 0.7–1.4) after 8 years of follow-up.[61,62] Consequently, insertion of a vena caval filter does not influence duration of anticoagulation.

Other markers for recurrence

Factor VIII,[47,56,63,64] factor IX,[47] factor XI,[47,65] homocysteine,[47,66,67] thrombin generation,[68–70] the activated partial thromboplastin time,[71] family history of VTE,[72] and age at diagnosis[7,27] have been evaluated, but the evidence that they are clinically important risk factors for recurrent VTE is generally weak.

Comparison of Different Durations of Anticoagulation for the Treatment of VTE and the Influence of Duration of Therapy on Risk of Recurrence

Randomized trials that have compared durations of anticoagulation for the treatment of VTE (patients with cancer-associated VTE were generally not included in these studies) can be divided into those that compared 2 time-limited (or finite) durations, and those that compared indefinite therapy (no scheduled time for treatment to be stopped) with a finite duration of therapy.

Different time-limited durations of therapy for VTE

Studies performed more than a decade ago established that shortening the duration of anticoagulation from 3[11,12] or 6[13] months to 4[11,12] or 6[13] weeks results in a doubling of the frequency of recurrent

VTE during follow-up of 1 to 2 years in most patients with VTE, and particularly those with unprovoked VTE. Whether extending the duration of treatment beyond 3 months reduces the risk of recurrence if anticoagulant therapy is then stopped has been less clear. This question is of greatest importance for patients with unprovoked VTE who have not been selected for indefinite anticoagulant therapy (see later discussion).

Four studies compared 3 months with either 6 or 12 months of anticoagulant therapy specifically in patients with unprovoked VTE,[21,22] or in patients with either unprovoked VTE or VTE provoked by a temporary risk factor.[15,73] All 4 studies found that the risk of recurrent VTE was very low while patients were receiving anticoagulant therapy, but increased markedly once treatment was stopped. The risk of recurrence during the total period of follow-up (during and after stopping therapy) was no lower (ie, was the same) in patients who stopped anticoagulants at 6 or 12 months compared with those who stopped treatment at 3 months (relative risk for recurrence 0.95, 95% CI 0.72–1.26).[10] These studies therefore suggest that (1) 3 months of anticoagulant therapy effectively treats the acute episode of VTE and reduces the risk of recurrent VTE to as low a value as can be achieved by a time-limited duration of therapy, and (2) treatment beyond 3 months prevents new episodes of VTE that are not directly related to the preceding episode.

The associated implications of these findings are that most patients with VTE, and most relevantly those with unprovoked proximal DVT or PE, should receive 3 months of anticoagulation to treat the acute event, and then a decision should be made to either stop treatment or to continue it indefinitely, with the option of subsequently stopping treatment if the patient's risk of bleeding becomes excessive (ie, the patient acquires risk factors for bleeding), or if the patient decides that the burden of anticoagulant therapy has become unacceptable.[10] After 3 months of treatment, if a patient's symptoms are continuing to improve, or the patient's preferences about indefinite therapy are uncertain, it is reasonable to defer the decision about indefinite therapy for some months (eg, until after 6 months of treatment).

Indefinite versus time-limited anticoagulant therapy for idiopathic VTE

Five randomized trials have evaluated long-term or indefinite warfarin therapy in patients with VTE.[17,20,23,24,54] Indefinite therapy was targeted to a standard intensity of anticoagulation (ie, international normalized ratio [INR] ~2.5) in

4 studies,[20,23,24,74] and to a low intensity in 2 studies.[17,23] Four studies compared indefinite therapy with a finite (short) course of warfarin,[17,20,24,74] and 1 study compared standard-intensity with low-intensity anticoagulation.[23]

In 3 trials, indefinite therapy was compared with stopping therapy in patients with unprovoked VTE who have completed at least 3 months of initial treatment.[17,20,24,54] The LAFIT study[20] enrolled patients with a first episode of proximal DVT or PE (patients with isolated distal DVT were not eligible), the PREVENT study[17] enrolled patients with 1 (62%) or more (38%) episodes of VTE and included those with isolated distal DVT (proportion unknown), and the PROLONG study[24,54] enrolled patients with a first episode of proximal DVT or PE who had a positive D-dimer result 1 month after stopping anticoagulant therapy. Long-term anticoagulant therapy was targeted to an INR of 2.5 (range INR 2.0–3.0) in the LAFIT and PROLONG studies, and was targeted to an INR of 1.75 (range INR 1.5–2.0) in PREVENT. The findings of the 3 studies were consistent and persuasive.[17,20,24] Allocation to long-term, standard-intensity anticoagulation reduced recurrent VTE by about 90% (intention-to-treat analysis) and, in those who remained on anticoagulant therapy (inclusive of times when anticoagulation was subtherapeutic), the reduction in recurrence was closer to 95%.[20,24] Recurrence rates in patients who stopped anticoagulant therapy were high and consistent with the previously noted estimates of 10% at 1 year, and 30% at 5 years, for patients with unprovoked proximal DVT or PE. Long-term anticoagulant therapy was associated with about a doubling of the frequency of major bleeding, with an absolute rate of major bleeding of 1% to 2% per year.[17,20,24,54,75] The overall benefit associated with long-term anticoagulant therapy resulted in the 2 studies that performed interim analyses being stopped early.[17,20]

The DURAC 2 study showed that, in patients with a second episode of VTE (not exclusively unprovoked events), consistent with the 3 previously noted studies, indefinite standard-intensity therapy reduced the risk of recurrence by more than 90% compared with just treating patients for 6 months.[74] The ELATE study, which randomized patients with 1 or more episodes of unprovoked VTE to indefinite therapy with either a target INR of 1.75 or INR 2.5, showed that standard-intensity therapy reduced the risk of recurrence by two-thirds compared with low-intensity therapy, and that the rate of major bleeding was low, and similar at about 1% per patient-year in the 2 groups.[23] The rates of recurrence with low-intensity therapy were similar in the PREVENT and ELATE studies, consistent with a risk reduction of about 75% compared with control. In combination, the results of these 5 studies also suggest that indefinite standard-intensity therapy in these settings (patient populations with a high risk for recurrence) reduces the composite (combined) outcome of recurrent VTE and major bleeding, and all-cause mortality.[10,76]

In addition to these 5 studies, a single-center study compared 6 and 24 months of warfarin therapy in a total of 64 patients with unprovoked proximal DVT or PE.[25] Although the small sample size precluded definitive comparisons, the longer duration of therapy also appeared to be of benefit in this study.[25]

Patient Preference and Indefinite Anticoagulant Therapy

When deciding to either stop anticoagulants (eg, after 3 months of therapy) or to continue treatment indefinitely, patient preferences must be considered because the burden associated with anticoagulant therapy differs markedly among individuals. For example, although anticoagulant therapy has been reported to be associated with a median utility of 0.92 (where 0 is equivalent to death and 1.0 is equivalent to perfect health), this utility was 0.77 or lower for a quarter of patients, and was 0.98 or higher for another quarter of patients (ie, rated as better than not being on anticoagulant therapy, which had a median utility of 0.96).[77] Consistent with these large differences in patients' perceptions, irrespective of whether the risk of recurrent VTE was assumed to be high or low, 25% of patients always wanted to stop treatment and another 23% of patients always wanted to stay on treatment in this study.[77]

Risk of Bleeding During Long-term Warfarin Therapy

If anticoagulant therapy is expected to be associated with a marked and unavoidable risk of bleeding in individual patients (ie, risk of bleeding that cannot be reduced), extended therapy may not be indicated despite a high risk for recurrence. In this assessment, it is the absolute increase in the risk of major bleeding (ie, expressed as percent per patient-years) that is most relevant. Of factors that have been evaluated as risk factors for major bleeding during anticoagulant therapy, the following seem to have the greatest potential to be clinically useful markers of increased risk: older age, particularly after 75 years; previous gastrointestinal bleeding, particularly if not associated with a reversible cause; previous noncardioembolic stroke;

chronic renal or hepatic insufficiency; active cancer, particularly if metastatic; concomitant antiplatelet therapy (which can usually be avoided) or thrombocytopenia; other serious acute or chronic illness; history of recurrent falls that cause trauma (eg, marked bruising); and poor control of anticoagulant therapy (eg, necessitating frequent INR testing or associated with frequent results of INR >5.0).[23,78–84] Several studies have reported clinical prediction rules designed to stratify the risk of bleeding during anticoagulant therapy in individual patients.[80,81,84–86] Other than checking that patients would have been eligible for the trials that established a role for long-term therapy, there is currently no validated way to estimate and balance an individual's increase in risk of bleeding on anticoagulant therapy with their increase in risk of recurrence if anticoagulant therapy is stopped, so that patients who should benefit from long-term therapy can be selected. To add to the complexity, risk factors for bleeding may also be risk factors for recurrence. For example, in the ELATE study, which compared low-with standard-intensity anticoagulant therapy, patients with risk factors for bleeding at enrollment had a higher risk of recurrence during follow-up, and risk factors for bleeding appeared to increase rather than decrease the benefits of standard-intensity compared with low-intensity therapy.[23] In patients with good anticoagulant control who do not have risk factors for bleeding (eg, unprovoked VTE), reasonable estimates are that the annual risk of major bleeding after the first 3 months of treatment is expected to be about 1% (increase of ˜0.6%) per year in those less than 65 years old, and about 2% (increase of ~1.2%) per year in those 65 to 75 years old.[10,75,87] However, because the risk of bleeding increases substantially after 75 years of age,[78,84,86] and because there is no convincing evidence that advanced age increases the risk of recurrent VTE, advanced age (eg, >75 years) is a relative contraindication to indefinite anticoagulation for the treatment of VTE.

Recommended Duration of Anticoagulation in Individual Patients

Based largely on the preceding analysis of risk factors for recurrent thrombosis and bleeding, and on the findings of studies that compared different durations and intensities of anticoagulation, an approach to selecting duration of anticoagulation for individual patients with VTE is outlined in **Table 1**. Because the presence of a reversible risk factor for VTE, lack of a provoking factor, or

Table 1
Recommendations for duration of anticoagulant therapy for VTE

Risk Factor for VTE	Durations of Treatment (Target INR 2.5, Range 2.0–3.0)
Transient risk factor[a]	3 mo
Unprovoked If also: isolated distal DVT; or a first proximal DVT or PE and a moderate or higher risk of bleeding[d]; or an informed patient's preference is to stop therapy	Indefinite[b] 3 mo
Active malignancy If also: a very high risk of bleeding[d]; isolated distal DVT; or an additional major transient risk factor for VTE[a]	Indefinite[c] Consider stopping therapy at 3 mo or when cancer becomes inactive

[a] Transient risk factors include major factors, such as surgery with general anesthesia, plaster cast immobilization of a leg, or hospitalization, all within the past month, and minor factors, such as estrogen therapy, pregnancy, prolonged travel (eg, longer than 8 hours), less-marked leg injury, or the previously noted major factors when they occur 1 to 3 months before diagnosis of VTE.
[b] Decision should be reviewed annually to consider whether the patient's risk of bleeding has increased, or whether patient preference had changed. Additional factors favoring indefinite therapy include more than 1 episode of unprovoked VTE; PE versus proximal DVT at presentation; male sex; positive D-dimer test during, or 1 month after, stopping anticoagulant therapy.
[c] Preferably with low-molecular-weight heparin for at least the first 3 months.
[d] Risk factors for bleeding include age 65 years or older, particularly after 75 years; previous noncardioembolic stoke; previous bleeding (eg, gastrointestinal), particularly if there was not a reversible cause; active peptic ulcer disease; renal impairment; anemia; thrombocytopenia; liver disease; diabetes mellitus; use of antiplatelet therapy (to be avoided) or thrombocytopenia; poor patient compliance; poor control of anticoagulation; structural lesion (including tumor) expected to be associated with bleeding; or recurrent falls. One or 2 risk factors suggests moderate risk of bleeding, and 3 or more risk factors suggests high risk.

cancer, at the time of thrombosis has the greatest prognostic influence on the risk of recurrence, this assessment carries most weight.

VTE associated with a reversible risk factor
For patients whose VTE is associated with a major reversible risk factor, such as recent surgery, stopping anticoagulant therapy after 3 months of treatment is expected to be associated with a subsequent risk of recurrent VTE of about 3% in the first year and about 10% in 5 years.[6,8,11,12,14,15,17,22,28] For patients whose VTE is associated with a minor reversible risk factor, such as a soft tissue injury to the leg, a prolonged flight, or estrogen therapy, stopping anticoagulant therapy after 3 months of treatment is expected to be associated with a subsequent risk of recurrent VTE of about 5% in the first year and about 15% in 5 years.[16,19,88] These rates of VTE are not high enough to justify treatment for longer than 3 months.

Unprovoked VTE
For patients with unprovoked proximal DVT or PE, stopping anticoagulant therapy after 3 or more months of treatment is expected to be associated with a subsequent risk of recurrent VTE of about 10% in the first year and about 30% in 5 years.[8,13,15,21] This rate is high enough, and the benefits of long-term anticoagulant therapy are sufficiently established by randomized trials in this group,[17,20,24] to justify long-term anticoagulation in most such patients. Although there is evidence that that female sex,[41] normal D-dimer levels 1 month after stopping therapy,[19,57,59] absence of residual DVT on ultrasound,[50,51] and absence of the postthrombotic syndrome[30] identify patients with unprovoked proximal DVT or PE who have a lower than average risk of recurrence, in the opinion of this author, no factor (or combination of factors[30]) is currently well enough validated as a negative predictor to justify routinely stopping anticoagulant therapy at the end of 3 months of treatment in such patients. However, the risk of recurrence is about half in patients with distal DVT compared with those with proximal DVT or PE,[13,15,26] so 3 months of anticoagulation is recommended for unprovoked isolated distal DVT.[10] If anticoagulant therapy is expected to be associated with a high risk of bleeding because of risk factors for bleeding or lack of access to

Box 1
Principles and recommendations for maintenance warfarin therapy

Interval between INR measurements

- Gradually increase interval from every 2 to 3 days in the first week to every 2 to 4 weeks (eg, after 6 weeks).[89]
- Decrease interval between testing if the patient becomes ill or if a medication is added or stopped.[89,92]
- Decrease interval if INR results become unstable.

Dosing of warfarin

- Average daily warfarin dose is about 6 mg at age 50 years and about 3.5 mg at age 80 years.[93]
- If warfarin maintenance dose needs to be increased or decreased, steps of 10% are usually suitable. This change can be made by calculating the total dose of warfarin given in the preceding week and adjusting the total dose for the next week(s) by 10%; this often translates into a change in the total week's dose of 2.5 to 5.0 mg of warfarin.[89]
- If INR is more than 5.0, 1 or 2 doses of warfarin should be withheld in addition to reducing the maintenance warfarin dose. If INR is more than 5.0 and the patient has risk factors of bleeding, or INR is more than 10.0, 1 to 2.5 mg of oral vitamin K should also be given.[89,90,94–96]

Delivery of anticoagulant monitoring

- A systematic process for monitoring warfarin therapy should be used that includes patient education and explicit patient and health care provider responsibility for each stage of the process (eg, patient attends a designated laboratory for INR testing, INR results are communicated to health care providers at pre-specified time [eg, same or following day], INR results are recorded in the patient's anticoagulation record, warfarin dose is selected, warfarin dose and timing of next INR measurement are communicated to the patient).[89,91]
- If anticoagulant response has become unstable, look for and try to correct why this has occurred (eg, erratic diet and vitamin k intake, new or intermittent medications, confusion about dosing, comorbid illness, poor compliance). Consider obtaining help from family members (eg, receiving dosage instructions) or the patient's pharmacy (eg, warfarin doses added to a daily dosing box or to blister packs).
- If unstable anticoagulant response persists, and particularly if daily warfarin dose is small or the patient's diet is erratic, a small supplemental dose of vitamin K (eg, 80 to 200 μg daily) can be tried. This may make fluctuations in dietary vitamin K less marked.[89,97,98]
- Assessment of risk factors for bleeding should be ongoing so that avoidable factors can be corrected (eg, inappropriate antiplatelet therapy), and anticoagulants can be stopped if the associated risks start to exceed the benefits.
- Self-testing, or self-dosing, is appropriate in selected well-educated and motivated patients.[89,99]
- Computer programs can facilitate selection of warfarin dose, tracking of INR and warfarin dosing, and communication of warfarin dosing to patients (eg, via mail).[89,100]

Interruption of warfarin for invasive procedures

- After 1 month, and particularly after 3 months, of anticoagulant therapy for VTE, short interruptions of warfarin (eg, 5 days) are well tolerated (ie, associated with a low risk of recurrence) provided patients have not undergone a procedure that is associated with VTE (eg, surgery).[101,102]
- Patients who have had a procedure that is associated with VTE (eg, surgery with general anesthetic) should receive supplemental VTE prophylaxis (eg, a heparin preparation) after the event until their INR increases, or is expected to have increased (eg, ~3 days), to an INR of more than 1.5.[101,102]
- If supplemental VTE prophylaxis is indicated, dosing of the heparin preparation depends on factors such as risk of bleeding after the surgical procedure, how long patients have already been treated, interval before warfarin can be restarted, and how quickly the INR rises in response to warfarin. In general, heparin should be started at a dose that is recommended for VTE prophylaxis in high-risk patients (eg, ~5000 units of low-molecular-weight heparin in 24 hours); if this dose is increased, this should not occur until ongoing hemostasis is confirmed (eg, postoperative day 2); dose can be increased in several steps (eg, initially increase to ~5000 units of low-molecular-weight heparin twice daily, for an average-weight person), rather than from prophylactic to full-therapeutic doses.
- During long-term phase of therapy, interruptions of warfarin rarely require insertion of a filter into the inferior vena cava.

appropriate anticoagulant monitoring, patients with a first unprovoked proximal DVT or PE should only be treated for 3 months. Patients who find anticoagulant therapy a substantial burden may also decide against indefinite therapy.

Cancer-associated VTE

Patients with active cancer generally should remain on long-term anticoagulant therapy (preferably low-molecular-weight heparin for at least the initial 3 months) because the risk of recurrent VTE is expected to be higher than 10% within a year of stopping treatment.[10]

LONG-TERM MONITORING AND ADJUSTMENT OF WARFARIN

Many factors modify the anticoagulant response to warfarin therapy and, therefore, there are marked differences in the dose of warfarin required to achieve an INR of 2.0 to 3.0, both among patients and in the same patient over time.[89,90] Consequently, warfarin dosing needs to be adjusted in response to ongoing INR measurements to maximize the proportion of time that patients are in the target INR range. Good anticoagulant control is important because (1) subtherapeutic anticoagulation (particularly INR <1.5) increases recurrent VTE, (2) supratherapeutic anticoagulation (particularly INR >5.0) increases bleeding, and (3) poor anticoagulant control increases the burden of anticoagulant therapy and discourages patients and health care providers from continuing warfarin therapy when it is indicated.[89,91] Principals and management strategies that facilitate optimal long-term anticoagulation are summarized in **Box 1**. Achieving optimal control of warfarin therapy requires commitment from patients and health care providers; access to dedicated anticoagulant clinics can greatly facilitate this process.[89,91]

SUMMARY

The duration of therapy should be individualized based on the increased risk of recurrent VTE if treatment is stopped and the increased risk of bleeding if treatment is continued. The risk of recurrence is low if thrombosis was provoked by a reversible risk factor such as surgery (ie, 3% within 1 year, and 10% within 5 years, of stopping therapy); 3 months of treatment is usually adequate for such patients. The risk of recurrence is high if thrombosis was associated with active cancer, particularly if it is metastatic and being treated with chemotherapy (ie, 20% within 1 year of stopping therapy); indefinite anticoagulant therapy, with low-molecular-weight heparin for at least the first 3 months, is often indicated for such patients. Risk of recurrence is intermediate if thrombosis was an unprovoked proximal DVT or PE (ie, 10% within 1 year, and 30% within 5 years, of stopping therapy); indefinite anticoagulant therapy is often

appropriate for such patients. High risk of bleeding, and patient dislike of being on anticoagulants, favors treating for only 3 months. New anticoagulants may improve the risk/benefit ratio of anticoagulant therapy and should reduce the burden of therapy.

REFERENCES

1. Hutten BA, Prins M, Gent M, et al. Incidence of recurrent thromboembolic and bleeding complications among patients with venous thromboembolism in relation to both malignancy and achieved international normalized ratio: a retrospective analysis. J Clin Oncol 2000;18:3078–83.
2. Merli G, Spiro TE, Olsson CG, et al. Subcutaneous enoxaparin once or twice daily compared with intravenous unfractionated heparin for treatment of venous thromboembolic disease. Ann Intern Med 2001;134:191–202.
3. Palareti G, Legnani C, Lee A, et al. A comparison of the safety and efficacy of oral anticoagulation for the treatment of venous thromboembolic disease in patients with or without malignancy. Thromb Haemost 2000;84:805–10.
4. Piovella F, Crippa L, Barone M, et al. Normalization rates of compression ultrasonography in patients with a first episode of deep vein thrombosis of the lower limbs: association with recurrence and new thrombosis. Haematologica 2002;87:515–22.
5. Prandoni P, Lensing AW, Piccioli A, et al. Recurrent venous thromboembolism and bleeding complications during anticoagulant treatment in patients with cancer and venous thrombosis. Blood 2002; 100:3484–8.
6. Prandoni P, Lensing AW, Cogo A, et al. The long-term clinical course of acute deep venous thrombosis. Ann Intern Med 1996;125:1–7.
7. Heit JA, Mohr DN, Silverstein MD, et al. Predictors of recurrence after deep vein thrombosis and pulmonary embolism: a population-based cohort study. Arch Intern Med 2000;160:761–8.
8. Palareti G, Legnani C, Cosmi B, et al. Risk of venous thromboembolism recurrence: high negative predictive value of D-dimer performed after oral anticoagulation is stopped. Thromb Haemost 2002;87:7–12.
9. Prandoni P, Lensing AW, Buller HR, et al. Deep-vein thrombosis and the incidence of subsequent symptomatic cancer. N Engl J Med 1992;327: 1128–33.
10. Kearon C, Kahn SR, Agnelli G, et al. Antithrombotic therapy for venous thromboembolic disease. American College of Chest Physicians evidence-based clinical practice guidelines (8th edition). Chest 2008;133:454S–545S.

11. Research Committee of the British Thoracic Society. Optimum duration of anticoagulation for deep-vein thrombosis and pulmonary embolism. Lancet 1992;340:873—6.

12. Levine MN, Hirsh J, Gent M, et al. Optimal duration of oral anticoagulant therapy: a randomized trial comparing four weeks with three months of warfarin in patients with proximal deep vein thrombosis. Thromb Haemost 1995;74:606—11.

13. Schulman S, Rhedin A-S, Lindmarker P, et al. A comparison of six weeks with six months of oral anticoagulant therapy after a first episode of venous thromboembolism. N Engl J Med 1995; 332:1661—5.

14. Pini M, Aiello S, Manotti C, et al. Low molecular weight heparin versus warfarin in the prevention of recurrences after deep vein thrombosis. Thromb Haemost 1994;72(2):191—7.

15. Pinede L, Ninet J, Duhaut P, et al. Comparison of 3 and 6 months of oral anticoagulant therapy after a first episode of proximal deep vein thrombosis or pulmonary embolism and comparison of 6 and 12 weeks of therapy after isolated calf deep vein thrombosis. Circulation 2001;103:2453—60.

16. Baglin T, Luddington R, Brown K, et al. Incidence of recurrent venous thromboembolism in relation to clinical and thrombophilic risk factors: prospective cohort study. Lancet 2003;362:523—6.

17. Ridker PM, Goldhaber SZ, Danielson E, et al. Long-term, low-intensity warfarin therapy for prevention of recurrent venous thromboembolism. N Engl J Med 2003;348:1425—34.

18. Spiezia L, Bernardi E, Tormene D, et al. Recurrent thromboembolism in fertile women with venous thrombosis: incidence and risk factors. Thromb Haemost 2003;90:964—6.

19. Baglin T, Palmer CR, Luddington R, et al. Unprovoked recurrent venous thrombosis: prediction by D-dimer and clinical risk factors. J Thromb Haemost 2008;6:577—82.

20. Kearon C, Gent M, Hirsh J, et al. A comparison of three months of anticoagulation with extended anticoagulation for a first episode of idiopathic venous thromboembolism. N Engl J Med 1999;340:901—7.

21. Agnelli G, Prandoni P, Santamaria MG, et al. Three months versus one year of oral anticoagulant therapy for idiopathic deep vein thrombosis. N Engl J Med 2001;345:165—9.

22. Agnelli G, Prandoni P, Becattini C, et al. Extended oral anticoagulant therapy after a first episode of pulmonary embolism. Ann Intern Med 2003;139: 19—25.

23. Kearon C, Ginsberg JS, Kovacs MJ, et al. Comparison of low-intensity warfarin therapy with conventional-intensity warfarin therapy for long-term prevention of recurrent venous thromboembolism. N Engl J Med 2003;349:631—9.

24. Palareti G, Cosmi B, Legnani C, et al. D-dimer testing to determine the duration of anticoagulation therapy. N Engl J Med 2006;355:1780—9.

25. Farraj RS. Anticoagulation period in idiopathic venous thromboembolism. How long is enough? Saudi Med J 2004;25:848—51.

26. Hansson PO, Sorbo J, Eriksson H. Recurrent venous thromboembolism after deep vein thrombosis: incidence and risk factors. Arch Intern Med 2000;160:769—74.

27. Murin S, Romano PS, White RH. Comparison of outcomes after hospitalization for deep vein thrombosis or pulmonary embolism. Thromb Haemost 2002;88:407—14.

28. Schulman S, Wahlander K, Lundström T, et al. THRIVE III Investigators. Secondary prevention of venous thromboembolism with the oral direct thrombin inhibitor ximelagatran. N Engl J Med 2003;349:1713—21.

29. Douketis JD, Kearon C, Bates S, et al. Risk of fatal pulmonary embolism in patients with treated venous thromboembolism. JAMA 1998;279: 458—62.

30. Rodger MA, Kahn SR, Wells PS, et al. Identifying unprovoked thromboembolism patients at low risk for recurrence who can discontinue anticoagulant therapy. CMAJ 2008;179:417—26.

31. Kniffin WD Jr, Baron JA, Barrett J, et al. The epidemiology of diagnosed pulmonary embolism and deep venous thrombosis in the elderly. Arch Intern Med 1994;154:861—6.

32. Schulman S, Lindmarker P, Holmstrom M, et al. Post-thrombotic syndrome, recurrence, and death 10 years after the first episode of venous thromboembolism treated with warfarin for 6 weeks or 6 months. J Thromb Haemost 2006;4:734—42.

33. Bell WR, Simon TL. Current status of pulmonary embolic disease: pathophysiology, diagnosis, prevention, and treatment. Am Heart J 1982;103: 239—61.

34. Stein PD, Henry JW. Prevalence of acute pulmonary embolism among patients in a general hospital and at autopsy. Chest 1995;108:978—81.

35. Kearon C. Natural history of venous thromboembolism. Circulation 2003;107:I22—30.

36. Goldhaber SZ, Visni L, De Rosa M. Acute pulmonary embolism: clinical outcomes in the International Cooperative Pulmonary Embolism Registry (ICOPER). Lancet 1999;353:1386—9.

37. Heit JA, Silverstein MD, Mohr DN, et al. Predictors of survival after deep vein thrombosis and pulmonary embolism: a population-based, cohort study. Arch Intern Med 1999;159:445—53.

38. Ribeiro A, Lindmarker P, Juhlin-Dannfelt A, et al. Echocardiography Doppler in pulmonary embolism: right ventricular dysfunction as a predictor of mortality rate. Am Heart J 1997;134:479—87.

39. Naess IA, Christiansen SC, Romundstad P, et al. Incidence and mortality of venous thrombosis: a population-based study. J Thromb Haemost 2007;5:692–9.

40. Beyth RJ, Cohen AM, Landefeld CS. Long-term outcomes of deep-vein thrombosis. Arch Intern Med 1995;155:1031–7.

41. McRae S, Tran H, Schulman S, et al. Effect of patient's sex on risk of recurrent venous thromboembolism: a meta-analysis. Lancet 2006;368: 371–8.

42. Lijfering WM, Veeger NJ, Middeldorp S, et al. A lower risk of recurrent venous thrombosis in women compared with men is explained by sex-specific risk factors at time of first venous thrombosis in thrombophilic families. Blood 2009;114: 2031–6.

43. Segal JB, Brotman DJ, Necochea AJ, et al. Predictive value of factor V Leiden and prothrombin G20210A in adults with venous thromboembolism and in family members of those with a mutation: a systematic review. JAMA 2009;301:2472–85.

44. Palareti G, Legnani C, Cosmi B, et al. Predictive value of D-dimer test for recurrent venous thromboembolism after anticoagulation withdrawal in subjects with a previous idiopathic event and in carriers of congenital thrombophilia. Circulation 2003;108:313–8.

45. Lindmarker P, Schulman S, Sten-Linder M, et al. The risk of recurrent venous thromboembolism in carriers and non-carriers of the G1691A allele in the coagulation factor V gene and the G20210A allele in the prothrombin gene. Thromb Haemost 1999;81:684–9.

46. Eichinger S, Pabinger I, Stumpflen A, et al. The risk of recurrent venous thromboembolism in patients with and without factor V Leiden. Thromb Haemost 1997;77(4):624–8.

47. Christiansen SC, Cannegieter SC, Koster T, et al. Thrombophilia, clinical factors, and recurrent venous thrombotic events. JAMA 2005;293: 2352–61.

48. Schulman S, Svenungsson E, Granqvist S. Anticardiolipin antibodies predict early recurrence of thromboembolism and death among patients with venous thromboembolism following anticoagulant therapy. Am J Med 1998;104:332–8.

49. Kearon C, Ginsberg JS, Anderson DR, et al. Comparison of 1 month with 3 months of anticoagulation for a first episode of venous thromboembolism associated with a transient risk factor. J Thromb Haemost 2004;2:743–9.

50. Prandoni P, Lensing AW, Prins MH, et al. Residual venous thrombosis as a predictive factor of recurrent venous thromboembolism. Ann Intern Med 2002;137:955–60.

51. Siragusa S, Malato A, Anastasio R, et al. Residual vein thrombosis to establish duration of anticoagulation after a first episode of deep vein thrombosis: the Duration of Anticoagulation based on Compression UltraSonography (DACUS) study. Blood 2008;112:511–5.

52. Prandoni P, Prins MH, Lensing AW, et al. Residual thrombosis on ultrasonography to guide the duration of anticoagulation in patients with deep venous thrombosis: a randomized trial. Ann Intern Med 2009;150:577–85.

53. Cosmi B, Legnani C, Cini M, et al. D-dimer levels in combination with residual venous obstruction and the risk of recurrence after anticoagulation withdrawal for a first idiopathic deep vein thrombosis. Thromb Haemost 2005;94:969–74.

54. Cosmi B, Legnani C, Tosetto A, et al. Use of D-dimer testing to determine duration of anticoagulation, risk of cardiovascular events and occult cancer after a first episode of idiopathic venous thromboembolism: the extended follow-up of the PROLONG study. J Thromb Thrombolysis 2009; 28:381–8.

55. Eichinger S, Minar E, Bialonczyk C, et al. D-dimer levels and risk of recurrent venous thromboembolism. JAMA 2003;290:1071–4.

56. Shrivastava S, Ridker PM, Glynn RJ, et al. D-dimer, factor VIII coagulant activity, low-intensity warfarin and the risk of recurrent venous thromboembolism. J Thromb Haemost 2006;4:1208–14.

57. Poli D, Antonucci E, Ciuti G, et al. Combination of D-dimer, F1+2 and residual vein obstruction as predictors of VTE recurrence in patients with first VTE episode after OAT withdrawal. J Thromb Haemost 2008;6:708–10.

58. Tait RC, Lowe GD, McColl MD, et al. Predicting risk of recurrent venous thrombosis using a 5-point scoring system including fibrin D-dimer. J Thromb Haemost 2007;5(Suppl 2):0-M-060.

59. Verhovsek M, Douketis JD, Yi Q, et al. Systematic review: D-dimer to predict recurrent disease after stopping anticoagulant therapy for unprovoked venous thromboembolism. Ann Intern Med 2008; 149:481–90, W94.

60. Bruinstroop E, Klok FA, Van De Ree MA, et al. Elevated D-dimer levels predict recurrence in patients with idiopathic venous thromboembolism: a meta-analysis. J Thromb Haemost 2009;7:611–8.

61. Decousus H, Leizorovicz A, Parent F, et al. A clinical trial of vena caval filters in the prevention of pulmonary embolism in patients with proximal deep-vein thrombosis. N Engl J Med 1998;338: 409–15.

62. PREPIC Study Group. Eight-year follow-up of patients with permanent vena cava filters in the prevention of pulmonary embolism: the PREPIC (Prevention du Risque d'Embolie Pulmonaire par

Interruption Cave) randomized study. Circulation 2005;112:416—22.

63. Kryle P, Minar E, Hirschl M, et al. High plasma levels of factor VIII and the risk of recurrent venous thromboembolism. N Engl J Med 2000;343:457—62.

64. Kraaijenhagen RA, in't Anker PS, Koopman MM, et al. High plasma concentration of factor VIIIc is a major risk factor for venous thromboembolism [see comments]. Thromb Haemost 2000;83:5—9.

65. Weltermann A, Eichinger S, Bialonczyk C, et al. The risk of recurrent venous thromboembolism among patients with high factor IX levels. J Thromb Haemost 2003;1:28—32.

66. Eichinger S, Stumpflen A, Hirschl M, et al. Hyperhomocysteinemia is a risk factor of recurrent venous thromboembolism. Thromb Haemost 1998;80:566—9.

67. Den Heijer M, Willems HP, Blom HJ, et al. Homocysteine lowering by B vitamins and the secondary prevention of deep vein thrombosis and pulmonary embolism: a randomized, placebo-controlled, double-blind trial. Blood 2007;109:139—44.

68. Hron G, Kollars M, Binder BR, et al. Identification of patients at low risk for recurrent venous thromboembolism by measuring thrombin generation. JAMA 2006;296:397—402.

69. van HV, Christiansen SC, Luddington R, et al. Elevated endogenous thrombin potential is associated with an increased risk of a first deep venous thrombosis but not with the risk of recurrence. Br J Haematol 2007;138:769—74.

70. Besser M, Baglin C, Luddington R, et al. High rate of unprovoked recurrent venous thrombosis is associated with high thrombin-generating potential in a prospective cohort study. J Thromb Haemost 2008;6:1720—5.

71. Hron G, Eichinger S, Weltermann A, et al. Prediction of recurrent venous thromboembolism by the activated partial thromboplastin time. J Thromb Haemost 2006;4:752—6.

72. Hron G, Eichinger S, Weltermann A, et al. Family history for venous thromboembolism and the risk for recurrence. Am J Med 2006;119:50—3.

73. Campbell IA, Bentley DP, Prescott RJ, et al. Anticoagulation for three versus six months in patients with deep vein thrombosis or pulmonary embolism, or both: randomised trial. Br Med J 2007;334:674—7.

74. Schulman S, Granqvist S, Holmström M, et al. The duration of oral anticoagulant therapy after a second episode of venous thromboembolism. N Engl J Med 1997;336:393—8.

75. Ost D, Tepper J, Mihara H, et al. Duration of anticoagulation following venous thromboembolism: a meta-analysis. JAMA 2005;294:706—15.

76. Kearon C. Indefinite anticoagulation after a first episode of unprovoked venous thromboembolism: yes. J Thromb Haemost 2007;5:2330—5.

77. Locadia M, Bossuyt PM, Stalmeier PF, et al. Treatment of venous thromboembolism with vitamin K antagonists: patients' health state valuations and treatment preferences. Thromb Haemost 2004;92:1336—41.

78. Palareti G, Leali N, Coccheri S, et al. Bleeding complications of oral anticoagulant treatment: an inception-cohort, prospective collaborative study (ISCOAT). Lancet 1996;348:423—8.

79. Beyth RJ, Quinn LM, Landefeld S. Prospective evaluation of an index for predicting the risk of major bleeding in outpatients treated with warfarin. Am J Med 1998;105:91—9.

80. Kuijer PMM, Hutten BA, Prins MH, et al. Prediction of the risk of bleeding during anticoagulant treatment for venous thromboembolism. Arch Intern Med 1999;159:457—60.

81. Beyth RJ, Quinn L, Landefeld CS. A multicomponent intervention to prevent major bleeding complications in older patients receiving warfarin. A randomized, controlled trial. Ann Intern Med 2000;133:687—95.

82. Dentali F, Douketis JD, Lim W, et al. Combined aspirin-oral anticoagulant therapy compared with oral anticoagulant therapy alone among patients at risk for cardiovascular disease: a meta-analysis of randomized trials. Arch Intern Med 2007;167:117—24.

83. Schulman S, Beyth RJ, Kearon C, et al. Hemorrhagic complications of anticoagulant and thrombolytic treatment: American College of Chest Physicians evidence-based clinical practice guidelines (8th edition). Chest 2008;133:257S—98S.

84. Gage BF, Yan Y, Milligan PE, et al. Clinical classification schemes for predicting hemorrhage: results from the National Registry of Atrial Fibrillation (NRAF). Am Heart J 2006;151:713—9.

85. Ruiz-Gimenez N, Suarez C, Gonzalez R, et al. Predictive variables for major bleeding events in patients presenting with documented acute venous thromboembolism. Findings from the RIETE Registry. Thromb Haemost 2008;100:26—31.

86. Palareti G, Cosmi B. Bleeding with anticoagulation therapy - who is at risk, and how best to identify such patients. Thromb Haemost 2009;102:268—78.

87. Segal JB, Streiff MB, Hoffman LV, et al. Management of venous thromboembolism: a systematic review for a practice guideline. Ann Intern Med 2007;146:211—22.

88. Prandoni P, Noventa F, Ghirarduzzi A, et al. The risk of recurrent venous thromboembolism after discontinuing anticoagulation in patients with acute proximal deep vein thrombosis or pulmonary embolism. A prospective cohort study in 1,626 patients. Haematologica 2007;92:199—205.

89. Ansell J, Hirsh J, Hylek E, et al. Pharmacology and management of the vitamin K antagonists: American

College of Chest Physicians evidence-based clinical practice guidelines (8th edition). Chest 2008; 133:160S–98S.

90. Schulman S. Clinical practice. Care of patients receiving long-term anticoagulant therapy. N Engl J Med 2003;349:675–83.

91. Garcia DA, Witt DM, Hylek E, et al. Delivery of optimized anticoagulant therapy: consensus statement from the Anticoagulation Forum. Ann Pharmacother 2008;42:979–88.

92. Holbrook AM, Pereira JA, Labiris R, et al. Systematic overview of warfarin and its drug and food interactions. Arch Intern Med 2005;165:1095–106.

93. Garcia D, Regan S, Crowther M, et al. Warfarin maintenance dosing patterns in clinical practice: implications for safer anticoagulation in the elderly population. Chest 2005;127:2049–56.

94. Crowther MA, Ageno W, Garcia D, et al. Oral vitamin K versus placebo to correct excessive anticoagulation in patients receiving warfarin: a randomized trial. Ann Intern Med 2009;150:293–300.

95. Dentali F, Ageno W, Crowther M. Treatment of coumarin-associated coagulopathy: a systematic review and proposed treatment algorithms. J Thromb Haemost 2006;4:1853–63.

96. Dezee KJ, Shimeall WT, Douglas KM, et al. Treatment of excessive anticoagulation with phytonadione (vitamin K): a meta-analysis. Arch Intern Med 2006; 166:391–7.

97. Sconce E, Avery P, Wynne H, et al. Vitamin K supplementation can improve stability of anticoagulation for patients with unexplained variability in response to warfarin. Blood 2007;109: 2419–23.

98. Rombouts EK, Rosendaal FR, Van Der Meer FJ. Daily vitamin K supplementation improves anticoagulant stability. J Thromb Haemost 2007;5: 2043–8.

99. Heneghan C, Alonso-Coello P, Garcia-Alamino JM, et al. Self-monitoring of oral anticoagulation: a systematic review and meta-analysis. Lancet 2006;367:404–11.

100. Poller L, Keown M, Ibrahim S, et al. An international multicenter randomized study of computer-assisted oral anticoagulant dosage vs. medical staff dosage. J Thromb Haemost 2008;6:935–43.

101. Kearon C, Hirsh J. Management of anticoagulation before and after elective surgery. N Engl J Med 1997;336(21):1506–11.

102. Douketis JD, Berger PB, Dunn AS, et al. The perioperative management of antithrombotic therapy: American College of Chest Physicians evidence-based clinical practice guidelines (8th edition). Chest 2008;133:299S–339S.

Venous Thromboembolism in Pregnancy

Paul E. Marik, MD, FCCM, FCCP

KEYWORDS

- Pregnancy • Venous thromboembolism
- Pulmonary embolus • Deep venous thrombosis
- Thrombophilia • Low molecular weight heparin

The incidence of venous thromboembolism (VTE) is estimated at 0.76 to 1.72 cases per 1000 pregnancies[1,2] Current estimates of mortality are 1.1 to 1.5 deaths per 100,000 deliveries in the United States and European countries.[1,2] In women of reproductive age, more than half of all venous thrombotic events are related to pregnancy.[3] Approximately 60% to 80% of all VTEs related to pregnancy are deep venous thrombosis (DVT). Compared with nonpregnant women, the risk of venous thrombotic events is increased fivefold during pregnancy and 60-fold in the first 3 months after delivery.[3] Similarly, the risk of pulmonary embolism (PE) is increased twofold during pregnancy and up to 30-fold in the postpartum period (defined as the first 3 months after delivery).[3] DVTs occur with equal frequency during each trimester. Approximately one-third of pregnancy-related DVTs and half of pregnancy-related PEs occur after delivery. Most cases of postpartum DVT occur within the first 4 weeks after delivery, most frequently in the second week,[3] although the risk remains elevated for up to 3 months postpartum (**Fig. 1**).

RISK FACTORS FOR VTE

Pregnancy is a hypercoagulable state. Fibrin generation is increased; fibrinolytic activity is decreased. Levels of coagulation factors II, VII, VIII, and X are all increased; free protein S levels are decreased, and acquired resistance to activated protein C is common.[4] Uncomplicated pregnancy is accompanied by substantial hemostatic activation as indicated by increased markers of coagulation activation, such as prothrombin fragment F1 +2 and D-dimer.[5] Plasminogen activator inhibitor type 1 (PAI-1) levels increase fivefold, while PAI-2 produced by the placenta increases dramatically during the third trimester.[6] In addition to coagulation activation and inhibition of fibrinolysis, there is a substantial reduction in venous flow velocity in the lower limbs in pregnancy; flow decreases approximately 50% by 25 to 29 weeks gestation and remains reduced for approximately 6 weeks after delivery.[7,8]

The most important risk factor for VTE in pregnancy is a history of previous thrombosis; 15% to 25% of thromboembolic events in pregnancy are recurrent events. Inherited thrombophilias and the antiphospholipid syndrome also amplify the risk for VTE during pregnancy and the pospartum period.[2] Risk factors for VTE during pregnancy are listed in **Table 1**.

HERITABLE THROMBOPHILIA AND VTE DURING PREGNANCY AND THE PUERPERIUM

A thrombophilia is defined as a disorder of hemostasis that predisposes an individual to a thrombotic event.[9] The prevalence of the inherited thrombophilias varies across populations (**Table 2**).[9–11] Recent data suggest that up to 50% of VTEs in pregnancy are associated with

Disclosure: Dr Marik certifies that he has no relationship including consultation, paid speaking, grant support, equity, patients or royalties from any company that makes products relevant to this manuscript.
Division of Pulmonary and Critical Care Medicine, EVMS Internal Medicine, Eastern Virginia Medical School, HH Suite 410, 825 Fairfax Avenue, Norfolk VA 23507, USA
E-mail address: marikpe@evms.edu

Clin Chest Med 31 (2010) 731–740
doi:10.1016/j.ccm.2010.06.004

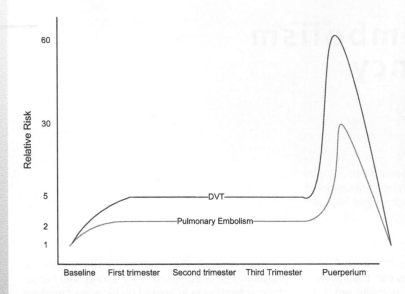

Fig. 1. The relative risk of deep venous thrombosis (DVT) and pulmonary embolism (PE) during pregnancy and the puerperium. Compared with nonpregnant women, the risk of venous thrombotic events is increased fivefold during pregnancy and 60-fold in the first 3 months after delivery.[3] Similarly, the risk of PE is increased twofold during pregnancy and up to 30-fold in the postpartum period (defined as the first 3 months after delivery).[3] Most cases of postpartum DVT occur within the first 4 weeks after delivery, most frequently in the second week,[3] although the risk remains elevated for up to 3 months postpartum.

an inherited or acquired thrombophilia.[12,13] Although inherited thrombophilias are common (affecting 15% of Western populations) and underlie approximately 50% of VTEs in pregnancy, VTE complicates only 0.1% of pregnancies. Furthermore, the absolute risk of VTE in pregnant patients with a thrombophilia is a modest 1% to 2%, with most events occurring postpartum. The rarity of VTE during pregnancy and postpartum, and the high prevalence of inherited thrombophilias, make universal screening of pregnant patients for thrombophilia cost-ineffective.[14,15]

When acute VTE occurs during pregnancy, thrombophilia screening is of limited value. It does not alter clinical management, and both pregnancy and thrombosis affect the circulating level of many of the coagulation factors. However, thrombophilia screening should be considered after anticoagulants have been stopped as the presence of a high-risk thrombophilia may indicate the need for thromboprophylaxis in subsequent pregnancies.

DIAGNOSING VTE

There is a striking predisposition for DVT to occur in the left leg (approximately 70% to 80% of cases). This may result from compression of the left iliac vein by the gravid uterus and the crossing right iliac artery.[16] DVT in pregnancy is also more likely to be proximal and massive than in nonpregnant patients. The incidence of DVT isolated in the iliac vein is thought to be relatively higher in pregnant women than in nonpregnant women. Isolated iliac vein thrombosis may present with abdominal pain, back pain, or swelling of the entire leg; however, patients may be totally asymptomatic.[17,18]

Clinical suspicion is critical to the diagnosis of VTE. In pregnancy this is complicated, because many of the classic signs and symptoms of DVT and PE, including leg swelling, tachycardia, tachypnea, and dyspnea, are present in normal pregnancies. Commonly used prediction rules for DVT and PE are not valid in pregnancy.[19] Chan and colleagues, however, have suggested that symptoms in the left leg, a calf circumference difference ≥2 cm, or leg symptoms in the first trimester identified pregnant patients whose pretest risk for DVT was high.[20] Though VTE is found in less than 10% of the pregnant women suspected of having it (compared with approximately 25% in studies of nonpregnant patients),[20,21] symptoms of VTE should always lead to objective testing as soon as possible, because missing the diagnosis may result in sudden death. Unless anticoagulation is contraindicated, low molecular weight heparin (LMWH) or unfractionated heparin (UFH) treatment is recommended until the diagnosis is excluded by objective testing.[22]

In pregnant patients with suspected DVT, workup begins with an assessment of pretest probability followed by compression ultrasound (CUS), a noninvasive test with a sensitivity of 97% and a specificity of 94% for diagnosing symptomatic, proximal DVT in the general population.[23] CUS appears to have a similar diagnostic accuracy in pregnant patients, with a false-negative rate of approximately 0.7%.[20,24,25] Patients with a negative test result should have a follow-up test within 7 days, because up to 25% of DVTs are diagnosed on serial CUS examinations.[20] CUS is less accurate for isolated calf and iliac vein thrombosis.[26] Magnetic resonance

Table 1
Risk factors for venous thromboembolism during pregnancy and the puerperium

Pre-existing Risk Factor	OR (95% CI)
Thrombophilia	See **Table 2**
Personal or family history of VTE	24.8 (17.1–36)
Obesity (BMI >30)	
Antepartum VTE	7.7 (3.2–19)
Postpartum VTE	10.8 (4.0–28.8)
Age >35 years	2.1 (2.0–2.3)
Smoking (10–30 cigarettes/d)	
Antepartum VTE	2.1 (1.3–3.4)
Postpartum VTE	3.4 (2.0–5.5)
Sickle cell disease	6.7 (4.4 –10.1)
Diabetes	2.0 (1.4 – 2.7)
Hypertension	1.8 (1.4–2.3)
New or Transient risk factor	
Twin pregnancy	2.6 (1.1 – 6.2)
Immobility	
Antepartum VTE	7.7 (3.2–19)
Postpartum VTE	10.8 (4.0–28.8)
In vitro fertilization	
Singleton	4.3 (2.0–9.4)
Twins	6.6 (2.1–21.0)
Caesarian section	
Routine without infection	1.3 (0.7–2.2)
Emergency without infection	2.7 (1.8–4.1)
Postpartum hemorrhage (>1000 mL)	
Without surgery	4.1 (2.3–7.3)
With surgery	12 (3.9 –36.9)
Infection	
Vaginal delivery	20.2 (6.4–63.5)
Any caesarian section	6.2 (2.4–16.2)
Pre-eclampsia	
Without IUGR	3.1 (1.8–5.3)
With IUGR	5.8 (2.1–16.0)

Abbreviations: BMI, body mass index; CI, confidence interval; IUGR, intrauterine growth retardation; OR, odds ratio; VTE, venous thromboembolism.
  Data from Refs.[2,25,85]

direct thrombus imaging (MRDTI), a test that has no radiation exposure and is not deleterious to the fetus, has a high sensitivity and specificity for the diagnosis of isolated iliac vein thrombosis.[18,27] Pulsed Doppler of the iliac vein and computed tomography (CT) scanning may be useful for detecting iliac vein thrombosis when magnetic resonance imaging (MRI) is not available.[28,29]

D-dimer levels increase with the progression of a normal pregnancy.[30] Furthermore, the interpretation of the D-dimer level depends upon which test is used to perform the assay and the cutoff values used. Current recommendations suggest that a D-dimer test should not be used as a stand-alone test to exclude DVT in pregnant patients.[31] Chan and colleagues reported that a negative SimplyRED assay (a red blood cell agglutination assay) (Agen Biomedical, Brisbane, Australia) when symptomatic DVT was suspected in the first and second trimester had a sensitivity of 100% for DVT, but the lower bound of the 95% confidence interval (CI) for sensitivity was relatively low (77%)[24] Chan and colleagues[24] also observed a low specificity for the SimplyRED assay. This finding reinforces the importance of confirming DVT with additional objective testing when a D-dimer test is positive.

Pregnant patients with a suspected PE require additional diagnostic imaging when CUS fails to detect a DVT. Chest radiographs exclude alternative diagnoses and guide further diagnostic testing. If alternative diagnoses (eg, pneumothoraces) are not identified by the chest radiograph, ventilation-perfusion (V/Q) lung scans or computed tomographic pulmonary angiography (CTPA) should be performed. In most centers, CTPA is preferred to VQ scanning in pregnant patients with suspected PE. CTPA does have some limitations. It results in suboptimal (nondiagnostic) images in 5% to 10% of nonpregnant subjects, often attributable to technical factors such as motion artifact or suboptimal contrast opacification of the pulmonary vessels. In pregnant patients, suboptimal CTPA is more likely because the hyperdynamic circulation and increased blood volume associated with pregnancy can result in less than ideal contrast opacification of the major pulmonary vessels.[32] Contrast injection protocols for CTPA should take the physiologic changes of pregnancy into account to improve diagnostic accuracy.[33]

Radiation dose is a consideration in selecting the most appropriate diagnostic technique. The calculated dose of radiation absorbed by the fetus is approximately 10 times higher with perfusion scintigraphy than CTPA (even if a half-dose scintigraphic technique is used), but the levels with both V/Q scanning and CTPA are well below the dose levels proposed for increased risk for congenital abnormalities.[34–36] The radiation dose for CTPA is associated with approximately 40 times greater radiation exposure to proliferating breast tissue during pregnancy.[34] Whether this translates into a measurable increase in breast cancer risk is unknown. The risks should be explained to

Table 2
Estimated prevalence rates for inherited thrombophilia and the risk (odds ratio) of thromboembolism during pregnancy in a European population

Thrombophilic Defect	Prevalence (%)	OR (95% CI)
Factor V Leiden heterozygous	2–7	8.3 (5.4–12.7)
Factor V Leiden homozygous	0.5–0.25	34.4 (9.9 –120.1)
Prothrombin G20210A heterozygous	2	6.8 (2.5 –18.8)
Prothrombin G20210A homozygous	Rare	26.4 (1.24 –559.3)
Antithrombin deficiency (<80% activity)	0.02–0.55	4.7 (1.3–16.9)
Protein C deficiency (<75% activity)	0.2–0.33	4.8 (2.2–10.6)
Protein S deficiency (<65% activity)	0.03–0.13	3.2 (1.5–6.9)
Methyltetrahydrofolate reductase Mutation (homozygous)	–	0.74 (0.22–2.48)
Antiphospholipid antibodies	18	15.8 (10.9–22.8)

Abbreviations: CI, confidence interval; OR, odds ratio.
   Data from Refs.[9–11]

patients, as those with a family history of breast cancer or those who have had a previous CTPA may choose lung perfusion scanning, despite the slightly higher risk to the fetus.

MANAGING VTE

The treatment and prophylaxis of VTE in pregnancy both center on the use of unfractionated heparin (UFH) or LMWH, because they do not cross the placenta and thus avoid the known risks of warfarin (the most commonly used treatment for VTE that does cross the placenta).[37]

Warfarin embryopathy is characterized by mid-face hypoplasia, stippled chondral calcification, scoliosis, short proximal limbs, and short phalanges; it affects 5% of fetuses exposed to the drug between 6 and 9 weeks gestation.[38] The use of warfarin in the second and early third trimester is associated with fetal intracranial hemorrhage and schizencephaly.[39–41]

For many years UFH was the standard anticoagulant used during pregnancy and into the puerperium; current guidelines now recommend LMWH.[21,22,37] Advantages of LMWH include a reduced risk of bleeding, predictable pharmacokinetics that allow weight-based dosing without the need for monitoring, and reduced risk for heparin-induced thrombocytopenia (HIT) and heparin-induced osteoporotic fractures.[21,42–44]

Management of isolated calf-vein thrombosis is controversial, and there are no established guidelines. However, as most ileo-femoral thromboses originate from calf-vein thromboses, therapeutic doses of LMWH should be considered in symptomatic patients who have no contraindications to anticoagulation. Vena caval filters (retrievable) should be considered only in patients for whom anticoagulation is contraindicated or for whom anticoagulation must be stopped because of bleeding or anticipated delivery (ie, within 2 weeks of delivery).[45,46]

Although LMWH is often administered once daily using a weight-adjusted dose regimen, renal excretion increases in pregnancy, thus decreasing the half-life of LMWH.[47,48] The decreased half-life is the basis of a recommendation for twice-daily weight-based dosing of LMWH.[21,22,37,49]

Once daily dosing is supported by a large multicenter case series in which 66% of pregnant women with VTE were treated with LMWH once daily. None developed recurrent thrombosis.[50] In a small randomized controlled trial (RCT), Narin and colleagues randomized 35 pregnant patients with DVT to enoxaparin 1 mg/kg twice daily or 1.5 mg/kg once daily. In this study there was no significant difference between groups in terms of recanalization (measured by CUS), post-thrombotic symptoms, or safety parameters.[51] These data suggest that once-daily dosing may be as safe and effective as a twice-daily dosing regimen. Clinical experience suggests that monitoring anti-Xa activity with dose adjustments is not required except in those patients at the extremes of body weight or those with altered renal function.[49,52]

Allergic skin complications caused by LMWH are considered rare and include pruritus, urticarial rashes, erythematous plaques and, rarely, skin necrosis. These reactions are reported to occur more commonly during long-term use in pregnant women.[53,54] Cross-reactivity occurs in about a third of women switched to another LMWH preparation. Limited experience with fondaparinux, a synthetic pentasaccharide (direct inhibitor of factor Xa), suggests that it may be a safe alternative in women with broad cross-reactivity among several LMWHs.[55] Although placental transfer of fondaparinux was not observed in a human cotyledon model,[56] limited clinical experience suggests that fondaparinux passes the placental barrier in vivo, resulting in low measurable anti-factor Xa activity in umbilical cord blood.

ANTICOAGULANT THERAPY DURING LABOR AND DELIVERY

Managing anticoagulation at the end of pregnancy is challenging, as the onset of labor is not predictable. Additionally, both vaginal and cesarean delivery are frequently done under regional anesthesia and are associated with blood loss. If spontaneous labor begins in fully anticoagulated women, neuraxial anesthesia should not be employed because of the risk of spinal hematoma.[21,57] This can be avoided by scheduling elective induction of labor or caesarian section. Women who continue taking LMWH should be advised that once in established labor, no further heparin should be administered.

LMWH cannot be expeditiously reversed. Because of the slow reversibility of LMWH, the difficulty in predicting onset of labor, and the relatively high chance of caesarean delivery in women with VTE, many obstetricians are reluctant to manage a woman all the way through pregnancy on LMWH. Although not validated by clinical studies, patients are commonly switched to subcutaneous UFH for the last few weeks of pregnancy. However, as the pharmacokinetics and pharmacodynamics of subcutaneous UFH are unpredictable during the third trimester of pregnancy, meticulous attention to monitoring of the activated partial thromboplastin time (aPTT) with dosage adjustment is required.[58] In addition, the pharmacokinetics of subcutaneous UFH and LMWH are quite similar and switching to UFH may not be beneficial.[59] These factors limit the benefit of this approach.

LMWH therapy may be resumed within 12 hours of delivery in the absence of persistent bleeding.[37] If neuraxial anesthesia has been used, therapeutic LMWH should be administered no earlier than 24 hours postoperatively/postpartum and then only when hemostasis is adequate.[60] Therapeutic anticoagulation with either LMWH or Coumadin is recommended for at least 6 weeks postpartum for a total duration of treatment (before and after delivery) of at least 6 months.[21] Neither warfarin nor heparin is secreted into breast milk, and both agents are therefore considered safe to use in

breast-feeding mothers.[61] The continuing risk of thrombosis should be assessed before treatment is discontinued. The post-thrombotic syndrome occurs in up to 60% of patients following acute proximal DVT and is a significant cause of morbidity.[62,63] Elastic compression stockings reduce the risk of the post-thrombotic syndrome by about 50% and should be worn on the affected leg for up to 2 years after the acute event.[22,63]

THROMBOLYTIC THERAPY

Although experience with thrombolytic therapy in pregnancy is limited, these agents may be life saving in patients with massive PE and severe hemodynamic compromise.[64] Despite the concern that thrombolytic therapy could lead to placental abruption, this complication has not been reported. Caesarian section or delivery within 10 days is considered a relative contraindication to thrombolytic therapy; however, successful thrombolysis has been reported within an hour after vaginal delivery and 12 hours after caesarian section.[65]

PULMONARY EMBOLISM IN LATE PREGNANCY/LABOR

Patients presenting with a pulmonary embolism in late pregnancy should be given supplemental oxygen and intravenous heparin and transferred to a major medical center with a high-risk maternal–fetal and cardiothoracic center. In hemodynamically stable patients, a temporary vena-caval filter should be placed once the diagnosis of pulmonary embolism has been confirmed.[45,46] When the patient goes into active labor or a caesarean section is contemplated, the heparin should be stopped (and reversed with protamine if necessary). Performing a caesarean section on a fully anticoagulated patient will predictably lead to uncontrolled bleeding and maternal death.

The management of the pregnant patient with massive PE at term or when the fetus is in distress is complex. A coordinated, individualized treatment strategy must be developed by the obstetrician, intensivist, cardiothoracic surgeon, anesthesiologist, and interventional radiologist and adapted to changing circumstances. Although thrombolytic therapy is considered to be strongly contraindicated in this circumstance, successful outcomes with the use of thrombolytic therapy for massive PE during labor have been reported.[66–68] Any surgical intervention should be undertaken only for maternal indications.[69] Patients who have suffered a massive PE tolerate positive pressure ventilation, general anesthesia, and blood loss very poorly, because these factors significantly compromise cardiac output and may lead to sudden death. Positive pressure ventilation increases right ventricular afterload and decreases preload (decreases venous return); this may result in severe hemodynamic compromise in a patient with massive PE and right ventricular failure. Caesarean section at this juncture carries a high risk of maternal death.[69,70] A caesarean section performed because of concern about fetal status is problematic, because fetal status is often a reflection of maternal status, and because a major surgical procedure performed on an unstable patient—the mother—may precipitate rapid deterioration. The exception to the requirement to pay primary attention to the mother is the perimortem caesarean, which is performed in an attempt to salvage the fetus, but which has also been documented to improve the effectiveness of cardiopulmonary resuscitation (CPR) for the mother. Should the interventional radiologist have the necessary expertise, pulmonary angiography with percutaneous mechanical clot fragmentation and placement of an inferior vena caval (IVC) filter may be attempted.[69,71] Should this approach not be feasible or fail, immediate cardiopulmonary bypass with surgical embolectomy followed by caesarean section (once the anticoagulation has been reversed) and placement of an IVC filter should be considered.

THROMBOPROPHYLAXIS DURING PREGNANCY AND THE PUERPERIUM

Despite the increased risk of VTE during pregnancy and the postpartum period, most women do not require thromboprophylaxis. In most cases, the risks of anticoagulation outweigh its benefits.

Women who would benefit from anticoagulation for prevention of thrombosis in pregnancy are those whose risk of VTE is greater than the risk of bleeding complications from heparin or LMWH (reported to be as high as 2%).[42,72]

Thromboprophylaxis could be considered in women who have had a previous VTE (both provoked and unprovoked). Such patients have a much higher risk of suffering recurrent VTE during pregnancy than women without a history of previous VTE[73,74] and an even higher risk of VTE in the puerperium. Antepartum and postpartum graduated elastic compression stockings are recommended for all women with previous VTE.[21] Similarly, postpartum pharmacologic thromboprophylaxis for at least 6 weeks (LMWH or warfarin) is recommended for all women with previous VTE.[21] The indications for antepartum pharmacologic prophylaxis are more controversial.[11,75] The risks and benefits of antepartum prophylaxis should be evaluated in each individual patient with the patient involved in the decision-making process. Pregnant women with multiple previous episodes of VTE (two or more) and those with higher-risk thrombophilias (eg, antithrombin deficiency, antiphospholipid syndrome, and homozygosity for prothrombin G20210A variant or factor V Leiden) should receive antenatal thromboprophylaxis (Table 3).[21] In a multicenter family study, Martinelli and colleagues demonstrated that the risk of first VTE during pregnancy and puerperium in double heterozygous carriers of factor V Leiden and prothrombin G20210A is low and similar to that of single carriers.[76] For pregnant women with a single idiopathic episode of VTE and those with a single previous VTE and a lower-risk thrombophilia, antenatal thromboprophylaxis is considered optional. Closer clinical surveillance

Table 3
Recommended antenatal prophylactic doses of low molecular weight heparin

	Enoxaparin	Dalteparin	Tinzaparin
Normal body weight (50–90kg)	40 mg/d	5000 U/d	4500 U/d
Body weight <50 kg	20 mg/d	2500 U/d	3500 U/d
Body weight >90 kg	40 mg 12 hourly	5000 U 12 hourly	4500 U 12 hourly
Higher prophylactic"dose[a]	0.5–1 mg/kg 12 hourly	50–100 IU/kg 12 hourly	4500 U 12 hourly

[a] Very high risk patients (antithrombin deficiency, antiphospholipid syndrome, multiple previous deep venous thromboses).
   Data from Bates SM, Greer IA, Pabinger I, et al. Venous thromboembolism, thrombophilia, antithrombotic therapy, and pregnancy. American College of Chest Physicians evidence-based clinical praactice guidelines (8th edition). Chest 2008;133:844S–86S; and Royal College of Obstetricians and Gynaecologists. Thromboprophylaxis during pregnancy, labour, and after vaginal delivery. Green Top Guideline No. 37. Available at: http://www.rcog.org.uk/resources/Public/pdf/Thromboprophylaxis_no037.pdf.

for VTE should be provided throughout pregnancy in those not receiving thromboprophylaxis.[21] In the absence of additional risk factors or thrombophilia, antenatal anticoagulation is not required for women whose previous VTE was not pregnancy-related or was associated with a risk factor that is no longer present.[73–75,77,78]

Data from retrospective studies suggest that women with antithrombin deficiency are at a high absolute risk of pregnancy-related VTE.[79] Antepartum prophylaxis should be strongly considered in these patients even when there is no personal history of VTE. As antithrombin is a cofactor for the activity of LMWH, the standard prophylactic dosing regimen of LMWH may be insufficient, and monitoring anti-Xa activity may be warranted in these patients. Thromboprophylaxis should also be considered in morbidly obese patients (body mass index BMI >40 kg/m^2) and those confined to bed, particularly when other risk factors are present. Aspirin is not recommended for thromboprophylaxis.[80]

Box 1
Risk assessment profile for thromboembolism in caesarean section

Low risk, early mobilization

Preterm cesarean delivery for uncomplicated pregnancy with no other risk factors

Moderate risk, LMWH or leg stockings

Age greater than 35 years

Obesity (BMI >30 kg/m^2)

Parity greater than threeGross varicose veins

Current infection

Preeclampsia

Immobility before operation (>4 days)

Major current illness

Emergency cesarean delivery in labor

High risk, LMWH + leg stockings

Presence of at least two risk factors (from moderate risk section)

Caesarean hysterectomy

Previous DVT or known thrombophilia

Data from Bates SM, Greer IA, Pabinger I, et al. Venous thromboembolism, thrombophilia, antithrombotic therapy, and pregnancy. American College of Chest Physicians evidence-based clinical practice guidelines (8th Edition). Chest 2008;133:844S–86S; and Chan WS, Chunilal S, Lee A, et al. A red blood cell agglutination D-dimer test to exclude deep venous thrombosis in pregnancy. Ann Intern Med 2007;147:165–70.

THROMBOPROPHYLAXIS FOLLOWING CAESAREAN SECTION

The risk of VTE after caesarean section may have been overestimated previously.[81,82] The pooled results from six studies demonstrate a postcaesarean DVT rate of 0.5% (95% CI, 0.1–1.4%),[83] a rate significantly lower than that of general surgical patients. These data suggests that low-risk patients who are able to ambulate immediately after surgery may not require DVT prophylaxis. Although there are no randomized controlled trials to guide thromboprophylaxis, the Royal College of Obstetricians and Gynecologists and the American College of Chest Physicians have published recommendations for risk assessment and thromboprophylaxis following caesarean section (**Box 1**).[21,84] The duration of thromboprophylaxis after caesarean section has not been studied. In the absence of such studies, it should be based on the individual patient's risk assessment. In high-risk patients for whom important risk factors persist following delivery, LMWH and compression stockings should be used for up to 4 to 6 weeks following delivery.[21]

SUMMARY

VTE is a common cause of morbidity and the most common cause of maternal death in Western nations. The classic signs and symptoms of VTE are common in normal pregnancy, and a high index of suspicion is required in all pregnant patients. Symptoms in the left leg, a calf circumference difference greater than or equal to 2 cm, and first trimester presentation of leg symptoms are highly predictive of DVT in pregnant patients. CUS is the diagnostic test of choice in patients with suspected DVT or PE. In patients with suspected PE and negative CUS, either perfusion scintigraphy or CTPA should be performed. Therapeutic doses of LMWH given once daily, are the preferred antepartum regimen in patients with proven VTE. Prophylactic doses of LMWH should be considered in patients with a previous VTE and a higher-risk thrombophilia. All patients who have had a previous VTE should use graduated compression stockings throughout pregnancy and the postpartum period, and should receive postpartum anticoagulant prophylaxis.

REFERENCES

1. Heit JA, Kobbervig CE, James AH, et al. Trends in the incidence of venous thromboembolism during pregnancy or postpartum: a 30-year population-based study. Ann Intern Med 2005;143:697–706.

2. James AH, Jamison MG, Brancazio LR, et al. Venous thromboembolism during pregnancy and the postpartum period: incidence, risk factors, and mortality. Am J Obstet Gynecol 2006;194:1311–5.

3. Pomp ER, Lenselink AM, Rosendaal FR, et al. Pregnancy, the postpartum period and prothrombotic defects: risk of venous thrombosis in the MEGA study. J Thromb Haemost 2008;6:632–7.

4. Brenner B. Haemostatic changes in pregnancy. Thromb Res 2004;114:409–14.

5. Eichinger S, Weltermann A, Philipp K, et al. Prospective evaluation of hemostatic system activation and thrombin potential in healthy pregnant women with and without factor V Leiden. Thromb Haemost 1999;82:1232–6.

6. Bremme KA. Haemostatic changes in pregnancy. Best Pract Res Clin Haematol 2003;16:153–68.

7. Macklon NS, Greer IA, Bowman AW. An ultrasound study of gestational and postural changes in the deep venous system of the leg in pregnancy. Br J Obstet Gynaecol 1997;104:191–7.

8. Macklon NS, Greer IA. The deep venous system in the puerperium: an ultrasound study. Br J Obstet Gynaecol 1997;104:198–200.

9. Haemostasis and Thrombosis Task Force. British Committee for Standards in Haematology, Investigation, and Management of Heritable Thrombophilia. Br J Haematol 2001;114:512–28.

10. Robertson L, Wu O, Langhorne P, et al. Thrombophilia in pregnancy: a systematic review. Br J Haematol 2006;132:171–96.

11. Nelson SM, Greer IA. Thrombophilia and the risk for venous thromboembolism during pregnancy, delivery, and puerperium. Obstet Gynecol Clin North Am 2006;33:413–27.

12. Greer IA. Thrombosis in pregnancy: maternal and fetal issues. Lancet 1999;353:1258–65.

13. Rosendaal FR. Venous thrombosis: a multicausal disease. Lancet 1999;353:1167–73.

14. Clark P, Twaddle S, Walker ID, et al. Cost-effectiveness of screening for the factor V Leiden mutation in pregnant women. Lancet 2002;359:1919–20.

15. Wu O, Robertson L, Twaddle S, et al. Screening for thrombophilia in high-risk situations: a meta-analysis and cost-effectiveness analysis. Br J Haematol 2005;131:80–90.

16. Ginsberg JS, Brill-Edwards P, Burrows RF, et al. Venous thrombosis during pregnancy: leg and trimester of presentation. Thromb Haemost 1992; 67:519–20.

17. Merhi Z, Awonuga A. Acute abdominal pain as the presenting symptom of isolated iliac vein thrombosis in pregnancy. Obstet Gynecol 2006;107:468–70.

18. Rodger MA, Avruch LI, Howley HE, et al. Pelvic magnetic resonance venography reveals high rate of pelvic vein thrombosis after cesarean section. Am J Obstet Gynecol 2006;194:436–7.

19. Wells PS, Anderson DR, Bormanis J, et al. Value of assessment of pretest probability of deep vein thrombosis in clinical management. Lancet 1997; 350:1795–8.

20. Chan WS, Lee A, Spencer FA, et al. Predicting deep venous thrombosis in pregnancy: out in "LEFt" field? Ann Intern Med 2009;151:85–92.

21. Bates SM, Greer IA, Pabinger I, et al. Venous thromboembolism, thrombophilia, antithrombotic therapy, and pregnancy. American College of Chest Physicians evidence-based clinical practice guidelines (8th edition). Chest 2008;133:844S–86S.

22. Royal College of Obstetricians and Gynaecologists. Thromboprophylaxis during pregnancy, labour, and after vaginal delivery. Green Top Guideline No. 37. Available at: http://www.rcog.org.uk/resources/Public/pdf/Thromboprophylaxis_no037.pdf. Accessed November 16, 2009.

23. Kearon C, Julian JA, Newman TE, et al. Noninvasive diagnosis of deep venous thrombosis. McMaster Diagnostic Imaging Practice Guidelines Initiative. Ann Intern Med 1998;128:663–77.

24. Chan WS, Chunilal S, Lee A, et al. A red blood cell agglutination D-dimer test to exclude deep venous thrombosis in pregnancy. Ann Intern Med 2007; 147:165–70.

25. Chunilal SD, Bates SM. Venous thromboembolism in pregnancy: diagnosis, management and prevention. Thromb Haemost 2009;101:428–38.

26. Eskandari MK, Sugimoto H, Richardson T, et al. Is color-flow duplex a good diagnostic test for detection of isolated calf vein thrombosis in high-risk patients? Angiology 2000;51:705–10.

27. Fraser DG, Moody AR, Morgan PS, et al. Diagnosis of lower-limb deep venous thrombosis: a prospective blinded study of magnetic resonance direct thrombus imaging. Ann Intern Med 2002;136:89–98.

28. Frede TE, Ruthberg BN, Frede TE, et al. Sonographic demonstration of iliac venous thrombosis in the maternity patient. J Ultrasound Med 1988;7:33–7.

29. Zerhouni EA, Barth KH, Siegelman SS. Demonstration of venous thrombosis by computed tomography. AJR Am J Roentgenol 1980;134:753–8.

30. Nolan TE, Smith RP, Devoe LD. Maternal plasma D-dimer levels in normal and uncomplicated pregnancies. Obstet Gynecol 1993;81:235–8.

31. Nijkeuter M, Huisman MV. Diagnosing pulmonary embolism in pregnancy: Is there a role for D-dimer as a stand-alone test? Crit Care Med 2006;34:2701–2.

32. King-Im JM, Freeman SJ, Boylan T, et al. Quality of CT pulmonary angiography for suspected pulmonary embolus in pregnancy. Eur Radiol 2008;18:2709–15.

33. Schaefer-Prokop C, Prokop M. CTPA for the diagnosis of acute pulmonary embolism during pregnancy. Eur Radiol 2008;18:2705–8.

34. Cook JV, Kyriou J. Radiation from CT and perfusion scanning in pregnancy. BMJ 2005;331:350.

35. International Commission on Radiological Protection. Publication 84. Annals of the International Commission on Radiological Protection 2000;30:1–43.

36. Nijkeuter M, Geleijns J, De RA, et al. Diagnosing pulmonary embolism in pregnancy: rationalizing fetal radiation exposure in radiological procedures. J Thromb Haemost 2004;2:1857–8.

37. Duhl AJ, Paidas MJ, Ural SH, et al. Antithrombotic therapy and pregnancy: consensus report and recommendations for prevention and treatment of venous thromboembolism and adverse pregnancy outcomes. Am J Obstet Gynecol 2007;197:457, e1–21.

38. Wesseling J, van Driel D, Heymans HS, et al. Coumarins during pregnancy: long-term effects on growth and development of school-age children. Thromb Haemost 2001;85:609–13.

39. Lee HC, Cho SY, Lee HJ, et al. Warfarin-associated fetal intracranial hemorrhage: a case report. J Korean Med Sci 2003;18:764–7.

40. Pati S, Helmbrecht GD. Congenital schizencephaly associated with in utero warfarin exposure. Reprod Toxicol 1994;8:115–20.

41. Forestier F, Daffos F, Capella-Pavlovsky M. Low molecular weight heparin (PK 10169) does not cross the placenta during the second trimester of pregnancy study by direct fetal blood sampling under ultrasound. Thromb Res 1984;34:557–60.

42. Greer IA, Nelson-Piercy C. Low molecularweight heparins for thromboprophylaxis and treatment of venous thromboembolism in pregnancy: a systematic review of safety and efficacy. Blood 2005;106:401–7.

43. Warkentin TE, Greinacher A, Koster A, et al. Treatment and prevention of heparin-induced thrombocytopenia. American College of Chest Physicians evidence-based clinical practice guidelines (8th edition). Chest 2008;133:340S–80S.

44. Pettila V, Leinonen P, Markkola A, et al. Postpartum bone mineral density in women treated for thromboprophylaxis with unfractionated heparin or LMW heparin. Thromb Haemost 2002;87:182–6.

45. Baglin TP, Brush J, Streff BM. Guidelines on the use of vena cava filters. British Committee for Standards in Haematology. Br J Haematol 2006;134:590–5.

46. Kocher M, Krcova V, Cerna M, et al. Retrievable Gunther Tulip Vena Cava Filter in the prevention of pulmonary embolism in patients with acute deep venous thrombosis in perinatal period. Eur J Radiol 2009;70:165–9.

47. Casele HL, Laifer SA, Woelkers DA, et al. Changes in the pharmacokinetics of the low-molecular-weight heparin enoxaparin sodium during pregnancy. Am J Obstet Gynecol 1999;181:1113–7.

48. Sephton V, Farquharson RG, Topping J, et al. A longitudinal study of maternal dose response to low molecular weight heparin in pregnancy. Obstet Gynecol 2003;101:1307–11.

49. Greer IA. Anticoagulants in pregnancy. J Thromb Thrombolysis 2006;21:57–65.

50. Voke J, Keidan J, Pavord S, et al. The management of antenatal venous thromboembolism in the UK and Ireland: a prospective multicentre observational survey. Br J Haematol 2007;139:545–58.

51. Narin C, Reyhanoglu H, Tulek B, et al. Comparison of different dose regimens of enoxaparin in deep vein thrombosis therapy in pregnancy. Adv Ther 2008; 25:585–94.

52. Rodie VA, Thomson AJ, Stewart FM, et al. Low molecular weight heparin for the treatment of venous thromboembolism in pregnancy: a case series. BJOG 2002;109:1020–4.

53. Bank I, Libourel EJ, Middeldorp S, et al. High rate of skin complications due to low-molecular-weight heparins in pregnant women. J Throm Haemo 2003;1:859–61.

54. Verdonkschot AE, Vasmel WL, Middeldorp S, et al. Skin reactions due to low molecular weight heparin in pregnancy: a strategic dilemma. Arch Gynecol Obstet 2005;271:163–5.

55. Gerhardt A, Zotz RB, Stockschlaeder M, et al. Fondaparinux is an effective alternative anticoagulant in pregnant women with high risk of venous thromboembolism and intolerance to low-molecular-weight heparins and heparinoids. Thromb Haemost 2007;97:496–7.

56. Lagrange F, Vergnes C, Brun JL, et al. Absence of placental transfer of pentasaccharide (Fondaparinux, Arixtra) in the dually perfused human cotyledon in vitro. Thromb Haemost 2002;87:831–5.

57. Kopp SL, Horlocker TT. Anticoagulation in pregnancy and neuraxial blocks. Anesthesiol Clin 2008; 26:1–22.

58. Brancazio LR, Roperti KA, Stierer R, et al. Pharmacokinetics and pharmacodynamics of subcutaneous heparin during the early third trimester of pregnancy. Am J Obstet Gynecol 1995;173:1240–5.

59. Morris TA, Jacobson A, Marsh JJ, et al. Pharmacokinetics of UH and LMWH are similar with respect to antithrombin activity. Thromb Res 2005;115: 45–51.

60. Horlocker TT, Wedel DJ, Benzon H, et al. Regional anesthesia in the anticoagulated patient: defining the risks (the second ASRA Consensus Conference on Neuraxial Anesthesia and Anticoagulation). Reg Anesth Pain Med 2003;28:172–97.

61. Ginsberg JS, Hirsh J, Turner DC, et al. Risks to the fetus of anticoagulant therapy during pregnancy. Thromb Haemost 1989;61:197–203.

62. McColl MD, Ellison J, Greer IA, et al. Prevalence of the post-thrombotic syndrome in young women with previous venous thromboembolism. Br J Haematol 2000;108:272–4.

63. Brandjes DP, Buller HR, Heijboer H, et al. Randomised trial of effect of compression stockings in patients with symptomatic proximal-vein thrombosis. Lancet 1997;349:759–62.

64. Leonhardt G, Gaul C, Nietsch HH, et al. Thrombolytic therapy in pregnancy. J Throm Haemo 2006; 21:271–6.

65. Stefanovic BS, Vasiljevic Z, Mitrovic P, et al. Thrombolytic therapy for massive pulmonary embolism 12 hours after cesarean delivery despite contraindication? Am J Emerg Med 2006;24:502–4.

66. Richards SR, Barrows H, O'Shaughnessy R. Intrapartum pulmonary embolus. A case report. J Reprod Med 1985;30:64–6.

67. Fagher B, Ahlgren M, Astedt B. Acute massive pulmonary embolism treated with streptokinase during labor and the early puerperium. Acta Obstet Gynecol Scand 1990;69:659–61.

68. Hall RJ, Young C, Sutton GC, et al. Treatment of acute massive pulmonary embolism by streptokinase during labour and delivery. Br Med J 1972;4:647–9.

69. Woodward DK, Birks RJ, Granger KA. Massive pulmonary embolism in late pregnancy. Can J Anaesth 1998;45:888–92.

70. Splinter WM, Dwane PD, Wigle RD, et al. Anaesthetic management of emergency caesarian section followed by pulmonary embolectomy. Can J Anaesth 1989;36:689–92.

71. Bechtel JJ, Mountford MC, Ellinwood WE. Massive pulmonary embolism in pregnancy treated with catheter fragmentation and local thrombolysis. Obstet Gynecol 2005;106:1158–60.

72. Lepercq J, Conard J, Borel-Derlon A, et al. Venous thromboembolism during pregnancy: a retrospective study of enoxaparin safety in 624 pregnancies. BJOG 2001;108:1134–40.

73. De Stefano V, Martinelli I, Rossi E, et al. The risk of recurrent venous thromboembolism in pregnancy and puerperium without antithrombotic prophylaxis. Br J Haematol 2006;135:386–91.

74. Pabinger I, Grafenhofer H, Kaider A, et al. Risk of pregnancy-associated recurrent venous thromboembolism in women with a history of venous thrombosis. J Throm Haemo 2005;3:949–54.

75. Brill-Edwards P, Ginsberg JS, Gent M, et al. Safety of withholding heparin in pregnant women with a history of venous thromboembolism. Recurrence of Clot in This Pregnancy Study Group. N Engl J Med 2000; 343:1439–44.

76. Martinelli I, Battaglioli T, De S, et al. The risk of first venous thromboembolism during pregnancy and puerperium in double heterozygotes for factor V Leiden and prothrombin G20210A. J Thromb Haemost 2008;6:494–8.

77. Simioni P, Tormene D, Prandoni P, et al. Pregnancy-related recurrent events in thrombophilic women with previous venous thromboembolism. Thromb Haemost 2001;86:929.

78. Royal College of Obstetricians and Gynaecologists. Thromboembolic disease in pregnancy and the puerperium: acute management. Green-Top Guideline No. 28. Available at: http://www.rcog.org.uk/resources/public/pdf/green_top_28_thromboembolic_minorrevision.pdf. Accessed November 16, 2009.

79. McColl MD, Ramsay JE, Tait RC, et al. Risk factors for pregnancy associated venous thromboembolism. Thromb Haemost 1997;78:1183–8.

80. Geerts WH, Bergqvist D, Pineo GF, et al. Prevention of venous thromboembolism: American College of Chest Physicians evidence-based clinical practice guidelines (8th edition). Chest 2008;133: 381S–453S.

81. Bonnar J. Can more be done in obstetric and gynecologic practice to reduce morbidity and mortality associated with venous thromboembolism? Am J Obstet Gynecol 1999;180:784–91.

82. Greer IA. Epidemiology, risk factors and prophylaxis of venous thromboembolism in obstetrics and gynaecology. Baillieres Clin Obstet Gynaecol 1997; 11:403–30.

83. Sia WW, Powrie RO, Cooper AB, et al. The incidence of deep vein thrombosis in women undergoing cesarean delivery. Thromb Res 2009;123: 550–5.

84. Royal College of Obstetrics and Gynaecology. Report of the RCOG working party on prophylaxis against thromboembolism in gynaecology and obstetrics. London: Royal College of Obstetrics and Gynaecology; 1995.

85. Jacobsen AF, Skjeldestad FE, Sandset PM. Ante- and postnatal risk factors of venous thrombosis: a hospital-based case–control study. J Throm Haemost 2008;6:905–12.

Chronic Thromboembolic Pulmonary Hypertension

William R. Auger, MD[a],*, Nick H. Kim, MD[a],
Terence K. Trow, MD[b]

KEYWORDS

- Chronic thromboemboli • Pulmonary hypertension
- Pulmonary thromboendarterectomy
- Pulmonary endarterectomy

Chronic thromboembolic pulmonary hypertension (CTEPH) is one of the few forms of pulmonary hypertension (PH) that can be cured surgically. It is critical that every patient presenting with PH have CTEPH excluded in order to avoid missing the chance to cure this otherwise fatal condition. This article discusses the epidemiology and predisposing factors of CTEPH, as well as the natural history of this disorder with and without treatment. Although an exact understanding of the mechanisms resulting in fibrosed thromboembolic residua is lacking, current research suggesting abnormalities in fibrin side chains rendering them resistant to lysis are reviewed. The proper preoperative assessment to diagnose CTEPH and to define surgical candidacy for pulmonary thromboendarterectomy (PTE) are discussed as well as technical aspects of the operation itself. Although PTE is the treatment approach of choice, some patients who are not surgical candidates for a variety of reasons have been treated with pulmonary arterial hypertension (PAH)–specific medical therapies. This article also reviews the current evidence from the literature for medical therapies in CTEPH.

CTEPH: EPIDEMIOLOGY AND PREDISPOSING FACTORS

The incidence of CTEPH following an acute pulmonary embolic event (or events) has not been adequately defined. Early characterization of patients with CTEPH resulted in the speculation that 0.1% to 0.5% of acute embolic survivors might develop this disease.[1] However, more recent data suggest that this estimate may be a significant understatement of how common CTEPH might be worldwide.[2] A recent prospective longitudinal study by Pengo and colleagues[3] reported a 2-year, cumulative incidence of 3.8% following a single episode of pulmonary embolism (median follow-up of 94.3 months in 223 patients) and 13.4% following recurrent venous thromboembolism. Another prospective series from Becattini and colleagues[4] suggested a lower incidence. Following 259 patients for an average period of 46 months, 2 patients were diagnosed with CTEPH (0.8%). For those patients in whom the pulmonary embolic event was considered to be idiopathic (n = 135), the incidence was 1.5%. In a larger group of patients, Miniati and colleagues[5] reported a CTEPH incidence of 1.3% in 320 pulmonary embolic survivors followed for a minimum of 1 year. If an incidence of 1% proves to be correct, and there is an estimated 200,000 pulmonary embolic survivors annually in the United States who are believed to have long-term survival potential,[6] up to 2000 patients would be expected to develop CTEPH. Available information suggests that this exceeds the number of patients with

[a] Division of Pulmonary and Critical Care Medicine, University of California, San Diego, 9300 Campus Point Drive, La Jolla, CA 92037, USA
[b] Pulmonary Vascular Disease Program, Department of Medicine, Yale University School of Medicine, Section of Pulmonary and Critical Care, LLCI 105D, 333 Cedar Street, PO Box 208057, New Haven, CT 06520-8057, USA
* Corresponding author.
E-mail address: bauger@UCSD.edu

Clin Chest Med 31 (2010) 741–758
doi:10.1016/j.ccm.2010.07.006

CTEPH diagnosed annually in the United States, suggesting that this disease remains underdiagnosed. Furthermore, because it is reported that 42% to 63% of patients with the established diagnosis of CTEPH have no previously documented acute venous thromboembolism,[2,7,8] it is likely that the number of CTEPH cases is even greater than is projected to follow known thromboembolic events.

In the absence of appropriate treatment, long-term survivorship of patients with chronic thromboembolic disease is poor. As in other forms of PH, early reports found survivorship for patients with chronic thromboembolic disease to be proportional to the degree of right ventricular dysfunction at the time of diagnosis. In one study, the 5-year survival rate in patients with CTEPH was 30% when the mean pulmonary artery pressure (mPAP) was greater than 40 mm Hg and 10% when it was greater than 50 mm Hg.[9] More recently, in a study of 49 patients with CTEPH receiving standard anticoagulation therapy alone, Lewczuk and colleagues[10] showed that an exercise capacity of less than 2 metabolic equivalents, an mPAP greater than 30 mm Hg, or the presence of significant chronic obstructive pulmonary disease appeared to predict a poor prognosis. Condliffe and colleagues,[8] in a multivariate analysis of 148 patients with distal, inoperable CTEPH, showed that walk distance and cardiac index (CI) were predictors of survivorship. Univariate analysis in this same group showed that patients in World Health Organization (WHO) functional class III or IV had greater than 3 times the mortality relative to those patients in functional class I or II. However, a recent study demonstrated that disease-modifying medical therapy provided to patients with CTEPH with inoperable disease resulted in improved survivorship and better prognosis.[11]

There seem to be several predisposing factors that place patients at risk for developing chronic thromboembolic disease. For those patients having survived 1 or more pulmonary embolic events, several clinical observations have been reported. The overall extent of pulmonary vascular obstruction at presentation may be important in the development of CTEPH. Pengo and colleagues[3] suggested that having larger perfusion defects at the time of the initial pulmonary embolus diagnosis was a risk factor for developing CTEPH. They also showed that a history of multiple pulmonary embolic events, a younger age at presentation, and an idiopathic pulmonary embolic event placed patients at greater risk. In a report in which massive pulmonary embolism was defined as greater than 50% obstruction of the pulmonary vascular bed, the incidence of CTEPH was 20.2% despite the use of thrombolytic therapy.[12] The presence of PH when an acute pulmonary embolism is diagnosed might be an important risk factor and should alert the clinician to the possibility that CTEPH may be a potential problem. In patients presenting with an acute pulmonary embolus, Ribeiro and colleagues[13] reported that those with pulmonary artery systolic pressures greater than 50 mm Hg were apt to experience persistent PH after 1 year.

There is also an association between certain medical conditions and the development of chronic thromboembolic disease. The presence of a thrombophilic state has been examined in patients with chronic thromboembolic disease. In the largest study investigating this issue, the prevalence of a hereditary thrombophilia (deficiencies of antithrombin III, protein C or protein S, or mutations of the genes that code for factor II and factor V) was not increased in samples analyzed in 46 patients with CTEPH or 64 patients with idiopathic pulmonary hypertension (IPAH) relative to 100 control subjects.[14] However along with a recent evaluation of 687 consecutive patients with CTEPH (N = 433) and nonthromboembolic PH (N = 254), this study found antiphospholipid antibodies to be more commonly associated with chronic thromboembolic disease.[15] Antiphospholipid antibodies were present in 20% of patients with CTEPH as reported by Wolf and colleagues[14]; Bonderman and colleagues[15] showed antiphospholipid antibodies or a lupus anticoagulant in 10% of their patients with CTEPH. In an earlier report, Bonderman and colleagues[16] also showed increased levels of factor VIII in 41% of 122 patients with CTEPH, levels that were substantially higher than those in control subjects and patients with nonthromboembolic PAH. The factor VIII levels remained increased following successful PTE surgery.

Several other medical conditions have been associated with an increased risk of developing CTEPH. In a report from 2005, Bonderman and colleagues[7] compared 109 consecutive patients with CTEPH with 187 patients who did not develop chronic thromboembolic disease after experiencing an acute pulmonary embolism. Multivariate analysis revealed that prior splenectomy, the presence of a ventriculoatrial shunt to treat hydrocephalus, and certain chronic inflammatory disorders, such as osteomyelitis and inflammatory bowel disease, were risk factors for CTEPH. A follow-up study gathering data in 687 patients with pulmonary hypertension from 4 European pulmonary vascular centers between 1996 and 2007 found the presence of ventriculoatrial shunts and infected pacemakers, prior splenectomy, previous and recurrent venous thromboembolism, thyroid replacement therapy, and a history of malignancy as risks factors associated with CTEPH.[15]

NATURAL HISTORY OF CHRONIC THROMBOEMBOLIC DISEASE AND CTEPH

The pathophysiologic mechanism whereby an acute pulmonary embolus evolves into the thromboembolic residua that becomes incorporated into the wall of the pulmonary vessel remains poorly understood. In most circumstances, with antithrombotic therapy, resolution of an acute pulmonary embolic burden is to a degree that normal pulmonary hemodynamics, gas exchange, and exercise tolerance are restored. However, complete anatomic recovery after acute pulmonary embolism may not occur, and the basis for incomplete thromboembolic resolution and what constitutes a pathologic state is largely unknown. The presence of coexisting cardiopulmonary disease, the initial embolic burden, and the age of the thrombus at the time of embolization may all contribute. Under normal physiologic conditions, Rosenhek and colleagues[17] showed that the pulmonary artery has increased fibrinolytic capabilities compared with the aorta. This seems to be based on higher levels of tissue plasminogen activator (TPA) expression versus plasminogen activator inhibitor (PAI-1). However, a TPA–PAI-1 imbalance that would favor incomplete thrombus dissolution has not been found to be operational in patients with CTEPH.[18] More recently, preliminary data suggest that certain patients may have fibrinogen variants that render them resistant to lysis.[19,20] As previously noted, identifiable thrombophilic tendencies in patients with CTEPH have included increased factor VIII levels and the presence of antiphospholipid antibodies and/or a lupus anticoagulant.[14–16]

Adding to the uncertainties surrounding the natural history of CTEPH is the observation that extensive mechanical obstruction of the central pulmonary vasculature as the sole basis for increase of the pulmonary vascular resistance (PVR), whether because of recurrent embolic events or in situ pulmonary artery thrombosis, seems to occur in a minority of individuals. There is evidence to suggest that the progressive increase in PVR in most patients results from pathologic changes in the distal pulmonary vascular bed, and, to a large extent, in those lung regions not involved with chronic thromboemboli. Supporting this observation, Moser and Bloor[21] studied lung biopsy findings obtained at the time of thromboendarterectomy surgery and showed the presence of several histopathologic changes in the microvasculature similar to those seen in other forms of small vessel PH. In addition, clinical observations have shown that there is a poor correlation between the scintigraphic and angiographic extent of central thromboembolic obstruction and the severity of hemodynamic compromise.[22,23] In patients with sequential perfusion scans available for review, PH has progressed in the absence of perfusion scan change or clinical evidence of embolic recurrence. Although speculative, circulating vasoconstrictors, immune-related events, local upregulation of vascular growth factors, or an individual genetic predisposition may, individually or in some combination, be operative in the development of the observed hypertensive pulmonary arteriopathy.[24–30]

CLINICAL PRESENTATION

Establishing the diagnosis of CTEPH can be difficult. The presenting signs and symptoms can be difficult to distinguish from other common cardiopulmonary conditions. Box 1 lists the common presenting symptoms in CTEPH. Because of the nonspecificity of these symptoms, patients with CTEPH are often misdiagnosed, resulting in misdirected therapies and significant delays in seeking appropriate medical and surgical treatment.[1] These symptoms are caused by a combination of hemodynamic and ventilatory derangements directly caused by CTEPH. The chronic increase in right ventricular afterload causes ventricular remodeling and dysfunction. The timeframe in which this occurs varies depending on the individual, and may be dependent on both thrombus burden and host factors.[3,13,24,28–30] The right ventricular dysfunction then leads to compromised cardiac output and insufficient tissue perfusion, especially during exertion or times of stress. In cases with little or no resting PH, significant ventilatory dead space can contribute to a patient's complaint of dyspnea.[31] Accordingly, patients with symptomatic

---

Box 1
Presenting symptoms of CTEPH
Dyspnea
Fatigue
Nonproductive cough
Chest discomfort
Palpitations
Lightheadedness with exertion or with bending forward
Syncope
Hemoptysis (more common with CTEPH than PAH)

chronic thromboembolic disease should be evaluated for thromboendarterectomy surgery even in the absence of significant PH.

Another barrier to timely diagnosis of CTEPH results from the frequent absence of a documented history of venous thromboembolism. Up to 60% of patients with CTEPH lack a clinical history of either deep venous thrombosis or pulmonary embolic disease.[2,7,8,32] As a result, chronic thromboembolic disease as a diagnostic possibility in the evaluation of a patient with pulmonary hypertension can be inappropriately dismissed.

Recent advancements in the treatment of PAH may have contributed to misdiagnoses and delayed referral of patients with CTEPH for pulmonary endarterectomy (PEA). Because the preferred treatment of CTEPH remains surgery, it is imperative that all patients with PH receive proper workup and consideration for this unique and potentially curative form of PH.[33] An improper evaluation for CTEPH can lead to the assumption that the patient has PAH. Treating for presumed PAH may result not only in a poor or uncertain clinical response but also a missed opportunity for effective treatment. The expansion of medical therapies for PAH has heralded an increase in off-label treatment of CTEPH, with resultant delays in referral for surgical consideration.[34]

PREOPERATIVE EVALUATION

The possibility of CTEPH should be considered in all patients with PH, regardless of age, gender, or comorbidities. This is particularly important if the cause of PH seems to be isolated to the pulmonary vasculature and common secondary causes have been excluded.[35] The presence of even 1 persistent segmental defect on perfusion scan should raise a suspicion for chronic thromboembolic disease.

The preoperative evaluation of patients with suspected chronic thromboembolic disease serves 4 important functions: (1) to accurately determine that chronic thromboembolic disease is the basis for the PH; (2) to determine whether the chronic thromboembolic lesions are amenable to endarterectomy; (3) to evaluate for significant comorbidities that may affect the decision to proceed with surgery, or which may require additional surgical intervention at the time of a thromboendarterectomy (such as coexisting coronary artery disease); and (4) to establish the extent of pulmonary hemodynamic compromise that may affect the perioperative risks.

The typical physical examination findings in CTEPH mirror that seen in other types of PAH. The unique finding present in 30% of CTEPH cases, although not pathognomonic, is the presence of pulmonary flow murmur(s) or bruits heard over the lung fields in the area of proximal pulmonary artery narrowing.[36] These flow murmurs may be audible in large vessel pulmonary vasculitis and pulmonary artery sarcomas that narrow the proximal pulmonary vessels, but would not be found in patients with PAH. As with PAH, signs of resting tachycardia, jugular venous distention, right ventricular heave, S3 gallop, hepatomegaly, ascites, edema, and peripheral cyanosis all suggest advanced disease and poor cardiac function. Hoarseness can be a sign of left recurrent laryngeal nerve compression from an enlarged left pulmonary artery (Ortner sign). Select patients with chronic thromboembolic disease who are not pulmonary hypertensive can be symptomatic from increased ventilatory dead space and may have a relatively normal physical examination.[31]

Chest radiographs in CTEPH can appear similar to chest radiographs in PAH. The right heart contour enlargement and proximal pulmonary artery prominence are seen with PH. However, patients with CTEPH can also have numerous opacities, ranging from reticular, nodular, and even cavitary patterns, not typically seen with PAH. These opacities represent scars from previous pulmonary emboli. Paucity of vasculature or oligemia in lung regions distal to proximally occluded pulmonary arteries can also be observed (**Fig. 1**). Pulmonary function tests are recommended in the routine workup of PH, and are useful in identifying those patients with obstructive or restrictive lung physiology. Lung volume measurement in some patients with CTEPH may reveal a mild to moderate restrictive defect that seems to be related to parenchymal scarring from prior infarcted lung.[37]

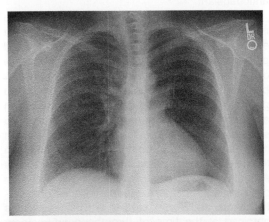

Fig. 1. Chest radiograph: right upper opacity is the normal region. (*Courtesy of* the University of California, San Diego, Pulmonary Thromboendarterectomy [PTE] Program, La Jolla, CA; with permission.)

Electrocardiogram findings, as in PAH, serve a limited diagnostic role. The patterns associated with right ventricular hypertrophy and right atrial enlargement correlate with hemodynamics. The presence of atrial fibrillation or flutter is notable both in terms of its contribution to worsening symptoms from PH and the likelihood for postoperative arrhythmia.[38] A transthoracic echocardiogram is usually the first test to suggest PH. In addition to the qualitative or quantitative assessment of PH provided by expertly performed transthoracic echocardiography, this study can detect other potentially complicating cardiac disorders.[39] The evaluation of left heart function, valvular structures, and interrogation for the presence of an atrial septal defect (especially a patent foramen ovale) provides useful information for patients with CTEPH considered potential candidates for surgery. If present and of such severity to warrant surgical correction, coronary bypass surgery, valve repair or replacement, and surgical closure of an atrial septal defect can be performed at the same setting of an endarterectomy without negatively affecting the length of the surgical procedure.[38] Accordingly, patients who are at risk for coronary atherosclerosis or age 45 years

or greater are recommended to have a screening left heart catheterization and coronary angiography as part of their evaluation for thromboendarterectomy surgery.

The imaging guidelines for differentiating between CTEPH and PAH are evolving. At some centers of excellence for pulmonary vascular diseases, the availability of better, faster, computed tomography (CT) and magnetic resonance technologies is driving a paradigm shift away from perfusion scanning and selective pulmonary arteriograms.[40,41] However, there are substantive diagnostic pitfalls involved with these more advanced technologies. In a recent report from Tunariu and colleagues,[42] CT angiography was shown to be less sensitive than ventilation perfusion (VQ) scanning in detecting CTEPH. Also, conditions such as in situ pulmonary arterial thrombi[43] and pulmonary artery sarcoma[44] can lead to a false-positive diagnosis of chronic thromboembolic disease if based solely on CT findings. Accordingly, the VQ scan remains a valuable screening test in differentiating PAH from CTEPH.[45] Large (segmental or larger), and persistent perfusion defect(s) unmatched by ventilation on VQ scintigraphy (**Fig. 2**) provides impetus to proceed with

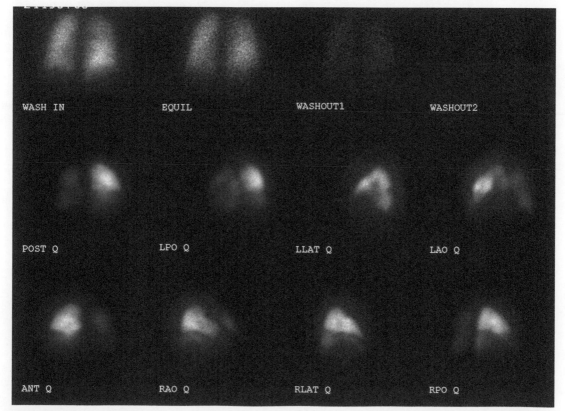

Fig. 2. VQ scan: perfusion is limited to the right upper lobe (upper 2 are ventilation; bottom 8 are perfusion images). (*Courtesy of* the University of California, San Diego, Pulmonary Thromboendarterectomy [PTE] Program, La Jolla, CA; with permission.)

more definitive diagnostic testing such as conventional pulmonary angiography. In most centers, this study remains the gold standard for the diagnosis of chronic thromboembolic disease, with chest CT and magnetic resonance imaging (MRI) providing complementary information if needed. CT can be especially helpful to evaluate the mediastinum, pulmonary venous structures, and for tumor involvement of the pulmonary vessels; conditions that can create large perfusion defects on VQ and mimic chronic thromboembolic disease.

The typical angiographic defects in chronic thromboembolic disease have been well described: proximal obstruction, abrupt narrowing, luminal irregularity, pouch defects, webs, or bands (Fig. 3A).[46] It is important to differentiate these findings from defects seen with acute pulmonary embolism, namely intraluminal filling defects. Chronic defects in segmental or more proximal

pulmonary arteries are accessible to an experienced surgeon.

Severity of PH is assessed and confirmed by right heart catheterization. These hemodynamic data are the critical remaining complements to the radiographic data in order to determine candidacy for PTE and to prognosticate perioperative risk. Right heart catheterization can be performed at the time of selective pulmonary arteriogram. The hemodynamic information obtained before arteriography assists in determining the volume of contrast needed to get adequate, high-quality images. A patient with low cardiac output requires smaller contrast volumes to clearly outline the pulmonary arteries, thereby reducing the risks associated with contrast, especially in patients with marginal renal function or low cardiac output. As in PAH, the severity of CTEPH is not dependent on the level of pulmonary arterial pressure, but

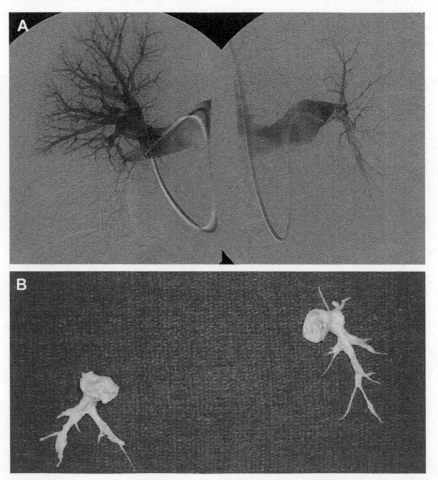

Fig. 3. (A) Pulmonary arteriogram: proximal pouch and abrupt narrowing. (B) PEA specimen: right interlobar and lower lobe specimen (left); entire left PA occlusion removed (right). (Courtesy of the University of California, San Diego, Pulmonary Thromboendarterectomy [PTE] Program, La Jolla, CA; with permission.)

rather on right ventricular function as assessed by cardiac output and right atrial pressure.

Preoperative PVR in CTEPH has been a strong and consistent predictor of postoperative risk, regardless of the center performing the thromboendarterectomy. Hartz and colleagues[47] reported that a preoperative PVR more than 1100 $dyn \cdot s \cdot cm^{-5}$ was associated with 41% mortality, compared with less than 6% if PVR was less than 1100 $dyn \cdot s \cdot cm^{-5}$. Dartevelle and colleagues[48] reported an increased postoperative mortality of 20% for patients with preoperative PVR of more than 1200 $dyn \cdot s \cdot cm^{-5}$ compared with 4% mortality if the preoperative PVR was less than 900 $dyn \cdot s \cdot cm^{-5}$. Similarly, based on 500 consecutive PTE cases, Jamieson and colleagues[32] reported an increased mortality of 10.1% for patients with preoperative PVR of more than 1000 $dyn \cdot s \cdot cm^{-5}$, compared with just 1.4% mortality if the preoperative PVR was less than 1000 $dyn \cdot s \cdot cm^{-5}$. However, this does not imply that patients with a high PVR should be discouraged from an attempted thromboendarterectomy. Those patients with CTEPH with marked PVR increase are often in profound right heart failure, have limited treatment alternatives, and typically have the greatest potential to benefit from this surgery. Therefore, severe PH is not a contraindication for PTE and selected patients should be referred for surgical consideration without delay.

Although randomized controlled data are lacking, many centers recommend a preoperative *inferior vena cava* (IVC) filter before planned PTE surgery. Although an attempt is made to resume anticoagulation early after PTE, the filter should provide an added protection against recurrent pulmonary embolism should significant postoperative bleeding delay anticoagulation. The safety of retrievable IVC filters for PTE is unknown; its potential benefit should be weighed against the risks of an added procedure (retrieval) and interruption of anticoagulation early after PTE surgery. All patients with CTEPH should receive lifelong therapeutic anticoagulation.

PTE SURGERY AND POSTOPERATIVE OUTCOMES

PTE surgery, or what is increasingly referred to as PEA surgery,[49] is the preferred treatment of selected patients with chronic thromboembolic disease. The presence of surgically accessible chronic thromboembolic lesions, as judged by the diagnostic studies discussed earlier, is the principal criterion in determining whether a patient is a candidate for surgery. The experience and capabilities of the surgical team also determine what will

be considered accessible lesions. Beyond this technical assessment, the decision to proceed with surgery is affected by the probability that pulmonary hemodynamic benefit will result following an endarterectomy, and the presence of comorbidities (eg, severe intrinsic lung disease, or poor left ventricular function) that might preclude an improvement in functional status. Outcomes seem to be best when surgery is performed by surgeons at a center with expertise in the care and management of patients with CTEPH; when there is a relative correlation between preoperative PVR and the extent of accessible chronic thromboembolic disease; when the preoperative PVR is less than 1000 $dyn \cdot s \cdot cm^{-5}$; and when certain coexisting medical conditions are absent (eg, splenectomy and ventriculoatrial shunts).[8,32,47,48,50,51]

Most patients who undergo PTE surgery have symptomatic PH with PVRs in excess of 300 $dyn \cdot s \cdot cm^{-5}$. At centers reporting their experience with patients having operable CTEPH, mean PVRs in the range of 500 to 1100 $dyn \cdot s \cdot cm^{-5}$ are typical.[48,50,52–59] However, certain patients with chronic thromboembolic disease may experience cardiopulmonary symptoms with exertion and demonstrate normal or minimally abnormal resting pulmonary hemodynamics. Often these patients have unilateral, main *pulmonary artery* (PA) occlusion with a chronic thromboembolus and are symptomatic from increased dead space ventilation. Despite the absence of hemodynamic compromise, endarterectomy surgery should be offered in an effort to restore lung perfusion and to prevent possible lung injury from long-term obstruction of the pulmonary vascular bed.

A detailed description of this surgical procedure can be found in several recent manuscripts.[52,60,61] Surgical success is based on the concept that a true endarterectomy, not an embolectomy, is necessary. Organized thromboembolic material is fibrotic and incorporated into the native vascular intima (see **Fig. 3**B). An adequate endarterectomy involves identification of this pseudointima and meticulously establishing a dissection plane to free the thrombotic residua from the native vessel wall. Considerable surgical experience with this procedure is required to identify the correct operative plane. The removal of nonadherent, partially organized thrombus within the lumen of the central pulmonary arteries is ineffective in reducing right ventricular afterload, whereas creation of a dissection plane too deep in the vessel wall poses the risk of PA perforation and massive pulmonary hemorrhage following discontinuation of cardiopulmonary bypass. Optimal exposure of the pulmonary vasculature intima therefore becomes critically important to the outcome of this procedure.

Cardiopulmonary bypass with periods of circulatory arrest provides this exposure in a bloodless operative field. The significant back bleeding resulting from bronchial arterial blood flow, which can be profound in the setting of longstanding pulmonary arterial obstruction, is mitigated with interruption of cardiopulmonary bypass (ie, circulatory arrest periods). It is during these circulatory arrest periods that dissection of thromboembolic residua from the lobar, segmental, and, to a degree, subsegmental arteries can be achieved.

Maintaining tissue integrity during intermittent circulatory arrest periods becomes the next critical challenge for surgical success. Although standard flow for cardiopulmonary bypass is practiced, deep hypothermia is established where the patient is systemically cooled to 18 to 20°C. Measures designed to minimize tissue injury during circulatory arrest periods include hemodilution to a hematocrit in the range of 18% to 25% in an effort to decrease blood viscosity during hypothermia and to optimize capillary blood flow. Additional cerebral protection is provided by surrounding the head with an ice-cooled blanket; following aortic cross-clamping, thiopental is administered until the electroencephalogram becomes isoelectric; and phenytoin is administered intravenously during the cooling period to reduce the risk of perioperative seizure activity. Myocardial protection is amplified with the administration of a single dose of cold cardioplegic solution following cross-clamping, and wrapping the heart in a cooling jacket.

Modifications of this approach intended to avoid deep hypothermia and/or circulatory arrest have been described and include the use of normothermic cardiopulmonary bypass or moderate hypothermia (28–32°C), aortic bronchial artery occlusion with a balloon catheter, antegrade cerebral artery perfusion with and without total circulatory arrest, and application of negative pressure in the left ventricle.[56,62–64] Implementation of these modifications was primarily designed to avoid deep hypothermic circulatory arrest and the potential for neurologic complications that may occur when the period of circulatory arrest exceeds 20 to 25 minutes. It has not yet been demonstrated that any of these modifications provides substantive benefit compared with the traditional technique.

For most patients undergoing PTE surgery, the restoration of blood flow to previously occluded lung regions results in an immediate reduction in PVR, with a consequent increase in cardiac output. This immediate hemodynamic benefit from surgery has been reported by numerous groups throughout the world,[11,48,50,52–59] noting that even normalization of the PA pressure and PVR can be achieved. A corresponding improvement in right ventricular function and cardiac remodeling has also been shown to occur after endarterectomy.[65–67] Similarly encouraging reports have consistently shown that this immediate hemodynamic benefit is sustained for months to years following PTE surgery. This benefit is accompanied by substantial gains in gas exchange and reversal of dead space ventilation,[68,69] functional status and exercise ability,[70,71] and quality of life.[11,72–76] Most patients initially in New York Heart Association (NYHA) functional class III or IV return postoperatively to NYHA class I or II functional class and are able to resume normal activities.[11,74,75]

In-hospital mortality following PTE surgery have steadily declined in the past decades. Patient series of widely different numbers have reported postoperative mortalities from 4% to 15%.[11,48,50,52–59] However, with experience and larger-volume programs, mortalities less than 7% are typical, with most programs experiencing a decline in mortality as experience accumulates.[50,52,56] Several factors seem to have contributed to this outcome, including a clearer understanding of the natural history of the disease, better diagnostic techniques, more selective surgical referral, and advances in operative and postoperative care. Attributable causes of death following PTE surgery are variable and similar to those associated with other open-heart procedures. Cardiac arrest, multiorgan failure, uncontrollable mediastinal bleeding, sepsis syndrome, and massive pulmonary hemorrhage are among the causes of death cited.[47,48,52,55–58] In larger patient series, residual PH with right heart dysfunction, and acute lung injury represent the major causes for postoperative deaths.[32,56,57]

Long-term survivorship after hospital discharge has also been shown to be significantly better than could be expected in the absence of appropriate surgical intervention.[9] Examining a cohort of 532 patients followed for up to 19 years after endarterectomy, in which all causes of death were included, Archibald and colleagues[75] showed a 75% probability of survivorship beyond 6 years. Similar results have been reported by Freed and colleagues who reported conditional survival as 92.5% at 5 years and 88.3% at 10 years following hospital discharge.[76] Saouti and colleagues[53] described overall 1-, 3-, and 5- year survival rates of 93.1%, 91.2%, and 88.7% in a group of 72 patients undergoing an endarterectomy.

SMALL VESSEL DISEASE IN CTEPH

The concern regarding concomitant small vessel disease in CTEPH stems from 3 timely issues: (1) not all patients benefit from PTE as a result of significant concomitant small vessel disease,

(2) advances in medical therapies for the treatment of PAH are focusing on treating other secondary types of PH including CTEPH, and (3) defining the small vessel contribution to CTEPH may improve the approach to establishing operability and help formulate a preoperative classification system.

Although most patients with CTEPH undergoing PTE improve their PH and long-term outcomes, approximately 10% to 15% of patients undergoing PTE experience significant postoperative residual PH, as defined as a PVR of more than 500 $dyn \cdot s \cdot cm^{-5}$. It is unknown how many patients with a milder degree of residual PH develop late problems not as a result of recurrent thromboembolic disease but from their small vessel disease. The postoperative PVR of more than 500 $dyn \cdot s \cdot cm^{-5}$ is an important benchmark; in the series of 500 PTE cases reported from the University of California at San Diego (UCSD), the mortality difference between postoperative PVR greater or less than 500 $dyn \cdot s \cdot cm^{-5}$ was 30.6% compared with 0.9%, respectively.

The potential causes of postoperative residual PH are numerous. In experienced PTE centers, incomplete endarterectomy of proximal material is an unlikely cause. If an inexperienced surgeon attempted the initial surgery, this possibility needs to be considered by analyzing the specimen with the preoperative angiographic and perfusion scan data. In select cases of incomplete PTE or recurrent disease, repeating the PTE should be considered.[77] The more likely cause of residual PH in most cases is from concomitant small vessel disease. **Table 1** outlines the 3 possible scenarios described in the pathology literature and their plausible mechanisms.[21,78] Histopathologic similarities observed within the small vessels have suggested comparisons with PAH regarding the potential pathogenesis and possibility for targeted medical treatment. However, understanding the basis for the small vessel component in CTEPH, and even the formation of chronic thromboembolic material, remains rudimentary and in need of elucidation.

A better preoperative tool for the assessment of small vessel disease in CTEPH is required. The mere presence of small vessel disease is not predictive of PTE benefit because most patients studied have such lesions and yet most patients benefit from PTE. The critical distinction lies in the relative contribution of the small vessel disease to the overall PH; a 2-compartment problem in CTEPH, consisting of mechanical large vessel obstruction and varying degrees of small vessel remodeling. The current preoperative evaluations are good at identifying the former, but not the latter. Although efforts are ongoing to try to divine preoperatively those who may have significant component of inoperable disease, no single test seems reliable, nor validated, to base treatment decisions on at this time.[79–81] The solution may come in the form of genetic screening, biomarker, physiologic parameter, novel imaging, or a combination of these. With the ability to discern the degree of coexisting small vessel disease in patients with CTEPH, a better preoperative classification system can be developed.

Table 1
Possible mechanisms contributing to distal inoperable microvascular disease in CTEPH

Mechanism	Vascular Pathology	Features
1	Predominant obstructions of small subsegmental elastic pulmonary arteries	Occlusions of small arteries with stenoses, webs, and bands; Similarity/overlap with IPAH
2	Classic pulmonary arteriopathy of small muscular arteries and arterioles distal to nonobstructed elastic pulmonary arteries	Intimal proliferation and/or increased media thickness, plexiform lesions; Endothelial dysfunction possibly related to increased pressure and flow
3	Pulmonary arteriopathy of small muscular arteries and arterioles distal to partially or totally obstructed elastic pulmonary arteries	Endothelial dysfunction possibly related to poor perfusion and/or bronchial-to-pulmonary vascular anastomoses

From Galie N, Kim NHS. Pulmonary microvascular disease in chronic thromboembolic pulmonary hypertension. Proc Am Thorac Soc 2006;3:571–6; with permission.

MEDICAL THERAPIES FOR CTEPH

Whenever possible, the definitive, and potentially life-saving, therapy for CTEPH is surgical PTE. Attempts at medical PAH-specific therapy for this disease should never be used in an attempt to avoid or delay evaluation for surgically operable disease.[1] It is of concern that use of PAH-specific therapy before referral to the UCSD center has steadily increased in recent years,[34] and that this practice did not result in any discernible advantage in preoperative or postoperative hemodynamics.

Nonetheless, there are certain situations in which the use of PAH-specific therapies may be considered. These situations include (1) surgically inaccessible disease, (2) surgically accessible disease in those with comorbidities making the risk benefit ratio unfavorable for PTE, (3) those with accessible disease who refuse to undergo PTE, (4) before operations as a bridge in those with severe right ventricle (RV) dysfunction or severely increased PVR, (5) persistent PAH from distal small vessel arteriopathy despite PTE,[82] and (6) those with limited central disease but with PH out of proportion to the central clot burden who are therefore unlikely to benefit from PTE.[1,83] Although the indications for PAH-specific therapy have not been clearly established in these circumstances, this article gives a summary of the experience to date with such treatments for CTEPH.

Endothelin Receptor Antagonism

There is biologic plausibility for a role of endothelin-1 (ET-1) excess in CTEPH. Kim and colleagues[84] explored a rat model using PA ligation that demonstrated increased intimal, medial, and adventitial thickening of the small (<100 μm) pulmonary arteries, and increased endothelin A and B receptor staining was also observed. Similarly, in a canine model using repeated ceramic bead embolization, PVR, and mPAP increased at 8 months with concomitant increases in plasma and vessel wall ET-1.[25] In humans undergoing PTE for CTEPH big ET-1 plasma levels were increased, as were ET_B receptor mRNA transcripts and protein levels compared with age matched controls.[27] Furthermore, ET-1 levels in CTEPH have been shown to correlate closely with hemodynamics and clinical severity in one cohort of 35 patients with CTEPH.[85] This finding has led to several small open-label trials of bosentan in CTEPH,[86–90] showing improvements in a variety of endpoints including 6-minute walk distance (6 MWD), hemodynamics, WHO functional class, and N-terminal pro-brain natiuretic peptide (NT-pro-BNP) levels [Table 2]. Seyfarth and colleagues[91] described a longer-term experience in 12 patients with CTEPH on bosentan for 2 years, suggesting sustained benefit in 6 MWD and RV performance as assessed by the total ejection isovolume (TEI) index on echocardiographic follow-up. In addition, the Bo-CTEPH study suggested quality-of-life improvements in a 6 month follow-up.[92] An open-label, nonrandomized, placebo-controlled study by Vassallo and colleagues[93] placed 17 patients with CTEPH on bosentan and 17 on placebo. They found statistically significant improvements in 6 MWD, Borg Dyspnea Index, and arterial partial pressure of oxygen (Pao_2) in the bosentan treated cohort. However, in the only large, double-blind, randomized controlled trial of bosentan in CTEPH (BENEFiT trial), although statistically significant improvements in PVR, total pulmonary resistance (TPR), and CI were all seen after 4 months, mean treatment effect for 6 MWD was only +2.2 m (not statistically significant).[94] More recently, Reesink and colleagues[95] examined the role of bosentan as a bridge to PTE and concluded that there were modest hemodynamic benefits in the treated group, but that individual factors predisposing to a beneficial response needed to be further studied. To our knowledge, no published data exist for the use of other endothelin receptor antagonists in CTEPH.

Phosphodiesterase 5 Inhibitors

Biologic plausibility also exists for this pathway in a piglet model of CTEPH used by Fadel and colleagues.[96] In this model, PA ligation resulted in decreased endothelial nitric oxide synthase function and protein after 5 weeks.

The acute administration of sildenafil in 9 patients with inoperable distal CTEPH resulted in consistently greater drops in PVR and mPAP and greater improvements in cardiac output than did nitric oxide.[97] Several small open-label trials of sildenafil in this disease have implied clinical benefit (**Table 3**).[98–101] A larger (n = 104) and longer-term study with sildenafil demonstrated significant improvements in 6 MWD, CI, and PVR at 3 months, with 6 MWD remaining improved at 12 months.[102] Suntharalingam and colleagues[103] subsequently published their double-blind, randomized, placebo-controlled experience in 19 subjects with inoperable CTEPH. They found no statistically significant difference in exercise capacity as measured by 6 MWD at 3 months but concluded that the study was underpowered to test that endpoint. Beneficial effects in WHO functional class, quality of life, CI, PVR, and NT-pro-BNP at 12 months were seen in the 17 patients who entered the open-label extension study after the first 3 months.

Table 2
Early uncontrolled open-label experience with bosentan in CTEPH

References	No. of Patients	6 MWD (m)	Cardiac Output (L/min)	CI (L/min/m²)	PVR (dyn s cm⁻⁵)	mPAP (mm Hg)	WHO Class (% Change >1)	NT-pro-BNP (pg/mL)	Time (mo)
Hughes et al[86]	20	+45[a]		+0.4[a]	−247[a]	−3	15		3
Bonderman et al[87]	16	+92[a]						−1620[a]	6
Hoeper et al[88]	19	+90	+0.7[a]	+0.4[a]	−303[a]	−6[a]	21	−716	3
Segovia et al[89]	6	+83[a]			−240[a]			−1169[a]	12
Hughes et al[90]	47	+49		+0.2[a]	−75	−1	17		12

[a] Indicates statistically significant change.

Table 3
Early open-label experience with sildenafil in CTEPH

References	No. of Patients	mPAP (mm Hg)	PVR (dyn s cm^{-5})	Peripheral Vascular Resistance Index (dyn s cm^{-5}/m^2)	Cardiac Output (L/min)	CI (L/min/m^2)	6 MWD (m)	NYHA (% improved)	Time (mo)
Ghofrani et al[98]	12	−7.7		−574[a]		+0.4[a]	+54[a]		6.5
Sheth et al[99]	6	−9[a]		−92		+0.17		83	1.5
Rossi et al[100]	9	−5[a]				+0.2	+37	44	6
Chapman et al[101]	11	−6	−188[a]				+200		2–12

[a] Indicates statistically significant change.

Prostanoid Therapies

Several small trials evaluating beraprost sodium, iloprost, trepostinil, and epoprostenol exist in the literature.

Nagaya and colleagues[104] examined 30 patients with PH, 16 of whom had CTEPH. In patients with CTEPH after 3 months of beraprost therapy, increases in maximal oxygen uptake, peak work load, and ventilatory response to CO_2 could be shown on cardiopulmonary exercise testing. Ono and colleagues[105] also studied the effect of beraprost in 43 patients with inoperable CTEPH. In this study, 20 patients received beraprost and 23 got standard therapy. PVR, mPAP, and NYHA functional class were all improved in the beraprost-treated group compared with the standard therapy group. Dario Vizza and colleagues[106] compared the effect of beraprost in 16 patients with distal inoperable CTEPH with 8 patients with idiopathic PAH and concluded that similar beneficial effects in 6 MWD and WHO functional class could be found.

Acutely, administration of aerosolized iloprost to 20 patients with CTEPH was found to have favorable effects on PVR, mPAP, and cardiac output.[107] However, subgroup analysis of the 57 patients with CTEPH included in 203 total patients in the double-blind, randomized, placebo-controlled Asthma Intervention Research (AIR) trial[108] did not seem to benefit in the 3-month study.[83,109] Kramm and colleagues[110] studied the role of iloprost immediately before PTE, found no significant vasodilatation, and cautioned about the significant systemic hypotension they encountered. The same group randomized 11 patients with persistent PH after PEA to iloprost and 11 to nebulized saline and found that iloprost demonstrated statistically significant improvements in CI, PVR, and mPAP without worsening systemic oxygenation.[111]

The use of subcutaneous treprostinil in CTEPH was retrospectively examined by Lang and colleagues.[112] Ninety-nine PAH (WHO group 1) and 23 CTEPH were included in their analysis. Overall, the investigators showed improvements in 6 MWD, Borg Dyspnea Index, and NYHA functional class. Although subgroup analysis of the patients with CTEPH was not formally offered, the investigators stated that "results were consistent across the spectrum of PH including CTEPH." The same group subsequently offered an open-label 1-year trial of trepostinil in 25 patients with CTEPH.[113] The average dose of treprostinil achieved was 21 ($\pm$5) ng/kg/min. Six-minute walk distance improved by 105 m and hemodynamics and brain natriuretic peptide (BNP) also showed considerable improvements. One recent study suggested synergistic effects of inhaled treprostinil added to sildenafil in CTEPH.[114]

Small studies of patients with CTEPH receiving intravenous (IV) epoprostenol suggest benefit. Nagaya and colleagues[115] administered this drug in 33 such patients awaiting PEA and showed a 28% PVR reduction, BNP decreases, and low operative mortality in those with the most severe form of CTEPH (8.3%). Bresser and colleagues[116] studied 9 patients who received IV epoprostenol and who eventually underwent PTE. Six patients treated for 2 to 26 months experienced improvement or stability with a similar mean reduction in PVR by 28%. Three patients deteriorated while on IV epoprostenol. Scelsi and colleagues[117] studied 11 patients with surgically untreatable CTEPH for 1 year. Epoprostenol was associated with improved clinical status, NYHA functional class improvement, increases in 6 MWD (99 m), and improved echocardiographic features. Twenty-seven consecutive patients with inoperable CTEPH were studied with endpoints of 6 MWD and hemodynamics at 3 months and survival for up to 3 years.[109] Improvements in 6 MWD, CI, and TPR were seen. After 20 ($\pm$8) months, 9 out of 18 patients had improved by 1 or more NYHA functional class. Survival at 1, 2, and 3 years was 73%, 59%, and 41% respectively.

Soluble Guanylate Cyclase Stimulators

The use of riociguat, a direct soluble guanylate cyclase stimulator, in CTEPH was recently reported by Ghofrani and colleagues.[118] Forty-two patients with CTEPH and 33 patients with PAH were enrolled in the open-label phase II trial. Overall improvements in 6 MWD, NT-pro-BNP levels, WHO functional class, and dyspnea scores were noted. A multicenter, international phase III trial is currently underway to evaluate the efficacy of riociguat in patients with inoperable CTEPH or residual PH after PTE.

SUMMARY

CTEPH develops in at least 1% of acute pulmonary emboli events and is likely underdiagnosed. Because evidence of an acute pulmonary embolus event is lacking in 42% to 63% of patients with CTEPH, it is likely that the number of CTEPH cases is even greater than is projected from known acute thromboembolic events. In the absence of appropriate treatment, the prognosis is poor, with survivorship dependent on the severity of right heart failure at the time of diagnosis. Risk factors for the development of CTEPH include the overall extent of the vascular obstruction on initial embolization, the presence of antiphospholipid antibodies, lupus anticoagulant, or increased factor VII levels, prior splenectomy, presence of ventriculoatrial shunts to treat hydrocephalus, and certain chronic inflammatory disorders such as inflammatory bowel disease, osteomyelitis, or an infected pacemaker. The pathophysiologic mechanism resulting in the evolution of an acute embolus into chronic thromboembolic residua is uncertain but may in part have to do with genetically determined variants in fibrin side chains that make them resistant to lysis. Mechanical obstruction of the central pulmonary vasculature as the sole basis for increases in PVR occurs in the minority of patients with CTEPH. Evidence supports the role of pathologic changes in the distal vascular bed, both in lung regions directly involved with chronic thromboemboli and in uninvolved lung regions. Why this occurs is unknown, but may involve circulating vasoconstrictors, immune-related events, local upregulation of vascular growth factors, and individual genetic predisposition. Clinical diagnosis can be difficult because patients present with nonspecific symptoms and often without a history of documented venous thromboembolism. A careful and thorough evaluation is needed to avoid misdiagnosis because presentations mimic IPAH in many instances. The possibility of CTEPH should be considered in all patients with PH. Examination findings, chest radiograph, electrocardiograph, and echocardiographic findings are nonspecific. Although CT angiography and MRI may provide complementary information, they often miss the eccentric lesions of CTEPH. Accordingly, the VQ scan remains the screening study of choice for CTEPH. Ultimately, a right heart catheterization should be performed to assess the severity of right ventricular dysfunction and to allow PVR calculation because the latter is a strong and consistent predictor of postoperative risk. Pulmonary angiography remains the imaging modality of choice to define surgical candidacy. PTE is the preferred treatment of selected patients with CTEPH and, in most patients, is life altering. All patients should be assessed for surgical candidacy, preferably at an experienced center. In patients not eligible for PTE, PAH-specific medical therapies can be considered, although the indications for them have not been clearly established. The literature supporting their use has been largely from open-label, small trials that are subject to inherent bias. In the only large, randomized, double-blinded, placebo-controlled trial of bosentan in this disorder, hemodynamic benefits compared with placebo could be shown, but without demonstrable benefit to exercise tolerance as measured by the 6 MWD. Further investigation is needed to more clearly define the role of PAH-specific therapies in this disorder.

REFERENCES

1. Auger WR, Fedullo PF. Chronic thromboembolic pulmonary hypertension. Semin Respir Crit Care Med 2009;30(4):471–83.
2. Lang IM. Chronic thromboembolic pulmonary hypertension – not so rare after all. N Engl J Med 2004;350:2236–8.
3. Pengo V, Lensing AW, Prins MH, et al. Incidence of chronic thromboembolic pulmonary hypertension after pulmonary embolism. N Engl J Med 2004; 350(22):2257–64.
4. Becattini C, Agnelli G, Pesavento R, et al. Incidence of chronic thromboembolic pulmonary hypertension after a first episode of pulmonary embolism. Chest 2006;130:172–5.
5. Miniati M, Simonetta M, Bottai M, et al. Survival and restoration of pulmonary perfusion in a long-term follow-up of patients after pulmonary embolism. Medicine (Baltimore) 2006;85:253–62.
6. Silverstein MD, Heit JA, Mohr DN, et al. Trends in the incidence of deep vein thrombosis and pulmonary embolism: a 25-year population-based study. Arch Intern Med 1998;158:585–93.
7. Bonderman D, Jakowitsch J, Adlbrecht C, et al. Medical conditions increasing the risk of chronic thromboembolic pulmonary hypertension. Thromb Haemost 2005;93:512–6.
8. Condliffe R, Kiely DG, Gibbs JS, et al. Prognostic and aetiological factors in chronic thromboembolic pulmonary hypertension. Eur Respir J 2009;33(2): 332–8.
9. Riedel M, Stanek V, Widimsky J, et al. Long-term follow-up of patients with pulmonary thromboembolism: late prognosis and evolution of hemodynamic and respiratory data. Chest 1982;81:151–8.
10. Lewczuk J, Piszko P, Jagas J, et al. Prognostic factors in medically treated patients with chronic pulmonary embolism. Chest 2001;119:818–23.
11. Condliffe R, Kiely DG, Gibbs SR, et al. Improved outcomes in medically and surgically treated chronic thromboembolic pulmonary hypertension. Am J Respir Crit Care Med 2008;177:1122–7.
12. Liu P, Meneveau N, Schiele F, et al. Predictors of long-term clinical outcome in patients with acute massive pulmonary embolism after thrombolytic therapy. Chin Med J 2003;116:503–9.
13. Ribeiro A, Lindmarker P, Johnsson H, et al. Pulmonary embolism: one-year follow-up with echocardiography Doppler and five-year survival analysis. Circulation 1999;99:1325–30.
14. Wolf M, Boyer-Neumann C, Parent F, et al. Thrombotic risk factors in pulmonary hypertension. Eur Respir J 2000;15:395–9.

15. Bonderman D, Wilkens H, Wakounig S, et al. Risk factors for chronic thromboembolic pulmonary hypertension. Eur Respir J 2009;33(2):325–31.
16. Bonderman D, Turecek PL, Jakowitsch J, et al. High prevalence of elevated clotting factor VIII in chronic thromboembolic pulmonary hypertension. Thromb Haemost 2003;90:372–6.
17. Rosenhek R, Korschineck I, Gharehbaghi-Schnell E, et al. Fibrinolytic balance of the arterial wall: pulmonary artery displays increased fibrinolytic potential compared with aorta. Lab Invest 2003;83:871–6.
18. Lang IM, Marsh JJ, Olman MA, et al. Parallel analysis of tissue-type plasminogen activator and type 1 plasminogen activator inhibitor in plasma and endothelial cells derived from patients with chronic pulmonary thromboemboli. Circulation 1994;90:706–12.
19. Morris TA, Marsh JJ, Chiles PG, et al. Fibrin derived from patients with chronic thromboembolic pulmonary hypertension is resistant to lysis. Am J Respir Crit Care Med 2006;173:1270–5.
20. Morris TA, Marsh JJ, Chiles PG, et al. High prevalence of dysfibrinogenemia among patients with chronic thromboembolic pulmonary hypertension. Blood 2009;114(9):1929–36.
21. Moser KM, Bloor CM. Pulmonary vascular lesions occurring in patients with chronic major vessel thromboembolic pulmonary hypertension. Chest 1993;103:685–92.
22. Ryan KL, Fedullo PF, Davis GB, et al. Perfusion scan findings understate the severity of angiographic and hemodynamic compromise in chronic thromboembolic pulmonary hypertension. Chest 1988;93:1180–5.
23. Azarian R, Wartski M, Collignon MA, et al. Lung perfusion scans and hemodynamics in acute and chronic pulmonary embolism. J Nucl Med 1997;38:980–3.
24. Du L, Sullivan CC, Chu D, et al. Signaling molecules in nonfamilial pulmonary hypertension. N Engl J Med 2003;348:500–9.
25. Kim H, Yung GL, Marsh JJ, et al. Endothelin mediates pulmonary vascular remodeling in a canine model of chronic embolic pulmonary hypertension. Eur Respir J 2000;15:640–8.
26. Firth AL, Yau J, White A, et al. Chronic exposure to fibrin and fibrinogen differentially regulates intracellular Ca2+ in human pulmonary arterial smooth muscle and endothelial cells. Am J Physiol Lung Cell Mol Physiol 2009;296:L979–86.
27. Bauer M, Wilkens H, Langer F, et al. Selective upregulation of endothelin B receptor gene expression in severe pulmonary hypertension. Circulation 2002;105:1034–6.
28. Thistlethwaite PA, Lee SH, Du LL, et al. Human angiopoietin gene expression is a marker for severity of pulmonary hypertension in patients undergoing pulmonary thromboendarterectomy. J Thorac Cardiovasc Surg 2001;122:65–73.
29. Tanabe N, Kimura A, Amano S, et al. Association of clinical features with HLA in chronic pulmonary thromboembolism. Eur Respir J 2005;25:131–8.
30. Yao W, Firth AL, Sacks RS, et al. Identification of putative endothelial progenitor cells (CD34+CD133+Flk-1+) in endarterectomized tissue of patients with chronic thromboembolic pulmonary hypertension. Am J Physiol Lung Cell Mol Physiol 2009;296:L870–8.
31. Kapitan KS, Clausen JL, Moser KM. Gas exchange in chronic thromboembolism after pulmonary thromboendarterectomy. Chest 1990;98:14–9.
32. Jamieson SW, Kapelanski DP, Sakakibara N, et al. Pulmonary endarterectomy: experience and lessons learned in 1,500 cases. Ann Thorac Surg 2003;76:1457–62.
33. McGoon M, Gutterman D, Steen V, et al. Screening, early detection, and diagnosis of pulmonary arterial hypertension: ACCP evidence-based clinical practice guidelines. Chest 2004;126:14S–34S.
34. Jensen KW, Kerr KM, Fedullo PF, et al. Pulmonary hypertensive medical therapy in chronic thromboembolic pulmonary hypertension before pulmonary thromboendarterectomy. Circulation 2009;120:1248–54.
35. Simonneau G, Robbins IM, Beghetti M, et al. Updated clinical classification of pulmonary hypertension. J Am Coll Cardiol 2009;54:S43–54.
36. Auger WR, Moser KM. Pulmonary flow murmurs: a distinctive physical sign found in chronic pulmonary thromboembolic disease [abstract]. Clin Res 1989;37:145A.
37. Morris TA, Auger WR, Ysrael MZ, et al. Parenchymal scarring is associated with restrictive spirometric defects in patients with chronic thromboembolic pulmonary hypertension. Chest 1996;10:399–403.
38. Thistlethwaite PA, Auger WR, Madani MM, et al. Pulmonary thromboendarterectomy combined with other cardiac operations: indications, surgical approach, and outcome. Ann Thorac Surg 2001;72:13–9.
39. Daniels LB, Krummen DE, Blanchard DG. Echocardiography in pulmonary vascular disease. Cardiol Clin 2004;22:383–99.
40. Heinrich M, Uder M, Tscholl D, et al. CT scan findings in chronic thromboembolic pulmonary hypertension: predictors of hemodynamic improvement after pulmonary thromboendarterectomy. Chest 2005;127:1606–13.
41. Kreitner KF, Kunz RP, Ley S, et al. Chronic thromboembolic pulmonary hypertension: assessment by magnetic resonance imaging. Eur Radiol 2007;17:11–21.
42. Tunariu N, Gibbs SJR, Win Z, et al. Ventilation-perfusion scintigraphy is more sensitive than

multidetector CTPA in detecting chronic thrombo-embolic pulmonary disease as a treatable cause of pulmonary hypertension. J Nucl Med 2007;48:680—4.

43. Moser KM, Fedullo PF, Finkbeiner WE, et al. Do patients with primary pulmonary hypertension develop extensive central thrombi? Circulation 1995;91:741—5.

44. Cox JE, Chiles C, Aquino SL, et al. Pulmonary artery sarcomas: a review of clinical and radiologic features. J Comput Assist Tomogr 1997;21:750—5.

45. Lisbona R, Kreisman H, Novales-Diaz J, et al. Perfusion lung scanning: differentiation of primary from thromboembolic pulmonary hypertension. AJR Am J Roentgenol 1985;144:27—30.

46. Auger WR, Fedullo PF, Moser KM, et al. Chronic major-vessel thromboembolic pulmonary artery obstruction: appearance at angiography. Radiology 1992;182:393—8.

47. Hartz RS, Byme JG, Levitsky S, et al. Predictors of mortality in pulmonary thromboendarterectomy. Ann Thorac Surg 1996;62:1255—9.

48. Dartevelle P, Fadel E, Mussot S, et al. Chronic thromboembolic pulmonary hypertension. Eur Respir J 2004;23:637—48.

49. Keogh AM, Mayer E, Benza RL, et al. Interventional and surgical modalities of treatment in pulmonary hypertension. J Am Coll Cardiol 2009;54:S67—77.

50. Bonderman D, Skoro-Sajer N, Jakowitsch J, et al. Predictors of outcome in chronic thromboembolic pulmonary hypertension. Circulation 2007;115:2153—8.

51. Tscholl D, Langer F, Wendler O, et al. Pulmonary thromboendarterectomy — risk factors for early survival and hemodynamic improvement. Eur J Cardiothorac Surg 2001;19:771—6.

52. Thistlethwaite PA, Kaneko K, Madani M, et al. Technique and outcomes of pulmonary endarterectomy surgery. Ann Thorac Cardiovasc Surg 2008;14(5):274—82.

53. Saouti N, Morshuis WJ, Heijmen RH, et al. Long-term outcome after pulmonary endarterectomy for chronic thromboembolic pulmonary hypertension: a single institution experience. Eur J Cardiothorac Surg 2009;35:947—52.

54. Ishida K, Masuda M, Tanaka H, et al. Mid-term results of surgery for chronic thromboembolic pulmonary hypertension. Interact Cardiovasc Thorac Surg 2009;9:626—9.

55. Ogino H, Ando M, Matsuda H, et al. Japanese single-center experience of surgery for chronic thromboembolic pulmonary hypertension. Ann Thorac Surg 2006;82:630—6.

56. Thomson B, Tsui SSL, Dunning J, et al. Pulmonary endarterectomy is possible and effective without the use of complete circulatory arrest - the UK experience in over 150 patients. Eur J Cardiothorac Surg 2008;33:157—63.

57. Rubens FD, Bourke M, Hynes M, et al. Surgery for chronic thromboembolic pulmonary hypertension - inclusive experience from a national referral center. Ann Thorac Surg 2007;83:1075—81.

58. D'Armini AM, Cattadori B, Monterosso C, et al. Pulmonary thromboendarterectomy in patients with chronic thromboembolic pulmonary hypertension: hemodynamic characteristics and changes. Eur J Cardiothorac Surg 2000;18:696—702.

59. Mellemkjaer S, Ilkjaer LB, Klaaborg KE, et al. Pulmonary endarterectomy for chronic thromboembolic pulmonary hypertension. Ten years experience in Denmark. Scand Cardiovasc J 2006;40:49—53.

60. Madani M, Jamieson SW. Technical advances of pulmonary endarterectomy for chronic thromboembolic pulmonary hypertension. Semin Thorac Cardiovasc Surg 2006;18:243—50.

61. Mayer E, Klepetko W. Techniques and outcome of pulmonary endarterectomy for chronic thromboembolic pulmonary hypertension. Proc Am Thorac Soc 2006;3:589—93.

62. Zund G, Pretre R, Niederhauser U, et al. Improved exposure of the pulmonary arteries for thromboendarterectomy. Ann Thorac Surg 1998;66:1821—3.

63. Christian Hagl, Khaladj N, Peters T, et al. Technical advances of pulmonary thromboendarterectomy for chronic thromboembolic pulmonary hypertension. Eur J Cardiothorac Surg 2003;23:776—81.

64. Mikus PM, Mikus E, Martin-Suarez S, et al. Pulmonary endarterectomy: an alternative to circulatory arrest and deep hypothermia: mid-term results. Eur J Cardiothorac Surg 2008;34:159—63.

65. Blanchard DG, Malouf PJ, Gurudevan SV, et al. Utility of right ventricular Tei index in the noninvasive evaluation of chronic thromboembolic pulmonary hypertension before and after pulmonary thromboendarterectomy. JACC Cardiovasc Imaging 2009;2:143—9.

66. Reesink HJ, Marcus JT, Tulevski II, et al. Reverse right ventricular remodeling after pulmonary endarterectomy in patients with chronic thromboembolic pulmonary hypertension: utility of magnetic resonance imaging to demonstrate restoration of the right ventricle. J Thorac Cardiovasc Surg 2007;133(1):58—64.

67. Iino M, Dymarkowski S, Chaothawee L, et al. Time course of reversed cardiac remodeling after pulmonary endarterectomy in patients with chronic pulmonary thromboembolism. Eur Radiol 2008;18:792—9.

68. Tanabe N, Okada O, Nakagawa Y, et al. The efficacy of pulmonary thromboendarterectomy on long-term gas exchange. Eur Respir J 1997;10:2066—72.

69. Van der Plas MN, Reesink HJ, Roos CM, et al. Pulmonary endarterectomy improves dyspnea by the relief of dead space ventilation. Ann Thorac Surg 2010;89:347–52.

70. Matsuda H, Ogino H, Minatoya K, et al. Long-term recovery of exercise ability after pulmonary endarterectomy for chronic thromboembolic pulmonary hypertension. Ann Thorac Surg 2006;82:1338–43.

71. Reesink HJ, van der Plas MN, Verhey NE, et al. Six-minute walk distance as parameter of functional outcome after pulmonary for chronic thromboembolic pulmonary hypertension. J Thorac Cardiovasc Surg 2007;133(2):510–6.

72. Zoia MC, D'Armini AM, Beccaria M, et al. Mid term effects of pulmonary thromboendarterectomy on clinical and cardiopulmonary function status. Thorax 2002;57:608–12.

73. Kramm T, Mayer E, Dahm M, et al. Long-term results after thromboendarterectomy for chronic pulmonary embolism. Eur J Cardiothorac Surg 1999;15:579–84.

74. Corsico AG, D'Armini AM, Cerveri I, et al. Long term outcome after pulmonary thromboendarterectomy. Am J Respir Crit Care Med 2008;178:419–24.

75. Archibald CJ, Auger WR, Fedullo PF, et al. Long-term outcome after pulmonary thromboendarterectomy. Am J Respir Crit Care Med 1999;160:523–8.

76. Freed DH, Thomson BM, Tsui SL, et al. Functional and hemodynamic outcome 1 year after pulmonary thromboendarterectomy. Eur J Cardiothorac Surg 2008;34:525–30.

77. Mo M, Kapelanski DP, Mitruka SN, et al. Reoperative pulmonary thromboendarterectomy. Ann Thorac Surg 1999;68:1770–6.

78. Yi ES, Kim H, Ahn H, et al. Distribution of obstructive intimal lesions and their cellular phenotypes in chronic pulmonary hypertension: a morphometric and immunohistochemical study. Am J Respir Crit Care Med 2000;162:1577–86.

79. Kim NHS, Fesler P, Channick RN, et al. Preoperative partitioning of pulmonary vascular resistance correlates with early outcome after thromboendarterectomy for chronic thromboembolic pulmonary hypertension. Circulation 2004;109:18–22.

80. Hardziyenka M, Reesink HJ, Bouma BJ, et al. A novel echocardiographic predictor of in-hospital mortality and mid-term haemodynamic improvement after pulmonary endarterectomy for chronic thromboembolic pulmonary hypertension. Eur Heart J 2007;28:842–9.

81. Skoro-Sajer N, Mittermayer F, Panzenboeck A, et al. Asymmetric dimethylarginine is increased in chronic thromboembolic pulmonary hypertension. Am J Respir Crit Care Med 2007;176:1154–60.

82. Galie N, Kim NHS. Pulmonary microvascular disease in chronic thromboembolic pulmonary hypertension. Proc Am Thorac Soc 2006;3:571–6.

83. Bresser P, Pepke-Zaba J, Jais X, et al. Medical therapies for chronic thromboembolic pulmonary hypertension. Proc Am Thorac Soc 2006;3:594–600.

84. Kim H, Yung GL, Konopka RG, et al. Pulmonary vascular remodeling distal to pulmonary artery ligation is accompanied by upregulation of endothelin receptors and nitric oxide synthase. Exp Lung Res 2000;26:287–301.

85. Reesink H, Meijer RC, Lutter R, et al. Hemodynamic and clinical correlates of endothelin-1 in chronic thrombembolic pulmonary hypertension. Circ J 2006;70:1058–63.

86. Hughes R, George P, Parameshwar J, et al. Bosentan in inoperable chronic thromboembolic pulmonary hypertension. Thorax 2005;60:707.

87. Bonderman D, Nowotny R, Skoro-Sajer N, et al. Bosentan therapy for inoperable chronic thromboembolic pulmonary hypertension. Chest 2005;128:2599–603.

88. Hoeper MM, Kramm T, Wilkens H, et al. Bosentan therapy for inoperable chronic thromboembolic pulmonary hypertension. Chest 2005;128(4):2363–7.

89. Segovia C, Ortiz UJC, Gomez Bueno M, et al. [Role of bosentan in patients with chronic venous thromboembolic pulmonary hypertension]. Med Clin (Barc) 2007;128(1):12–4 [in Spanish].

90. Hughes RJ, Jais X, Bonderman D, et al. The efficacy of bosentan in inoperable chronic thromoboembolic pulmonary hypertension: a 1 year follow-up study. Eur Respir J 2006;28(1):138–43.

91. Seyfarth HJ, Hammerschmidt S, Pankau H, et al. Long-term bosentan in chronic thromboembolic pulmonary hypertension. Respiration 2007;74:287–92.

92. Ulrich S, Speich R, Domenighetti G, et al. Bosentan therapy for chronic thromboembolic pulmonary hypertension. Swiss Med Wkly 2007;137:573–80.

93. Vassallo FB, Kodric M, Scarduelli C, et al. Bosentan for patients with chronic thrombembolic pulmonary hypertension. Eur J Intern Med 2009;20:24–9.

94. Jais X, D'Armini AM, Jansa P, et al. Bosentan for treatment of inoperable chronic thromboembolic pulmonary hypertension. J Am Coll Cardiol 2008;52(25):2127–34.

95. Reesink H, Surie S, Kloek JJ, et al. Bosentan as a bridge to pulmonary endarterectomy for chronic thromboembolic pulmonary hypertension. J Thorac Cardiovasc Surg 2010;139:85–91.

96. Fadel E, Mazmanian GM, Baudet B, et al. Endothelial nitric oxide synthase function in pig lung after chronic pulmonary artery obstruction. Am J Respir Crit Care Med 2000;162:1429–34.

97. Suntharalingam J, Hughes RJ, Goldsmith K, et al. Acute hemodynamic responses to inhaled nitric oxide and intravenous sildenafil in distal chronic thromboembolic pulmonary hypertension (CTEPH). Vascul Pharmacol 2007;46:449–55.

98. Ghofrani HA, Schermuly RT, Rose F, et al. Sildenafil for long-term treatment of non-operable chronic thromboembolic pulmonary hypertension. Am J Respir Crit Care Med 2003;167:1139–41.

99. Sheth A, Park JES, Ong YE, et al. Early hemodynamic benefit of sildenafil in patients with coexisting chronic thromboembolic pulmonary hypertension and left ventricular dysfunction. Vascul Pharmacol 2005;42:41–5.

100. Rossi R, Nuzzo A, Lattanzi A, et al. Sildenafil improves endothelial function in patients with pulmonary hypertension. Pulm Pharmacol Ther 2008;21:172–7.

101. Chapman TH, Wilde M, Sheth A, et al. Sildenafil therapy in secondary pulmonary hypertension: is there benefit in prolonged use? Vascul Pharmacol 2009;51:90–5.

102. Reichenberger F, Voswinckel R, Rutsch M, et al. Long-term treatment with sildenafil in chronic thromboembolic pulmonary hypertension. Eur Respir J 2007;30:922–7.

103. Suntharalingam J, Treacy CM, Doughty NJ, et al. Long-term use of sildenafil in inoperable chronic thromboembolic pulmonary hypertension. Chest 2008;134:229–36.

104. Nagaya N, Shimizu Y, Satoh T, et al. Oral beraprost sodium improves exercise capacity and ventilatory efficiency in patients with primary or thromboembolic pulmonary hypertension. Heart 2002;87: 340–5.

105. Ono F, Nagaya N, Okumura H, et al. Effect of orally active prostacyclin analogue on survival in patients with chronic thromboembolic pulmonary hypertension without major vessel obstruction. Chest 2003; 123:1583–8.

106. Dario Vizza C, Badagliacca R, Sciomer S, et al. Mid-term effects of beraprost, an oral prostacylin analogue, in the treatment of distal CTEPH: a case control study. Cardiology 2006;106: 168–73.

107. Krug S, Hammerschmidt S, Pankau H, et al. Acute improved hemodynamics following inhaled iloprost in chronic thrombembolic pulmonary hypertension. Respiration 2008;76:154–9.

108. Olchewski H, Simonneau G, Galie N, et al. Inhaled iloprost for severe pulmonary hypertension. N Engl J Med 2002;347:322–9.

109. Cabrol S, Souza R, Jais X, et al. Intravenous epoprostenol in inoperable chronic thromboembolic pulmonary hypertension. J Heart Lung Transplant 2007;26:357–62.

110. Kramm T, Eherle B, Krummenauer F, et al. Inhaled iloprost in patients with chronic thromboembolic pulmonary hypertension: effects before and after pulmonary thromboendarterectomy. Ann Thorac Surg 2003;76:711–8.

111. Kramm T, Eberle B, Guth S, et al. Inhaled iloprost to control residual pulmonary hypertension following pulmonary endarterectomy. Eur J Cardiothorac Surg 2005;28:882–8.

112. Lang I, Gomez-Sanches M, Kneussl M, et al. Efficacy of long-term subcutaneous treprostinil in pulmonary hypertension. Chest 2006;129:1636–43.

113. Skoro-Sajer N, Boderman D, Wiesbauer F, et al. Treprostinil for severe inoperable chronic thromboembolic pulmonary hypertension. J Thromb Haemost 2007;5:483–9.

114. Voswinckel R, Reichenberger F, Enke B, et al. Acute effects of the combination of sildenafil and inhaled treprostinil on haemodynamics and gas exchange in pulmonary hypertension. Pulm Pharmacol Ther 2008;21:824–32.

115. Nagaya N, Sasaki N, Ando M, et al. Prostacylin therapy before pulmonary thromboendarterectomy in patients with chronic thromboembolic pulmonary hypertension. Chest 2003;123(2):338–43.

116. Bresser P, Fedullo PF, Auger WR, et al. Continuous intravenous epoprostenol for chronic thromboembolic pulmonary hypertension. Eur Respir J 2004; 23:595–600.

117. Scelsi L, Ghio S, Campana C, et al. Epoprostenol in chronic thromboembolic pulmonary hypertension with distal lesions. Ital Heart J 2004;5(8):618–23.

118. Ghofrani HA, Hoeper MM, Hoefken G, et al. Riociguat dose titration in patients with chronic thromboembolic pulmonary hypertension (CTEPH) or pulmonary arterial hypertension (PAH) [abstract]. Am J Respir Crit Care Med 2009;179:A3337.

Mortality Risk Assessment and the Role of Thrombolysis in Pulmonary Embolism

Mareike Lankeit, MD[a], Stavros Konstantinides, MD[b],*

KEYWORDS

- Pulmonary embolism • Thrombolysis • Risk assessment
- Mortality risk

Acute venous thromboembolism remains a frequent disease, with an incidence that ranges between 23 and 69 cases per 100,000 population per year.[1,2] Of these patients, approximately one-third present with clinical symptoms of acute pulmonary embolism (PE) and two-thirds with deep venous thrombosis (DVT).[3] Unfortunately, morbidity and mortality associated with acute PE remain high despite the recent advances in noninvasive imaging modalities, notably computed tomographic pulmonary angiography, and of the highly effective therapeutic options currently available. Case fatality rates vary widely depending on the clinical severity of the thromboembolic episode,[4–7] but large recent registries and cohort studies suggest that approximately 10% of all patients with acute PE die during the first 1 to 3 months after diagnosis.[8,9] In the United States, venous thromboembolism may contribute to as many as 100,000 deaths each year.[10] Overall, 1% of all patients admitted to hospitals die of acute PE, and 10% of all hospital deaths are PE-related.[11–13] These facts emphasize the need to better implement our knowledge on the pathophysiology of the disease, recognize the determinants of death or major adverse events in the early phase of acute PE, and most importantly, identify those patients who necessitate prompt medical, surgical, or interventional treatment to restore the patency of the pulmonary vasculature.

DEFINING HIGH-RISK PE

Acute PE is not universally life threatening, but rather covers a wide spectrum of clinical severity and death risk. In various studies, early (30-day or in-hospital) mortality rates were reported to range between less than 1% and well over 50%, mostly depending on the baseline clinical profile of the patients studied.[4–9,14]

It is now well established that the principal pathophysiological factor that determines disease severity and consequently the patients' clinical course and risk of death over the short term is the presence or absence of right ventricular (RV) dysfunction and failure resulting from acute pressure overload.[15] Almost 4 decades ago, it was found that increased pulmonary artery pressure may develop in up to 60% to 70% of patients who suffer acute PE, particularly when the emboli obstruct more than one-third of the area of the pulmonary vasculature. It has repeatedly been emphasized, however, that the magnitude of pulmonary artery hypertension and, as a result, the extent of RV pressure overload, is only roughly (and unreliably) related to thrombus burden and the severity of anatomic obstruction.[16–18] This complexity is due to the involvement of numerous pathophysiological variables, which include platelet activation, pulmonary vasoconstriction, and sympathetic (inotropic) stimulation of the heart. Once the

[a] Department of Cardiology and Pulmonology, Georg August University of Göttingen, Germany
[b] Department of Cardiology, Democritus University of Thrace, University General Hospital, 68100 Alexandroupolis, Greece
* Corresponding author.
E-mail address: skonst@med.duth.gr

Clin Chest Med 31 (2010) 759–769
doi:10.1016/j.ccm.2010.06.007
0272-5231/10/$ – see front matter © 2010 Elsevier Inc. All rights reserved.

patient develops RV pressure overload, persistent myocardial ischemia (even in the absence of maintained coronary flow to the right ventricle), preexisting cardiovascular disease or other serious comorbidity, and the presence of a patent foramen ovale with right to left shunt and serious arterial hypoxemia, may further enhance the hemodynamic impact of the thromboembolic event.[19–23] The interplay of all these factors, each one of which, if present, may be more or less pronounced in the individual patient, determines the development and extent of acute RV dysfunction. This latter event may in turn initiate a vicious circle of increased myocardial oxygen demand, myocardial ischemia or even infarction, leftward septal displacement, and left ventricular preload reduction, which ultimately lead to cardiogenic shock and death.[15]

Based on these pathophysiological mechanisms and their impact on the patients' prognosis, it has been proposed that clinical assessment of PE severity should focus on PE-related early death risk rather than reflect the volume, shape, or distribution of intrapulmonary emboli as determined by various imaging modalities. Accordingly, the recently updated guidelines of the European Society of Cardiology have introduced the terms high-risk and non-high-risk (the latter including intermediate-risk and low-risk) PE in an attempt to replace potentially confusing definitions such as "massive," "nonmassive" or "submassive" PE, which may be used in a different sense among pathologists, radiologists, and clinicians caring for the patient.[24,25] According to this updated nomenclature, "clinically massive" high-risk PE indicates overt RV failure that results in refractory arterial hypotension and shock (ie, systolic blood pressure <90 mm Hg, or a pressure drop ≥40 mm Hg for at least 15 minutes). This condition accounts for almost 5% of all cases of acute PE and is associated with a high risk of in-hospital death, particularly during the first hours after admission.[5,26,27] On the other hand, in the absence of hemodynamic instability, patients are generally thought to have a favorable clinical outcome provided that the disease is diagnosed correctly and anticoagulation can be instituted without delay.[14,28]

RISK-ADJUSTED DIAGNOSTIC APPROACH TO PE

Numerous multistep algorithms have been proposed and prospectively validated for the diagnostic workup of normotensive patients with suspected PE. Recent algorithms are based on the superior diagnostic sensitivity and specificity of multidetector-row computed tomography (MDCT)/pulmonary angiography, and its ability to confirm and in particular safely exclude PE without the need for venous ultrasound as an intermediate step.[25,29–31] On the other hand, management of the hemodynamically unstable, hypotensive patient with suspected high-risk PE should, as in all emergency situations, direct the focus not on perfect diagnostic accuracy but rather on immediate availability of the diagnostic modality, and on whether it offers the ability to begin life-saving treatment as rapidly as possible. The latter treatment consists of recanalization of the pulmonary vasculature with thrombolytic agents or surgery/intervention to reverse RV pressure overload and failure. Clinical probability is usually high in this setting, and there is no rationale for performing a time-consuming D-dimer test in such a life-threatening situation. Thus, according to the algorithm proposed in recent guidelines,[25] if MDCT pulmonary angiography is not readily available or the transfer to the Radiology Department is deemed unsafe for the unstable patient, a bedside echocardiogram is the quickest and thus most appropriate imaging test for confirming the presence of acute RV failure. Additional information that can be obtained from ultrasound imaging includes the presence of large floating intracardiac thrombi, which indicate an imminent threat of recurrent, potentially fatal PE.[32] Finally, if RV dysfunction can be excluded, echocardiography may provide alternative explanations for the patient's hypotension and shock such as left ventricular failure due to cardiomyopathy or large myocardial infarction, critical valvular disease, pericardial tamponade, or aortic dissection. In mechanically ventilated patients, transesophageal echocardiography is a useful alternative to transthoracic imaging, permitting direct visualization of possible thrombi in the right atrium, foramen ovale, right ventricle, or the proximal segments of the common and right pulmonary artery.

Conventional pulmonary angiography is rarely necessary in acute high-risk PE. However, it may be a valuable diagnostic option in selected cases, particularly when the patient is already in the catheterization laboratory due, for example, to suspected myocardial infarction, or if catheter-based aspiration or fragmentation of the pulmonary thrombus is being considered.[33,34]

BENEFITS OF THROMBOLYSIS IN ACUTE PE

In view of the high early mortality and complication risk associated with high-risk PE,[5,26,27] existing guidelines[25,35] and the overwhelming majority of experts and clinicians agree that patients who present with persistent arterial hypotension or shock are in need of immediate pharmacologic or mechanical recanalization of the occluded pulmonary arteries.

In early reports dating back to 1971, streptokinase infusion over 72 hours resulted in a significant reduction of systolic pulmonary artery pressure, total pulmonary resistance, and the angiographic index of PE severity; in comparison, conventional heparin anticoagulation appeared to have no appreciable effect on these parameters during the first 3 days.[36] Subsequently, several randomized trials[37-44] published between 1973 and 1993 showed that thrombolytic therapy with urokinase, streptokinase, or alteplase was capable of reducing thromboembolic obstruction, as assessed by pulmonary angiography, more rapidly than endogenous thrombolysis aided by heparin anticoagulation. The short-term benefits of thrombolytic agents also extended to hemodynamic parameters and the improvement of RV function as determined by right heart catheterization or echocardiography. On the other hand, these trials were unable to show that thrombolysis may also improve the short- or long-term clinical outcome of patients with acute PE. Although this may partly be due to the small size of most of them,[38-43] the explanation probably lies in that they did not focus on patients at high risk of early PE-related death as possible candidates for thrombolytic treatment. In this regard, the hemodynamic benefits of thrombolysis over heparin alone are confined to the first few days after acute PE, and studies performed in the late 1960s indicated that endogenous thrombolysis supported by heparin anticoagulation was (also) capable of reversing pulmonary artery hypertension within a 3-week (or longer) period in most cases.[45] More recently, trials directly comparing thrombolysis with heparin and including follow-up angiographic or echocardiographic studies showed that 1 week after treatment, the improvement in the severity of vascular obstruction[37,43] and the reversal of RV dysfunction[46] no longer differed between thrombolysis-treated and heparin-treated patients. Thus, it is important to consider thrombolysis only in those cases in which a high probability of early (ie, within the first few hours or days after presentation) PE-related death is anticipated.

POTENTIAL RISKS OF THROMBOLYSIS

Pooled data from controlled thrombolysis trials in PE, which either compared thrombolysis with heparin alone or different thrombolytic regimens with each other,[37,41,43,47-54] revealed a 13% cumulative rate of major bleeding and a 1.8% rate of intracranial/fatal hemorrhage.[55] Major hemorrhage has been less common in the most recent (and largest) trials,[44,47] in agreement with the notion that thrombolysis-related bleeding rates may be lower when noninvasive imaging methods are used to diagnose PE. Noninvasive diagnostic strategies have increasingly been adopted over the past 10 years thanks to the technical advances in computed tomographic (CT) pulmonary angiography.[24] On the other hand, retrospective cohort studies and registries have suggested a 36% incidence of major bleeding events and a 4% rate of intracranial/fatal hemorrhage following thrombolysis for PE.[4,5,56,57] These rates may be inappropriately high, because registries are likely to include patients who have received thrombolysis despite the presence of formal contraindications.[5] At the same time, however, registry data may better reflect everyday clinical practice compared with controlled trials. In any case, all the results presented here highlight the importance of carefully selecting the candidates for thrombolysis in acute PE, being particularly cautious in those who appear hemodynamically stable at presentation.

CURRENT USE OF THROMBOLYSIS IN ACUTE PE WITH HIGH RISK FOR EARLY DEATH

Although the angiographic and hemodynamic benefits of thrombolysis are unequivocal, at least over the short term, the (presumed) favorable effects of thrombolysis on the clinical outcome of patients with PE have thus far not been convincingly demonstrated. As already mentioned, this partly relies on the fact that the majority of thrombolysis trials in PE were too small to address clinical end points. Even the most recent and largest of these trials failed to show a survival benefit,[44,47] possibly because they included "low-risk" patients whose mortality rate in the acute phase could not be further reduced by immediate recanalization.

Pooled data from 5 trials that included hemodynamically unstable patients have suggested a significant reduction of death or PE recurrence after thrombolysis in this group (from 19.0% to 9.4%; odds ratio [OR], 0.45; 95% confidence interval [CI], 0.22–0.92).[58] In this regard, hemodynamic instability is commonly defined as need for cardiopulmonary resuscitation, systolic blood pressure <90 mm Hg or a drop of systolic blood pressure by $\geq$40 mm Hg for $\geq$15 minutes with signs of end-organ hypoperfusion, or need for catecholamine infusion to maintain adequate organ perfusion and a systolic blood pressure $\geq$90 mm Hg. If PE is clinically suspected, such patients should immediately receive a weight-adjusted bolus of unfractionated heparin while awaiting the results of further diagnostic workup; as soon as PE is confirmed, thrombolysis should be administered without delay. As many as 92% of these patients may respond favorably to thrombolysis, judging by their clinical and echocardiographic improvement within the first 36 hours.[59] The greatest benefit is observed when treatment is initiated within 48 hours of symptom onset,[39] but thrombolysis can still be beneficial to patients who have had symptoms for as long as 6 to 14 days.[60] If thrombolysis is absolutely contraindicated or has failed, surgical embolectomy or catheter-based thrombus fragmentation and aspiration is a valuable alternative.[33,34] Thrombolysis may also be considered in patients with PE and free-floating thrombi in the right heart if the risk of open heart surgery is deemed extremely high.[61,62]

Validated and tested regimens of thrombolytic agents are shown in **Table 1**, which also reviews the absolute and relative contraindications to thrombolysis. Regarding the performance of various thrombolytic regimens in head-to-head comparisons, the Urokinase-Streptokinase Pulmonary Embolism Trial (USPET) documented

similar efficacy of urokinase (UK) and streptokinase (SK) infused over a period of 12 to 24 hours.[54] In more recent randomized comparison trials,[51,52] 100 mg of recombinant tissue plasminogen activator (rtPA) infused over 2 hours led to faster angiographic and hemodynamic improvement compared with UK infused over 12 or 24 hours at the rate of 4400 U/kg/h. However, the results no longer differed at the end of the UK infusion. Similarly, the 2-hour infusion of rtPA appeared to be superior to a 12-hour SK infusion (at 100,000 U/h), but no difference was observed when the same SK dosage was also given over 2 hours.[63,64] Furthermore, 2 trials that compared the 2-hour, 100-mg rtPA regimen with a short infusion (over 15 minutes) of 0.6 mg/kg rtPA reported a slightly faster improvement with the 2-hour regimen at the cost of slightly (nonsignificantly) higher bleeding rates.[49,65] Thus, the thrombolytic regimens tested to date appear to be more or less comparable in terms of efficacy, but long infusions periods of the older thrombolytics SK or UK should generally be avoided.

Table 1
Thrombolytic agents, regimens, and contraindications

Agent	Regimen		Contraindications to Thrombolysis[25]
Streptokinase[a]	250,000 U as a loading dose over 30 min, followed by 100,000 U per hour over 12–24 h		*Absolute*
	Accelerated regimen: 1.5 million IU over 2 h[b]		History of hemorrhagic stroke or stroke of unknown origin
Urokinase[a,c]	4400 U/kg body weight as a loading dose over 10 min, followed by 4400 U/kg/h over 12–24 h		Ischemic stroke in previous 6 months Central nervous system neoplasms
	Accelerated regimen: 3 million U over 2 h[b]		Major trauma, surgery, or head injury in previous 3 weeks
Alteplase[a]	100 mg over 2 h[d]		*Relative*
	Accelerated regimen: 0.6 mg/kg over 15 min		Transient ischemic attack in previous 6 months
Reteplase[a,e]	Two bolus injections of 10 U 30 min apart		Oral anticoagulation
Tenecteplase[f]	30–50 mg bolus over 5–10 s adjusted for body weight:		Pregnancy or first postpartum week
	<60 kg:	30 mg	Noncompressible puncture sites
	≥60 to <70 kg:	35 mg	Traumatic resuscitation
	≥70 to <80 kg:	40 mg	Refractory hypertension (systolic
	≥80 to <90 kg:	45 mg	blood pressure >180 mm Hg)
	≥90 kg:	50 mg	Advanced liver disease
			Infective endocarditis
			Active peptic ulcer

[a] Unfractionated heparin should not be infused together with streptokinase or urokinase; it can be given during alteplase or reteplase administration. Low molecular weight heparins have not been tested in combination with thrombolysis in patients with pulmonary embolism.
[b] Short (2-hour) infusion periods are generally recommended.
[c] Urokinase is available in some European countries, not in the United States.
[d] Food and Drug Administration–approved regimen.
[e] Off-label use of reteplase.
[f] Off-label use of tenecteplase; this is the regimen recommended for acute myocardial infarction. A recent randomized pilot trial[67] found it to be safe and effective in nonhigh-risk PE.
Adapted from Konstantinides S. Clinical practice. Acute pulmonary embolism. N Engl J Med 2008;359(26):2804–13; with permission.

Satisfactory hemodynamic results have also been obtained with double-bolus reteplase given as 2 injections (10 U) 30 minutes apart.[66] Furthermore, a multicenter randomized pilot trial demonstrated the feasibility and safety of tenecteplase, given as a weight-adjusted bolus corresponding to the regimen recommended for acute myocardial infarction, in acute nonhigh-risk PE.[67] However, neither reteplase nor tenecteplase are officially approved for treatment of PE at present.

POTENTIAL ROLE OF THROMBOLYSIS IN INTERMEDIATE-RISK (SUBMASSIVE) PE

At present, low molecular weight heparin or fondaparinux is considered adequate treatment for most normotensive patients with pulmonary embolism, whereas routine thrombolysis is generally not recommended as a first-line therapeutic option.[25,35] However, the results of the most recent randomized thrombolysis trial[47] can be interpreted as indicating that early thrombolysis may be considered in selected patients with "nonmassive," nonhigh-risk PE including, for example, those with comorbidities predisposing to an adverse outcome provided that these patients have no contraindications to thrombolytic treatment.

Who might then be a candidate for thrombolysis besides patients with high-risk PE? As already emphasized, RV dysfunction and failure is a crucial

pathophysiological event and the main determinant of prognosis in acute PE (**Fig. 1**). Therefore, its early detection and reversal before the patient develops hemodynamic instability and shock should have high priority in the management of the disease. Based on this concept, currently available tools and emerging strategies for identifying normotensive intermediate-risk patients with RV dysfunction and/or myocardial injury are discussed below. These tools might extend the indications for thrombolysis in acute PE in the future.

Diagnosis of RV Dysfunction in Normotensive Patients

Echocardiography is an imaging modality capable of detecting the changes occurring in the morphology and function of the right ventricle as a result of acute pressure overload. Several registries and cohort studies were able to demonstrate an association between various echocardiographic parameters and a poor in-hospital outcome in terms of PE-related death and complications.[14,28,44,68,69] The post hoc analysis of a large international registry further suggested that echocardiographically detected RV dysfunction is an independent predictor of adverse outcome in normotensive patients.[70] Nevertheless, the potential prognostic and, particularly, therapeutic

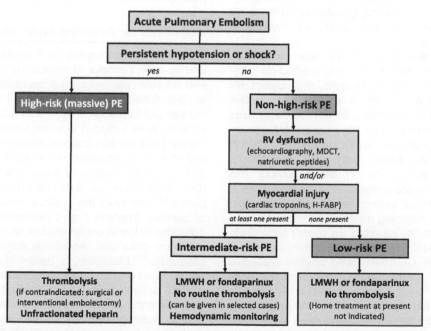

Fig. 1. Proposed risk-adjusted management algorithm for acute pulmonary embolism. H-FABP, heart-type fatty acid-binding protein; LMWH, low molecular weight heparin or fondaparinux; MDCT, multidetector-row computed tomography (pulmonary angiography); PE, pulmonary embolism; RV, right ventricle; UFH, unfractionated heparin.

implications of cardiac ultrasound findings for non-high-risk PE remain the subject of debate. The persisting uncertainty is mainly due to the lack of standardization of the echocardiographic criteria and the absence of adequately powered, controlled studies focusing on normotensive (rather than unselected) patients with PE.[71] Accordingly, a recent meta-analysis of 5 studies including a total of 475 normotensive patients with PE reported an only moderate overall negative (60%; 95% CI, 55%–65%) and positive (58%; 95% CI, 53%–63%) value of echocardiography for predicting early death, while also emphasizing the limitations due to the clinical and methodological diversity of the pooled publications.[72] The largest randomized thrombolysis trial in PE to date, which included 256 normotensive patients with RV dysfunction (mainly) detected by echocardiography, reported a significantly reduced incidence of the primary end point (30-day mortality or need for treatment escalation) in patients who underwent early thrombolysis as opposed to those treated with heparin alone. However, there was no significant influence of the type of treatment on mortality rates during the acute phase of PE.[47] It is thus likely that additional information beyond echocardiographic findings may be needed before the decision can be made to treat aggressively (with thrombolytic agents) a normotensive patient with acute PE. Recent preliminary reports suggest that the prognostic value of echocardiography can be improved if combined with biomarkers of myocardial injury.[73–75]

Four-chamber views of the heart on MDCT, which is currently the preferred method for diagnosing PE in most institutions, may detect RV enlargement due to PE. In a large retrospective series of 431 patients, 30-day mortality was 15.6% in patients with RV enlargement (reconstructed 4-chamber views), defined as right/left ventricular dimension ratio >0.9, on MDCT, compared with 7.7% in those without this finding.[76] A meta-analysis of 2 studies (with 2 different right/left ventricular diameter thresholds, 1.5 and 1.0) including a total of 191 normotensive patients with PE reported an overall 58% (95% CI, 51%–65%) negative predictive value and a 57% (95% CI, 49%–64%) positive predictive value of RV dilatation on CT for identifying early PE deaths.[72] Of course, these rates strongly depend on the characteristics of the populations studied, and a prospective evaluation of the prognostic value of CT indicators of RV dysfunction is still missing.

Natriuretic peptides are released as a result of cardiomyocyte stretch and are very sensitive indicators of neurohormonal activation due to ventricular dysfunction. The biologically active C-terminal peptide 77-108 (BNP) and the inactive N-terminal fragment 1-76 (NT-proBNP) are detectable in human plasma, and their levels have been determined and evaluated in patients presenting with acute PE.[77–80] In general, both BNP and NT-proBNP are characterized by very high prognostic sensitivity and a negative prognostic value, which is probably even higher than that of the cardiac troponins.[81] On the other hand, they exhibit a very low specificity and positive prognostic value in the range of 12% to 25%.[81] Furthermore, the optimal cut-off levels of BNP (or NT-proBNP) for distinguishing between a prognostically "favorable" versus "unfavorable" result in patients with PE have not yet been prospectively determined.[82] A recent meta-analysis of 13 studies found that 51% of the 1132 patients included had elevated BNP or NT-proBNP levels, and these were associated with an increased risk of early death (OR, 7.6; 95% CI, 3.4–17) and a complicated in-hospital course (OR, 6.8; 95% CI, 4.4–10).[83] Nevertheless, elevation of natriuretic peptides alone does not, by itself, justify more invasive treatment regimens. Evolving concepts of risk stratification suggest that the prognostic value of natriuretic peptides may be improved if they are combined with echocardiography,[73] or integrated into risk scores that also include clinical parameters and echocardiography.[84]

Biomarkers for Detecting Myocardial Injury

Elevated cardiac troponin I or T levels, a sensitive and specific indicator of myocardial cell damage and microscopic myocardial necrosis, are found in up to 50% of patients with acute PE.[85] Twenty studies published since 1998 with a total of 1985 patients were included in a meta-analysis, which showed that cardiac troponin elevation was associated with an increased risk of death (OR, 5.24; 95% CI, 3.28–8.38) and major adverse events (OR, 7.03; 95% CI, 2.42–20.43) in the acute phase.[86] However, the positive predictive value of cardiac troponin I or T elevation has been consistently low in cohort studies, so that troponin elevation does not necessarily indicate a poor prognosis.[81] Moreover, a recent meta-analysis that focused only on normotensive patients (a total of 1366 patients included in 9 studies) was unable to confirm the prognostic value of cardiac troponins in non-high-risk PE.[87] Thus, based on the available data, the current opinion is that troponin elevation alone does not suffice to risk-stratify normotensive patients with PE, and particularly to identify intermediate-risk patients who might necessitate early aggressive (for example, thrombolytic) treatment. A large ongoing randomized trial is currently investigating whether normotensive patients with RV dysfunction, detected by echocardiography or CT, plus evidence of myocardial injury indicated by a positive troponin test, may benefit from early thrombolytic treatment.[88]

Fatty acid–binding proteins (FABPs) are small cytoplasmic proteins that are abundant in tissues with active fatty acid metabolism, including the heart.[89] Heart-type FABP (H-FABP) is particularly important for myocardial homoeostasis, because 50% to 80% of the heart's energy is provided by lipid oxidation, and H-FABP ensures intracellular transport of insoluble fatty acids. Following myocardial cell damage, this small protein diffuses much more rapidly than troponins through the interstitial space and appears in the circulation as early as 90 minutes after symptom onset, reaching its peak within 6 hours.[90] These features make H-FABP an excellent candidate marker of myocardial injury,[91] and preliminary data suggested that it may provide prognostic information superior to that of cardiac troponins in acute PE.[92,93] These data were recently confirmed by a study focusing on nonhigh-risk patients with acute PE.[94]

Growth-differentiation factor 15 (GDF-15), a distant member of the transforming growth factor β cytokine family, is an emerging biomarker for patients with cardiovascular disease. In particular, GDF-15 appears capable of integrating information both on RV dysfunction and myocardial injury in patients with acute PE. In a cohort study of 123 consecutive patients with confirmed PE, elevated levels of GDF-15 on admission were strongly and independently related with an increased risk of death or major complications during the first 30 days after diagnosis. Moreover, the prognostic information provided by GDF-15 appeared to be additive to that of cardiac troponins and natriuretic peptides, and to echocardiographic findings of RV dysfunction. GDF-15 also emerged as an independent predictor of long-term mortality.[95]

THROMBOLYSIS IN CURRENT AND EMERGING CONCEPTS OF PE MANAGEMENT

Experts and recently updated guidelines agree that thrombolysis is indicated patients with acute PE who are at high risk for early death, that is, in patients presenting with arterial hypotension and shock or refractory hypoxemia. On the other hand, heparin (unfractionated or low molecular weight) or fondaparinux is adequate treatment for most normotensive patients with PE (see **Fig. 1**). Recombinant tissue plasminogen activator (alteplase), given as a 100-mg infusion over 2 hours, is considered the treatment of choice for patients with PE, although regimens using urokinase or streptokinase were also shown to be efficacious in the past. Reteplase and tenecteplase, if eventually approved for PE, may turn out to be practical alternatives. However, beyond the relatively small population of PE patients at high risk for death (5% of all patients) as a target population for thrombolysis, there is increasing awareness of the need for risk stratification of normotensive patients and the search for an intermediate-risk group (previously defined as having "submassive" PE).[96] Recent meta-analyses of cohort studies suggest that imaging of the right ventricle or biomarkers of myocardial injury alone may be insufficient for guiding therapeutic decisions. Instead, accumulating evidence appears to support strategies that combine the information provided by an imaging procedure (RV dysfunction on echocardiography or CT) with a biomarker test (RV myocardial injury indicated by elevated troponin I or T, or possibly H-FABP, GDF-15). Accordingly, a large multinational randomized trial has set out to determine whether normotensive, intermediate-risk patients with RV dysfunction, detected by echocardiography or CT, plus evidence of myocardial injury indicated by a positive troponin test, may benefit from early thrombolytic treatment (EudraCT number, 2006-005,328-18).[88] The primary efficacy end point is a clinical composite end point of all-cause mortality or hemodynamic collapse within the first 7 days. Safety end points are total strokes (intracranial hemorrhage or ischemic stroke) within 7 days, and major bleeds (other than intracranial hemorrhage) within 7 days. Six-month follow-up is also being conducted. This study, which is already underway in 12 European countries, plans to enroll a total of 1000 patients and will be completed in 2011.

REFERENCES

1. Silverstein MD, Heit JA, Mohr DN, et al. Trends in the incidence of deep vein thrombosis and pulmonary embolism: a 25-year population-based study. Arch Intern Med 1998;158(6):585–93.

2. Anderson FA Jr, Wheeler HB, Goldberg RJ, et al. A population-based perspective of the hospital incidence and case-fatality rates of deep vein thrombosis and pulmonary embolism. The Worcester DVT Study. Arch Intern Med 1991;151(5):933–8.

3. White RH. The epidemiology of venous thromboembolism. Circulation 2003;107(23 Suppl. 1):I4–8.

4. Goldhaber SZ, Visani L, De Rosa M. Acute pulmonary embolism: clinical outcomes in the International Cooperative Pulmonary Embolism Registry (ICOPER). Lancet 1999;353(9162):1386–9.

5. Kasper W, Konstantinides S, Geibel A, et al. Management strategies and determinants of outcome in acute major pulmonary embolism: results of a multicenter registry. J Am Coll Cardiol 1997;30(5):1165–71.

6. British Thoracic Society. Optimum duration of anticoagulation for deep-vein thrombosis and pulmonary embolism. Research Committee of the British Thoracic Society. Lancet 1992;340(8824):873–6.

7. Carson JL, Kelley MA, Duff A, et al. The clinical course of pulmonary embolism. N Engl J Med 1992;326(19):1240–5.

8. Aujesky D, Jimenez D, Mor MK, et al. Weekend versus weekday admission and mortality after acute pulmonary embolism. Circulation 2009;119(7): 962–8.

9. Laporte S, Mismetti P, Decousus H, et al. Clinical predictors for fatal pulmonary embolism in 15,520 patients with venous thromboembolism: findings from the Registro Informatizado de la Enfermedad TromboEmbolica venosa (RIETE) Registry. Circulation 2008;117(13):1711–6.

10. Internet Communication. Available at: http://www.surgeongeneral.gov/news/pressreleases/pr20080915.html. Accessed June 23, 2010.

11. Cohen AT, Agnelli G, Anderson FA, et al. Venous thromboembolism (VTE) in Europe. The number of VTE events and associated morbidity and mortality. Thromb Haemost 2007;98(4):756–64.

12. Cohen AT, Edmondson RA, Phillips MJ, et al. The changing pattern of venous thromboembolic disease. Haemostasis 1996;26(2):65–71.

13. Lindblad B, Sternby NH, Bergqvist D. Incidence of venous thromboembolism verified by necropsy over 30 years. BMJ 1991;302(6778):709–11.

14. Kasper W, Konstantinides S, Geibel A, et al. Prognostic significance of right ventricular afterload stress detected by echocardiography in patients with clinically suspected pulmonary embolism. Heart 1997;77(4):346–9.

15. Konstantinides S. Pulmonary embolism: impact of right ventricular dysfunction. Curr Opin Cardiol 2005;20(6):496–501.

16. Miller RL, Das S, Anandarangam T, et al. Association between right ventricular function and perfusion abnormalities in hemodynamically stable patients with acute pulmonary embolism. Chest 1998;113 (3):665–70.

17. McIntyre KM, Sasahara AA. Determinants of right ventricular function and hemodynamics after pulmonary embolism. Chest 1974;65(5):534–43.

18. McIntyre KM, Sasahara AA. The hemodynamic response to pulmonary embolism in patients without prior cardiopulmonary disease. Am J Cardiol 1971; 28(3):288–94.

19. Greyson C, Xu Y, Cohen J, et al. Right ventricular dysfunction persists following brief right ventricular pressure overload. Cardiovasc Res 1997;34(2): 281–8.

20. Schmitto JD, Doerge H, Post H, et al. Progressive right ventricular failure is not explained by myocardial ischemia in a pig model of right ventricular pressure overload. Eur J Cardiothorac Surg 2009;35(2): 229–34.

21. Chung T, Connor D, Joseph J, et al. Platelet activation in acute pulmonary embolism. J Thromb Haemost 2007;5(5):918–24.

22. Smulders YM. Pathophysiology and treatment of haemodynamic instability in acute pulmonary embolism: the pivotal role of pulmonary vasoconstriction. Cardiovasc Res 2000;48(1):23–33.

23. Konstantinides S, Geibel A, Kasper W, et al. Patent foramen ovale is an important predictor of adverse outcome in patients with major pulmonary embolism. Circulation 1998;97(19):1946–51.

24. Konstantinides S. Clinical practice. Acute pulmonary embolism. N Engl J Med 2008;359(26):2804–13.

25. Torbicki A, Perrier A, Konstantinides SV, et al. Guidelines on the diagnosis and management of acute pulmonary embolism: The Task Force for the Diagnosis and Management of Acute Pulmonary Embolism of the European Society of Cardiology (ESC). Eur Heart J 2008;29:2276–315.

26. Kucher N, Rossi E, De Rosa M, et al. Massive pulmonary embolism. Circulation 2006;113(4):577–82.

27. Stein PD, Henry JW. Prevalence of acute pulmonary embolism among patients in a general hospital and at autopsy. Chest 1995;108(4):978–81.

28. Grifoni S, Olivotto I, Cecchini P, et al. Short-term clinical outcome of patients with acute pulmonary embolism, normal blood pressure, and echocardiographic right ventricular dysfunction. Circulation 2000;101(24):2817–22.

29. Righini M, Le Gal G, Aujesky D, et al. Diagnosis of pulmonary embolism by multidetector CT alone or combined with venous ultrasonography of the leg: a randomised non-inferiority trial. Lancet 2008;371 (9621):1343–52.

30. Stein PD, Fowler SE, Goodman LR, et al. Multidetector computed tomography for acute pulmonary embolism. N Engl J Med 2006;354(22):2317–27.

31. van Belle A, Buller HR, Huisman MV, et al. Effectiveness of managing suspected pulmonary embolism using an algorithm combining clinical probability, D-dimer testing, and computed tomography. JAMA 2006;295(2):172–9.

32. Torbicki A, Galie N, Covezzoli A, et al. Right heart thrombi in pulmonary embolism: results from the International Cooperative Pulmonary Embolism Registry. J Am Coll Cardiol 2003;41(12):2245–51.

33. Eid-Lidt G, Gaspar J, Sandoval J, et al. Combined clot fragmentation and aspiration in patients with acute pulmonary embolism. Chest 2008;134(1): 54–60.

34. Kucher N, Goldhaber SZ. Mechanical catheter intervention in massive pulmonary embolism: proof of concept. Chest 2008;134(1):2–4.

35. Kearon C, Kahn SR, Agnelli G, et al. Antithrombotic therapy for venous thromboembolic disease: American College of Chest Physicians Evidence-Based Clinical Practice Guidelines (8th edition). Chest 2008;133(Suppl 6):454S–545.

36. Miller GA, Sutton GC, Kerr IH, et al. Comparison of streptokinase and heparin in treatment of isolated acute massive pulmonary embolism. Br Heart J 1971;33(4):616.

37. The urokinase pulmonary embolism trial. A national cooperative study. Circulation 1973;47(Suppl 2): II1–108.

38. Tibbutt DA, Davies JA, Anderson JA, et al. Comparison by controlled clinical trial of streptokinase and heparin in treatment of life-threatening pulmonary embolism. Br Med J 1974;1(904):343–7.

39. Ly B, Arnesen H, Eie H, et al. A controlled clinical trial of streptokinase and heparin in the treatment of major pulmonary embolism. Acta Med Scand 1978;203(6):465–70.

40. Marini C, Di Ricco G, Rossi G, et al. Fibrinolytic effects of urokinase and heparin in acute pulmonary embolism: a randomized clinical trial. Respiration 1988;54(3):162–73.

41. Levine M, Hirsh J, Weitz J, et al. A randomized trial of a single bolus dosage regimen of recombinant tissue plasminogen activator in patients with acute pulmonary embolism. Chest 1990;98(6):1473–9.

42. Tissue plasminogen activator for the treatment of acute pulmonary embolism. A collaborative study by the PIOPED Investigators. Chest 1990;97(3):528–33.

43. Dalla-Volta S, Palla A, Santolicandro A, et al. PAIMS 2: alteplase combined with heparin versus heparin in the treatment of acute pulmonary embolism. Plasminogen activator Italian multicenter study 2. J Am Coll Cardiol 1992;20(3):520–6.

44. Goldhaber SZ, Haire WD, Feldstein ML, et al. Alteplase versus heparin in acute pulmonary embolism: randomised trial assessing right-ventricular function and pulmonary perfusion. Lancet 1993;341(8844): 507–11.

45. Dalen JE, Banas JS Jr, Brooks HL, et al. Resolution rate of acute pulmonary embolism in man. N Engl J Med 1969;280(22):1194–9.

46. Konstantinides S, Tiede N, Geibel A, et al. Comparison of alteplase versus heparin for resolution of major pulmonary embolism. Am J Cardiol 1998;82 (8):966–70.

47. Konstantinides S, Geibel A, Heusel G, et al. Heparin plus alteplase compared with heparin alone in patients with submassive pulmonary embolism. N Engl J Med 2002;347(15):1143–50.

48. Kanter DS, Mikkola KM, Patel SR, et al. Thrombolytic therapy for pulmonary embolism. Frequency of intracranial hemorrhage and associated risk factors. Chest 1997;111(5):1241–5.

49. Sors H, Pacouret G, Azarian R, et al. Hemodynamic effects of bolus vs 2-h infusion of alteplase in acute massive pulmonary embolism. A randomized controlled multicenter trial. Chest 1994;106(3): 712–7.

50. Goldhaber SZ, Kessler CM, Heit JA, et al. Recombinant tissue-type plasminogen activator versus a novel dosing regimen of urokinase in acute pulmonary embolism: a randomized controlled multicenter trial. J Am Coll Cardiol 1992;20(1):24–30.

51. Meyer G, Sors H, Charbonnier B, et al. Effects of intravenous urokinase versus alteplase on total pulmonary resistance in acute massive pulmonary embolism: a European multicenter double-blind trial. The European Cooperative Study Group for Pulmonary Embolism. J Am Coll Cardiol 1992;19(2): 239–45.

52. Goldhaber SZ, Kessler CM, Heit J, et al. Randomised controlled trial of recombinant tissue plasminogen activator versus urokinase in the treatment of acute pulmonary embolism. Lancet 1988;2(8606): 293–8.

53. Verstraete M, Miller GA, Bounameaux H, et al. Intravenous and intrapulmonary recombinant tissue-type plasminogen activator in the treatment of acute massive pulmonary embolism. Circulation 1988;77 (2):353–60.

54. Urokinase-streptokinase embolism trial. Phase 2 results. A cooperative study. JAMA 1974;229(12): 1606–13.

55. Konstantinides S, Marder VJ. Thrombolysis in venous thromboembolism. In: Colman RW, Marder VJ, Clowes AW, et al, editors. Hemostasis and thrombosis. Philadelphia: Lippincott Williams and Wilkins; 2006. p. 1317–29.

56. Hamel E, Pacouret G, Vincentelli D, et al. Thrombolysis or heparin therapy in massive pulmonary embolism with right ventricular dilation: results from a 128-patient monocenter registry. Chest 2001;120(1):120–5.

57. Meyer G, Gisselbrecht M, Diehl JL, et al. Incidence and predictors of major hemorrhagic complications from thrombolytic therapy in patients with massive pulmonary embolism. Am J Med 1998;105(6): 472–7.

58. Wan S, Quinlan DJ, Agnelli G, et al. Thrombolysis compared with heparin for the initial treatment of pulmonary embolism: a meta-analysis of the randomized controlled trials. Circulation 2004;110 (6):744–9.

59. Meneveau N, Seronde MF, Blonde MC, et al. Management of unsuccessful thrombolysis in acute

massive pulmonary embolism. Chest 2006;129(4): 1043–50.

60. Daniels LB, Parker JA, Patel SR, et al. Relation of duration of symptoms with response to thrombolytic therapy in pulmonary embolism. Am J Cardiol 1997; 80(2):184–8.

61. Rose PS, Punjabi NM, Pearse DB. Treatment of right heart thromboemboli. Chest 2002;121(3):806–14.

62. Chartier L, Bera J, Delomez M, et al. Free-floating thrombi in the right heart: diagnosis, management, and prognostic indexes in 38 consecutive patients. Circulation 1999;99(21):2779–83.

63. Meneveau N, Schiele F, Metz D, et al. Comparative efficacy of a two-hour regimen of streptokinase versus alteplase in acute massive pulmonary embolism: immediate clinical and hemodynamic outcome and one-year follow-up. J Am Coll Cardiol 1998;31 (5):1057–63.

64. Meneveau N, Schiele F, Vuillemenot A, et al. Streptokinase vs alteplase in massive pulmonary embolism. A randomized trial assessing right heart haemodynamics and pulmonary vascular obstruction. Eur Heart J 1997;18(7):1141–8.

65. Goldhaber SZ, Agnelli G, Levine MN. Reduced dose bolus alteplase vs conventional alteplase infusion for pulmonary embolism thrombolysis. An international multicenter randomized trial. The Bolus Alteplase Pulmonary Embolism Group. Chest 1994;106(3): 718–24.

66. Tebbe U, Graf A, Kamke W, et al. Hemodynamic effects of double bolus reteplase versus alteplase infusion in massive pulmonary embolism. Am Heart J 1999;138(1 Pt 1):39–44.

67. Becattini C, Agnelli G, Salvi A, et al. Bolus tenecteplase for right ventricle dysfunction in hemodynamically stable patients with pulmonary embolism. Thromb Res 2010;125(3):e82–6.

68. Kucher N, Goldhaber SZ. Management of massive pulmonary embolism. Circulation 2005;112(2): e28–32.

69. Ribeiro A, Lindmarker P, Juhlin-Dannfelt A, et al. Echocardiography Doppler in pulmonary embolism: right ventricular dysfunction as a predictor of mortality rate. Am Heart J 1997;134(3):479–87.

70. Kucher N, Rossi E, De Rosa M, et al. Prognostic role of echocardiography among patients with acute pulmonary embolism and a systolic arterial pressure of 90 mm Hg or higher. Arch Intern Med 2005;165 (15):1777–81.

71. ten Wolde M, Sohne M, Quak E, et al. Prognostic value of echocardiographically assessed right ventricular dysfunction in patients with pulmonary embolism. Arch Intern Med 2004;164(15):1685–9.

72. Sanchez O, Trinquart L, Colombet I, et al. Prognostic value of right ventricular dysfunction in patients with haemodynamically stable pulmonary embolism:

a systematic review. Eur Heart J 2008;29(12): 1569–77.

73. Binder L, Pieske B, Olschewski M, et al. N-terminal pro-brain natriuretic peptide or troponin testing followed by echocardiography for risk stratification of acute pulmonary embolism. Circulation 2005;112 (11):1573–9.

74. Scridon T, Scridon C, Skali H, et al. Prognostic significance of troponin elevation and right ventricular enlargement in acute pulmonary embolism. Am J Cardiol 2005;96(2):303–5.

75. Kucher N, Wallmann D, Carone A, et al. Incremental prognostic value of troponin I and echocardiography in patients with acute pulmonary embolism. Eur Heart J 2003;24(18):1651–6.

76. Schoepf UJ, Kucher N, Kipfmueller F, et al. Right ventricular enlargement on chest computed tomography: a predictor of early death in acute pulmonary embolism. Circulation 2004;110(20):3276–80.

77. Kucher N, Printzen G, Doernhoefer T, et al. Low pro-brain natriuretic peptide levels predict benign clinical outcome in acute pulmonary embolism. Circulation 2003;107(12):1576–8.

78. Kucher N, Printzen G, Goldhaber SZ. Prognostic role of brain natriuretic peptide in acute pulmonary embolism. Circulation 2003;107(20):2545–7.

79. Pruszczyk P, Kostrubiec M, Bochowicz A, et al. N-terminal pro-brain natriuretic peptide in patients with acute pulmonary embolism. Eur Respir J 2003;22(4):649–53.

80. ten Wolde M, Tulevski II, Mulder JW, et al. Brain natriuretic peptide as a predictor of adverse outcome in patients with pulmonary embolism. Circulation 2003;107(16):2082–4.

81. Kucher N, Goldhaber SZ. Cardiac biomarkers for risk stratification of patients with acute pulmonary embolism. Circulation 2003;108(18):2191–4.

82. Giannitsis E, Katus HA. Risk stratification in pulmonary embolism based on biomarkers and echocardiography. Circulation 2005;112(11):1520–1.

83. Klok FA, Mos IC, Huisman MV. Brain-type natriuretic peptide levels in the prediction of adverse outcome in patients with pulmonary embolism: a systematic review and meta-analysis. Am J Respir Crit Care Med 2008;178(4):425–30.

84. Sanchez O, Trinquart L, Caille V, et al. Prognostic factors for pulmonary embolism: the PREP study, a prospective multicenter cohort study. Am J Respir Crit Care Med 2010;181(2):168–73.

85. Korff S, Katus HA, Giannitsis E. Differential diagnosis of elevated troponins. Heart 2006;92(7):987–93.

86. Becattini C, Vedovati MC, Agnelli G. Prognostic value of troponins in acute pulmonary embolism: a meta-analysis. Circulation 2007;116(4):427–33.

87. Jimenez D, Uresandi F, Otero R, et al. Troponin-based risk stratification of patients with acute nonmassive

pulmonary embolism: systematic review and meta-analysis. Chest 2009;136(4):974—82.

88. Lankeit M, Konstantinides S. Tenecteplase can be given to patients with intermediate-risk pulmonary embolism—but should it? Thromb Res 2009. [Epub ahead of print].

89. Storch J, Thumser AE. The fatty acid transport function of fatty acid-binding proteins. Biochim Biophys Acta 2000;1486(1):28—44.

90. Alhadi HA, Fox KA. Do we need additional markers of myocyte necrosis: the potential value of heart fatty-acid-binding protein. QJM 2004;97(4):187—98.

91. Pelsers MM, Hermens WT, Glatz JF. Fatty acid-binding proteins as plasma markers of tissue injury. Clin Chim Acta 2005;352(1-2):15—35.

92. Puls M, Dellas C, Lankeit M, et al. Heart-type fatty acid-binding protein permits early risk stratification of pulmonary embolism. Eur Heart J 2007;28(2):224—9.

93. Kaczynska A, Pelsers MM, Bochowicz A, et al. Plasma heart-type fatty acid binding protein is superior to troponin and myoglobin for rapid risk stratification in acute pulmonary embolism. Clin Chim Acta 2006;371(1—2):117—23.

94. Dellas C, Puls M, Lankeit M, et al. Elevated heart-type fatty acid-binding protein levels on admission predict an adverse outcome in normotensive patients with acute pulmonary embolism. J Am Coll Cardiol 2010;55(19):2150—7.

95. Lankeit M, Kempf T, Dellas C, et al. Growth differentiation factor-15 for prognostic assessment of patients with acute pulmonary embolism. Am J Respir Crit Care Med 2008;177(9):1018—25.

96. Lankeit M, Konstantinides S. Thrombolysis for hemodynamically stable patients with pulmonary embolism: still searching for the intermediate-risk group. Thromb Res 2009;124(6):647—8.

Interventional Therapies for Venous Thromboembolism: Vena Caval Interruption, Surgical Embolectomy, and Catheter-Directed Interventions

Victor F. Tapson, MD, FCCP, FRCP

KEYWORDS

- Pulmonary embolism • Deep venous thrombosis
- Vena caval filter • Catheter fragmentation
- Pharmacomechanical thrombolysis

Anticoagulation is effective in acute pulmonary embolism (PE), and clinical trial data strongly indicate that this approach improves mortality.[1,2] However, circumstances arise in patients with venous thromboembolism (VTE) in which anticoagulation is either insufficient or too dangerous. Other approaches must then be considered. The evidence base for alternative approaches is weaker than for anticoagulation, based on the paucity of prospective, randomized clinical trial data,[3] but they nonetheless must be considered. The indications, contraindications, and available data supporting these therapeutic methods are discussed.

VENA CAVAL INTERRUPTION
Background

Vena caval interruption is an important option for the management of selected patients with VTE. This procedure is accomplished via percutaneous image-guided insertion of the inferior vena caval filter (IVCF) device into the vena cava. Occasionally, in the setting of upper extremity thrombosis,

a superior vena caval filter is placed. Approximately 15% of patients with a diagnosis of deep vein thrombosis (DVT) undergo IVCF placement.[4] Unfortunately, most scientific publications mentioning this technique have been of retrospective, uncontrolled studies. Placement of an IVCF is indicated in the setting of chronic thromboembolic pulmonary hypertension.[3] The focus in this article, however, is the setting of acute PE.

There is substantial variability among filters, including their size, shape, and composition, but there are no randomized controlled clinical trials comparing the efficacy or safety of the different devices. Although the clinical significance of design differences has not been determined, any future prospective clinical trials should take them into consideration. Filter devices are shown in **Fig. 1**.

Indications for Filter Placement: Proven VTE

The primary indications for IVCF placement include contraindications to anticoagulation, significant bleeding during anticoagulation, and

Disclosures: None.
Division of Pulmonary and Critical Care Medicine, Room 351, Bell Building, Box 31175, Duke University Medical Center, Durham, NC, 27710, USA
E-mail address: tapso001@mc.duke.edu

Clin Chest Med 31 (2010) 771–781
doi:10.1016/j.ccm.2010.07.008

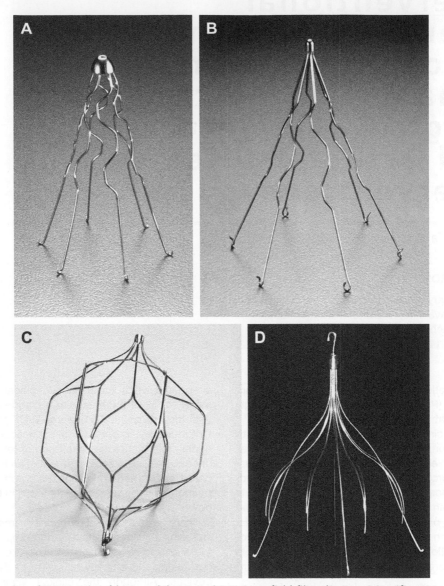

Fig. 1. Examples of IVCFs: A brief history. (*A*) Original 24F Greenfield filter (Boston Scientific, Watertown, MA, USA), first successful device used clinically, served as basis of most of the literature before 1990. (*B*) Low-profile titanium Greenfield filter (Boston Scientific); approximately 1991 to 1992; emphasizes trend to smaller filters for percutaneous delivery. (*C*) Optease retrievable filter (Cordis; Johnson & Johnson, Warren, NJ, USA), noncone-shaped. Hook is oriented to feet, so retrieval is from femoral approach (2003). (*D*) Celect filter (Cook Medical Inc., Bloomington, IN, USA). This is a late-generation retrievable filter, has a hook at the apex for jugular retrieval (2008). (*Courtesy of* John Kaufman MD. Oregon Health & Science University Hospital, Portland, OR.)

documented extension of DVT or recurrent PE while therapeutically anticoagulated.[3] These indications are listed in **Box 1**.

Filters are sometimes placed in the setting of massive PE (PE associated with hemodynamic compromise), or in other settings in which patients are deemed to be at high risk of death, particularly if thrombolytic therapy is contraindicated.[5,6] Among patients with hemodynamic compromise in the International Cooperative Pulmonary

Embolism Registry (ICOPER), insertion of an IVCF was associated with a reduction of early recurrent PE and death.[7] Subsequent epidemiologic data suggested that placement of an IVCF in patients presenting with acute PE (with or without symptomatic DVT) is associated with an approximate doubling of the frequency of VTE during follow-up; however, recurrent PE (1.3-fold increase) was less common than DVT (approximately 2.6-fold increase).[8] Potential indications

Box 1
Accepted indications for IVCF placement[a]

- Contraindications to anticoagulation[a,b]
- Bleeding complications during anti-coagulation[a,b]
- Extension of known thrombosis/recurrent PE during therapeutic anticoagulation
- Chronic thromboembolic pulmonary hypertension[a,b]

[a] American College of Chest Physicians (ACCP) recommendations.
[b] This recommendation does not require the presence of symptomatic deep venous thrombosis.

for IVCF placement that have been reported but not studied in controlled trials are listed in **Box 2**.

Randomized Clinical Trial Data

No prospective randomized trials have evaluated IVCF insertion as sole therapy (without concurrent anticoagulation) in patients with acute DVT or PE. In the Prevention du Risque d'Embolie Pulmonaire par Interruption Cave (PREPIC) study, filter placement was evaluated as an adjunct to anticoagulant therapy in a large randomized controlled trial of 400 patients with acute DVT who were deemed to be at high risk of acute PE. Results were reported at 2 years and 8 years of follow-up.[9,10] Several conclusions could be reached: filters did not change overall the frequency of VTE (DVT

Box 2
Other reported indications for vena caval filters[a]

- Inability or difficulty in achieving/maintaining therapeutic anticoagulation[b]
- High risk of complication of anticoagulation (eg, high fall risk)[b]
- Poor compliance with anticoagulation medications[b]
- Life-threatening pulmonary embolism
- Iliocaval DVT
- Thrombolysis for iliocaval venous thrombosis
- Large, free-floating proximal DVT
- Prophylactic indications (no established VTE; eg, major trauma when anticoagulation cannot be given)

[a] These have been reported but data are inadequate or conflicting and the evidence base is insufficient for an ACCP recommendation.
[b] These may be considered by some to be contraindications to anticoagulation, and thus, fit the ACCP recommendation.

and/or PE combined) and did not affect total mortality (relative risk [RR], 1.08 at 2 years; and RR, 0.95 at 8 years), although the rate of PE (symptomatic plus asymptomatic) was reduced at 12 days (RR, 0.4), 2 years (RR, 0.54), and at 8 years (RR, 0.41). Filters increased DVT at 2 years (RR, 1.8) and at 8 years (RR, 1.3; hazard ratio, 1.5; 95% confidence interval, 1.02 to 2.3) in the first report.[9] Despite more frequent DVT during follow-up and frequent evidence of thrombus occurring at the filter site in those with recurrent VTE (43% of cases), IVCF placement was not associated with a higher frequency of post-thrombotic syndrome (PTS). Finally, 2.5% (5 patients) in the nonfilter group and 1.0% (2 patients) in the filter group died of PE during the 8 year follow-up. Complications of filter placement were rare. The PREPIC study[9] included 145 patients (36% of total) with symptomatic acute PE and 52 patients (13% of total) with asymptomatic PE at enrollment in addition to their proximal DVT. Multivariable analyses did not find an association between presence of PE at study entry and frequency of PE at 2 years; however, such an association was present at the 8-year time point.[10] The primary concern in the setting of acute VTE is mortality over the short-term; the concern for subsequent DVT may be lessened in the current retrievable filter era, although this has not been proven.

It is not entirely clear why the incidence of DVT is increased after filter placement. Occlusion of the vena cava resulting from thrombosis or trapped emboli seems to be the most likely cause.[8,10] Filter contact with the vena cava has been shown to stimulate smooth muscle cell migration in the wall of the vessel, which could lead to caval stenosis.[11]

Prophylactic Indications for Filter Placement

Vena caval filters are sometimes placed for prophylactic indications; that is, the patient does not have VTE, but is at risk of developing it and cannot receive effective prophylaxis or is deemed to be at exceptionally high risk of developing VTE. Although retrospective case series have suggested that the placement of prophylactic IVCFs in trauma may reduce symptomatic and fatal PE, there are no randomized trials of prophylactic IVCF use in any patient group.[12]

The number of filter placements in the United States continues to increase.[8,13] It seems that about half of all vena caval filter placements are for prophylactic indications and a large proportion of the prophylactic filters placed are retrievable.[14,15]

Retrievable Filters: Implications and Available Data

The option of filter retrieval seems to have contributed to the increased frequency of placement. These filters are not only retrievable several months after placement; but removal at approximately 1 year after placement has proven successful and safe,[13] although less data are available with very late retrieval.

Because of the inadequate evidence base involving the use of IVCFs, particularly, the lack of clinical trial data for retrievable devices, a multidisciplinary group of physicians and researchers was convened in June 2007 by the Society of Interventional Radiology (SIR). A research agenda for IVCFs that included preclinical and health technology research, pilot clinical studies, and pivotal multicenter clinical trials was established and recently published.[6]

The panel proposed 32 clinical research topics, 8 basic science topics, and 6 organizational research topics. The potential study receiving the highest total score was a randomized controlled trial of prophylactic retrievable filters in trauma patients. The next 3 clinical topics selected by the expert panelists were, in order of decreasing priority, randomized trials of prophylactic filters in a wide range of patient populations with filter retrieval, filters in high-risk PE patient populations, and a multicenter prospective PREPIC-like trial of filters in anticoagulation candidates.[6] A summary of potential IVCF indications that were thought by the panel to merit additional study are listed in **Box 3**.

In spite of the apparent ease with which IVCFs can be placed and, more recently, retrieved, complications, although rare, can occur. These can be related to insertion, retrieval, or simply to the filter remaining in place. Studies conducted to date assessing retrievability have nearly all been retrospective and uncontrolled. Chung and Owen[16] reviewed results of 11 such studies and found variable retrieval success and IVCF complication rates. Successful retrieval occurred in 101 of 102 cases (99%) in one study and was as low as 77% in another.[16] The range of retrieval times was 2 to 345 days. Complications in this series of studies included PE despite filter placement (0%–2%), filter thrombi in 0% to 15%, and filter migration in up to 3% of cases.[16] These and other potential filter complications are listed in (**Box 4**).

In summary, the evidence base for IVCF placement/retrieval is inadequate, but the classic indications, (ie, contraindications to/complications from anticoagulation and progression of thrombosis/recurrent embolism on therapeutic

---

Box 3
Selected clinical research topics to consider: priority topics from the SIR multidisciplinary research consensus panel

- Randomized clinical trial (RCT) of prophylactic filters in trauma patients
- RCT of prophylactic filters in a wide range of patients; evaluate retrieval
- RCT of filters in high-risk PE populations
- Multicenter prospective PREPIC-like trial of IVCFs in anticoagulation candidates
- RCT of permanent versus retrievable filters
- Long-term follow-up study of retrievable filters
- RCT with clinically relevant practice changing endpoints: study prophylactic IVCF in a population at high risk of VTE and have early contraindication for anticoagulation: may compare permanent versus retrieved filters; need long-term follow-up, including PTS and PE
- Registry of IVCF outcomes
- Filter comparison trial
- Survey of practice patterns/preferences
- RCT studying specific populations with high anticipated rate of filter retrieval
- Risk factor stratification trial
- RCT of IVCFs in high-risk VTE cases and bleeding

Data from Kaufmann JA, Rundback JH, Kee ST, et al. Development of a research agenda for inferior vena cava filters: proceedings from a multidisciplinary research consensus panel. J Vasc Interv Radiol 2009;20:697–707.

Box 4
Potential IVCF complications

- Allergic reaction to contrast dye
- Insertion site bleeding/hematoma
- Dysrhythmia
- Air embolism
- Pneumothorax/hemothorax
- Guide-wire entrapment
- Incomplete filter opening
- DVT
- Stenosis of the vena cava
- Filter migration
- Filter fracture
- Infection at insertion site
- Insertion site thrombosis
- Arteriovenous fistula
- Extravascular penetration of guide wire
- Angulation/filter tilting
- Thrombosis of the vena cava
- Death from a complication (exceedingly rare)

anticoagulation) are deeply entrenched in clinical practice. The use of filters in massive PE and for certain prophylactic indications may seem to be based on sound clinical judgment but clinical trials should be conducted.

SURGICAL EMBOLECTOMY

Massive PE is a life-threatening condition with a high early mortality rate due to acute right ventricular (RV) failure and cardiogenic shock. It is generally accepted that systemic thrombolytic therapy is appropriate in the setting of proven PE associated with hemodynamic compromise in the absence of contraindications.[3] Other potential indications for thrombolysis, particularly PE associated with RV dilation and hypokinesis, have been the topic of opinion/debate for decades.[17] Administration of thrombolytic agents in settings including extensive PE by computed tomographic arteriography (CTA) or ventilation perfusion (VQ) scan, PE associated with severe hypoxemia, and extensive residual DVT with proven PE have likewise not been adequately studied, but clinicians are frequently faced with these scenarios. When a clinician thinks that aggressive therapy is indicated and thrombolytic therapy should be administered, despite contraindications, surgical embolectomy should be considered. Specifically, the American College of Chest Physicians (ACCP) recommends that in "selected highly compromised patients who are unable to receive thrombolytic therapy because of bleeding risk, or whose critical status does not allow sufficient time for systemic thrombolytic therapy to be effective, pulmonary embolectomy may be used if appropriate expertise is available." The recommendation is a weak one (grade 2C). In clinical practice, particularly when thrombolysis is administered by bolus, embolectomy does not generally offer faster results, because securing a thoracic surgeon and getting to the operating room takes time.

The procedure involves a median sternotomy, incision of the main pulmonary artery, and circulatory arrest with cardiopulmonary bypass. Unfortunately, since the first published report of open pulmonary embolectomy in 1924,[18] this operation has rarely been performed and is often reserved for patients already in cardiac arrest.[19] In 2 large PE registries, surgical embolectomy was used in only 1% of patients with massive PE and cardiogenic shock.[7,20] The in-hospital mortality rate following surgical embolectomy was approximately 30%.[7]

Later, some centers liberalized their criteria for acute pulmonary embolectomy and operated on patients with anatomically extensive PE and concomitant moderate-to-severe RV dysfunction despite preserved systemic arterial pressure. Aklog and colleagues[21] reported 29 consecutive patients who underwent embolectomy, all of whom had large central emboli in the right and/or left pulmonary artery, with some having true saddle embolism. All 26 patients who underwent preoperative echocardiography had moderate or severe RV dysfunction. Of these 29 patients, 26 (89%) survived surgery and were alive more than 1 month postoperatively, with a median follow-up of 10 months. The high survival rate of 89% (much higher than in other series) was attributed to improved surgical technique, rapid diagnosis and triage, and careful patient selection. Investigators involved with other recent small series also suggest that embolectomy before cardiac arrest is instrumental in offering the best chance of survival[22] and that operating in the setting of RV dysfunction without true hemodynamic compromise further increases the chance for survival.[23] Unfortunately, it is unclear what the survival rates would have been in these series without embolectomy. Although it is feasible that patients with extensive PE and RV dysfunction could be randomized to embolectomy versus thrombolytic therapy, embolectomy candidates often have contraindications to thrombolytic agents, making such a study difficult. The better question might be whether such patients could be randomized to early embolectomy, or to thrombolytic agents versus anticoagulation with or without IVCF placement. Because of the critical nature of these patients' condition and the rapid decision-making often required, such studies would be extremely difficult to accomplish. It seems that embolectomy results are optimal when performed in centers with experience If pulmonary embolectomy is to be considered, appropriate expertise should be available.[3]

Clinicians involved with the care of patients with extensive/massive PE should discuss the potential clinical scenarios with their surgical colleagues in advance, so that treatment can be expedited in the most seamless manner when these patients present.

CATHETER-DIRECTED INTERVENTIONS
Background and Indications

As with systemic thrombolysis and surgical embolectomy, clinical trial data for percutaneous catheter intervention for acute PE are insufficient for formulating strong recommendations. The potential for an aggressive approach with, perhaps, a lower bleeding risk than systemic thrombolysis and the avoidance of cardiopulmonary bypass makes these interventional approaches attractive to consider in patients who are compromised enough to meet criteria for thrombolysis or embolectomy. The focus of this section is to examine these approaches in the setting of acute PE.

It was demonstrated more than 2 decades ago that simple infusion of a thrombolytic agent directly into the pulmonary artery offered no benefit over systemic delivery.[24] Several investigators have, however, found that directed mechanical techniques, such as the suctioning or fragmentation of large proximal emboli[25] or the combined pharmacomechanical approach with intraembolic infusion of thrombolytic agents into such clots,[26,27] might have more benefit and potential safety than simply infusing thrombolytic agents via a peripheral vein or dripping them into the pulmonary artery. The 2008 ACCP recommendations did not provide a discussion of the various techniques but recommended the following: "in selected highly compromised patients who are unable to receive thrombolytic therapy because of bleeding risk, or whose critical status does not allow sufficient time for systemic thrombolytic therapy to be effective, we suggest use of interventional catheterization techniques if appropriate expertise is available (Grade 2C)."[3] As with the comparison with open embolectomy, systemic thrombolysis by bolus administration is faster than catheter techniques; although intensive care unit admission is advised, moving the patient is not essential, and systemic thrombolysis generally works quickly. Nonetheless, there are potential advantages to the catheter approach. The recently published European Society of Cardiology Task Force guidelines indicates that "catheter embolectomy or fragmentation of proximal pulmonary arterial clots may be considered as an alternative to surgical treatment in high-risk PE patients when thrombolysis is absolutely contraindicated or has failed."[28]

Currently, the indication is for a catheter-directed procedure in proven PE with hemodynamic compromise or a severity level (significant hypoxemia or RV dysfunction by echocardiogram) that would merit consideration of systemic lysis or embolectomy; that is, a patient deemed at high risk of death. The presence of a contraindication to systemic thrombolytic agents increases the practicality of a catheter-directed approach. Of 304 patients from the ICOPER who received PE systemic thrombolysis, 66 (22%) experienced major bleeding and 9 (3%) experienced intracranial bleeding.[7] No randomized controlled clinical trials have compared surgical embolectomy with catheter embolectomy.

The General Approach to Catheter-Directed Embolectomy

The presence of acute PE should be proven by CTA or VQ scan before the procedure; alternatively, pulmonary arteriography can be performed in the interventional radiology laboratory in a patient with a high clinical suspicion of PE who is compromised enough to consider treating aggressively. Hemodynamic and electrocardiographic monitoring should be undertaken. In patients with massive PE, the amount of contrast material should be reduced. Because most compromised patients have large proximal emboli, manual injection of 10 to 15 mL of contrast agent is generally sufficient to document emboli. Power injection of larger volumes is generally not necessary and may be dangerous in the setting of RV failure. A large proximal embolus is shown in **Fig. 2**, before catheter-directed lysis with local thrombolytic therapy.

Specific Catheter-Directed Techniques

Regardless of which approach is used, expertise is required. In most hospitals, the interventional radiologist performs catheter-directed embolectomy, and the level of interest and clinical expertise is variable. The optimal embolectomy catheter should be easily maneuverable, effective at suctioning, fragmenting, or infusing a thrombolytic

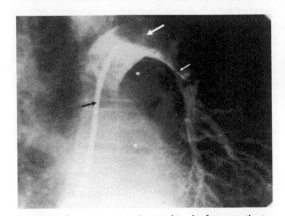

Fig. 2. Pulmonary arteriography before catheter-directed lysis in massive pulmonary embolism. Contrast is delivered via the arteriography catheter (*black arrow*). A large proximal embolus (*large white arrow*) is demonstrated before thrombolytic infusion. The thrombolytic agent is infused via a perfusion catheter with multiple exit ports (*smaller white arrow*). The patient had a brain tumor, and low-dose tissue plasminogen activator (10 mg) was infused without complications. Hypotension and severe hypoxemia subsequently resolved. (*Courtesy of* Victor Tapson MD, Durham, NC.)

agent, and should be safe, so as to avoid pulmonary arterial/cardiac perforation and mechanical hemolysis. Catheter-based techniques that have been clinically reported are listed in **Table 1**. The therapeutic tips of various catheter-directed embolectomy devices are shown in **Fig. 3**.

Aspiration embolectomy

The Greenfield suction embolectomy catheter (Boston Scientific/Meditech; Watertown, MA, USA) was introduced in 1969,[29] and it remains the only device with Food and Drug Administration approval specifically for acute PE. This 10F steerable catheter has a 5 to 7 mm plastic suction cup at its tip. Major disadvantages are that it requires insertion by venotomy via the femoral or jugular vein without a guidewire, and the device and embolus must be removed as a unit through the surgical venotomy. This device has been used effectively in extracting pulmonary emboli in up to 83% of patients, with a significant improvement in hemodynamics and a 30-day mortality rate of 30%.[30]

Catheter-directed embolus fragmentation

Various catheter devices have been used to break apart large proximal emboli by direct mechanical action. Most results reported on these devices have also included local thrombolysis; therefore, the efficacy of thrombus fragmentation without thrombolysis is unclear. Mechanical fragmentation using conventional cardiac catheters[31] or modified pulmonary catheters with rotational or other macerating devices[32] has evolved over the past 2 decades. Satisfactory results from case reports and consecutive, usually single-center series

have been reported, but these devices have never been rigorously evaluated in clinical trials.

A rotatable modified 5F pigtail catheter (Cook Medical Inc; Europe; Bjaeverskov, Denmark) has been effectively used for clot fragmentation. A central guidewire acts as the axis around which the catheter rotates to fragment large emboli, which embolize distally in the pulmonary circulation. In 20 patients with massive PE treated with this technique, the recanalization rate was 33% and survival was 80%. The catheter was shown to be more effective when used with thrombolytic therapy.[33,34]

Catheter-based rheolysis

The Amplatz thrombectomy device (Bard-Microvena; White Bear Lake, MN, USA) is a 7F catheter device that houses an impeller mounted on a drive shaft that rotates at 150,000 revolutions per minute, creating a vortex of circulating blood, pulling emboli toward the impeller and macerating them.[35] The remaining embolic particles and blood are expelled through side ports. This catheter cannot be used with a guidewire, so a 10F guide catheter is advanced close to the embolus and the device is introduced through the catheter. This rheolytic technique has been successfully used with and without concomitant thrombolysis. Hemoptysis has occurred with the Amplatz device, although the reason is unclear. The recirculation of pulverized embolus and blood causes transient mechanical hemolysis.

The Aspirex device (Straub Medical; Wangs, Switzerland) was designed for percutaneous interventional treatment of PE in large pulmonary arteries.[27,32] The central core of the catheter

---

Table 1
Catheter-based embolectomy techniques

Technique	Examples	Manufacturer
Aspiration	Greenfield embolectomy device[a]	Boston Scientific; Watertown, MA, USA
Fragmentation	Rotatable pigtail catheter	Cook Medical Inc., Europe; Bjaeverskov, Denmark; The Netherlands
Mechanical rheolysis	Amplatz device Aspirex device[b] Hydrolyser[b] AngioJet[b] Oasis device	Bard-Microvena; White Bear Lake, MN, USA Straub Medical; Wangs, Switzerland Cordis; Warren, NJ, USA Possis; Minneapolis, MN, USA Boston Scientific; Watertown, MA, USA
Local thrombolysis[a]	tPA (alteplase) Urokinase (Abbokinase)	Genentech (Roche); Basel, Switzerland Abbott Laboratories; Abbott Park, IL, USA
Angioplasty/ stenting	Wallstent Gianturco Z stents	Schneider Europe AG; Bülach, Switzerland Cook Europe; Bjaeverskov, Denmark

[a] >100 cases reported.
[b] >20 cases reported.

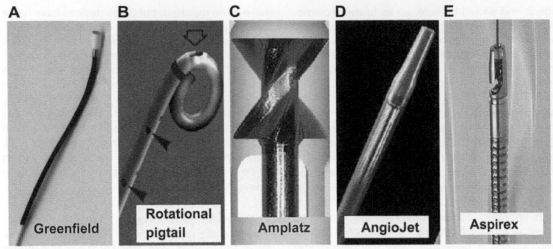

Fig. 3. Catheter embolectomy: Tips of catheter devices used. (*A*) Steerable Greenfield pulmonary embolectomy catheter (10F). (*B*) Pigtail rotational catheter (5F). (*C*) Amplatz thrombectomy device; the protected impeller is connected to the drive shaft. (*D*) Rheolytic AngioJet Xpeedior catheter (6F). (*E*) Aspirex 11-flex catheter device. (*Modified from* Kucher N. Catheter embolectomy for acute pulmonary embolism. Chest 2007;132:657–63; with permission.)

system is a high-speed (40,000 revolutions per minute) rotational coil, which creates negative pressure through the aspiration port at the catheter tip and macerates and removes aspirated embolic material. The device is introduced via a 12F sheath into the internal jugular or femoral vein. A group of investigators from Mexico recently reported results with this device in 18 patients with acute PE. They were deemed to have "massive PE" based on angiographic evidence of an embolus in a main pulmonary branch or in 2 or more lobar branches, together with RV dysfunction. Of the 18 patients, 8 (44%) had systolic blood pressures less than 90 mm Hg, and only 2 of 18 received concomitant local thrombolysis. One patient died from acute PE, and intracerebral hemorrhage occurred in another patient who recovered with minor neurologic deficit. There were no other complications. All patients received heparin, and an IVCF device was placed in 15 of 18 patients (83.3%). Thrombectomy has also been performed with this device in cases of massive DVT and IVCF thrombosis.[36]

The Hydrolyser (Cordis; Warren, NJ, USA) is a 7F catheter with a large side hole near the distal tip. The larger catheter lumen is used for aspiration of the fragmented clots and blood, and the smaller lumen is the injection channel. High-velocity injection through the smaller lumen creates lower pressure dynamics in the larger lumen and a vortex, causing fragmentation and aspiration of the clots by the pressure gradient. This device has been used with and without thrombolytic therapy.[37–39]

Hemoptysis has been reported after the procedure.[37]

The AngioJet 6F Xpeedior rheolytic thrombectomy catheter (Possis; Minneapolis, MN, USA) is a double-lumen catheter percutaneously introduced via the common femoral vein into the main pulmonary trunk or the affected pulmonary artery.[40,41] One lumen serves to deliver high-pressure saline jets into the thrombus, and the other effluent lumen serves for clot removal using a localized pressure region (Venturi effect) that attracts the thrombus for fragmentation into small particles. The fragmented debris are then pushed out through the evacuation line as a result of the retrograde high-pressure saline jets, finally transporting them into a collection bag.

Early experience with this catheter in a small group of 8 patients suggested that the AngioJet device with adjunctive low-dose urokinase was more rapidly effective than local thrombolysis alone.[40] Subsequently, results in 25 patients treated with the device have been reported.[41] Of these, 8 were deemed to be in severe shock, 12 in moderate hemodynamic compromise, and 5 in mild hemodynamic compromise. Significant improvement in obstruction, perfusion, and Miller indices were observed overall as well as in each subgroup (all *P* values<0.001). Improvement in these parameters was confirmed in patients (n = 8) treated with local fibrinolysis and also in those who did not receive concomitant thrombolysis (n = 17, *P*<.05). Four patients died in hospital; all other patients but 1 were safely discharged after an appropriate hospital stay, and all were alive at long-term follow-up (median 61 months). Another study of 30 patients with PE and hemodynamic compromise is being conducted with the AngioJet device in Switzerland. Very unstable patients with life-threatening massive PE for whom the time delays to transport them to the catheterization laboratory are unacceptable are being excluded.[42]

The Oasis catheter (Boston Scientific/Medi-Tech) also uses the Venturi effect, creating a vortex with resulting fragmentation and aspiration of emboli.[43] Few clinical data are available.

Catheter-directed thrombolysis
Catheter-directed thrombolytic therapy with intrapulmonary administration of a fairly low dose of a thrombolytic agent has been reported in several small studies and case reports.[26,44–47] As described, simply infusing thrombolytic agents directly into the pulmonary artery seems to offer no benefit over infusion via a peripheral vein.[24] The technique necessitates the positioning of an infusion catheter within the embolus, with injection of a bolus of thrombolytic drug followed by a continuous infusion. The following intrapulmonary thrombolytic regimens have been used in combination with a therapeutic infusion of unfractionated heparin in patients with massive PE: 250,000 international units [IU]/h urokinase over 2 hours followed by 100,000 IU/h urokinase for 12 to 24 hours and a 10-mg bolus of alteplase followed by infusion of 20 mg/h over 2 hours or 100 mg over 7 hours.[25] Short-acting, newer generation fibrinolytic drugs, such as reteplase (2.5–5 units) or tenecteplase (5–10 mg), may be considered. A pulmonary arteriogram showing extensive proximal PE with a guide catheter and infusion catheter in place is seen in **Fig. 2**.

Balloon angioplasty and stenting procedures
Successful balloon angioplasty of obstructing acute emboli has been reported.[48] Too few data are available to speculate on efficacy and safety, and because of other available catheterization techniques, it is rarely undertaken. Pulmonary arterial stents have been used successfully in the experimental animal model setting[49] as well as in isolated patient cases.[50] Self-expanding stents have been used in the setting of massive PE and failed thrombolysis or failed thrombus fragmentation.[50,51] It would seem that this approach, if used, should be reserved for cases of acute PE in which other aggressive measures have failed.

Complications of Catheter-Directed Embolectomy
Complications include those resulting from anticoagulation and contrast dye, including bleeding, contrast-induced nephropathy, and anaphylactic reactions to iodine contrast. Potential vascular access complications include bleeding, hematoma, arteriovenous fistula, and pseudoaneurysm. Major bleeding rates range from 0% to 17%.[25] Arrhythmias may occur when advancing the catheter through the right heart. The most serious complication resulting from these catheter-directed procedures is perforation or dissection of a pulmonary artery, causing massive pulmonary hemorrhage and immediate death. The risk of perforation increases with smaller vessels.[25] Other serious complications include pericardial tamponade. To minimize the risk of perforation or dissection, embolectomy procedures should only be performed in the main and lobar pulmonary artery branches and not attempted in smaller vessels.

Device-related complications include hemorrhage and mechanical hemolysis. Acute pancreatitis due to mechanical hemolysis has been reported.[52]

Summary: Catheter-Directed Embolectomy
There are no randomized, controlled data supporting catheter-based techniques, but they have been used clinically with some success. Overall success rates range from 67% to 100%,[25] but these rates suffer from significant potential reporting bias. Catheter-based embolectomy can be considered when systemic thrombolysis and surgical embolectomy cannot be performed. It is impossible to determine the superiority of a particular catheter-based technique because of the lack of comparative and randomized trial data. Many patients treated with fragmentation techniques have also received thrombolytic agents, making results and comparisons more difficult. At present, local expertise and familiarity with a particular device should guide the clinician when a catheter-based procedure seems to be indicated.

SUMMARY
Although anticoagulation offers the most appropriate therapeutic approach for most patients with acute DVT and PE, there are clearly scenarios in which anticoagulation is contraindicated or the risk of death is deemed too high for anticoagulation alone. Although the evidence base for alternative approaches is weaker than for anticoagulation, the options discussed may

still be considered in individual patients. Future clinical trials must address these issues and supplement the inadequacies of the current evidence base.

REFERENCES

1. Barritt DW, Jordan SC. Anticoagulant drugs in the treatment of pulmonary embolism: a controlled trial. Lancet 1960;1:1309–12.
2. Alpert JS, Smith R, Carlson J, et al. Mortality in patients treated for pulmonary embolism. JAMA 1976;236:1477–80.
3. Kearon C, Kahn SR, Agnelli G, et al. Antithrombotic therapy for venous thromboembolic disease. American college of chest physicians evidence-based clinical practice guidelines. (8th edition). Chest 2008;133:454S–545S.
4. Jaff MR, Goldhaber SZ, Tapson VF. High utilization rate of vena cava filters in deep vein thrombosis. Thromb Haemost 2005;93:1117–9.
5. Greenfield LJ, Proctor M. Filter complications and their management. Semin Vasc Surg 2000;13:213–6.
6. Kaufmann JA, Rundback JH, Kee ST, et al. Development of a research agenda for inferior vena cava filters: proceedings from a multidisciplinary research consensus panel. J Vasc Interv Radiol 2009;20: 697–707.
7. Goldhaber SZ, Visani L, De Rosa M, et al. Acute pulmonary embolism: clinical outcomes in the international cooperative pulmonary embolism registry (ICOPER). Lancet 1999;353:1386–9.
8. White RH, Zhou H, Kim J, et al. A population-based study of the effectiveness of IVC filter use among patients with venous thromboembolism. Arch Intern Med 2000;160:2033–41.
9. Decousus H, Leizorovicz A, Parent F, et al. A clinical trial of vena caval filters in the prevention of pulmonary embolism in patients with proximal deep-vein thrombosis. N Engl J Med 1998;338:409–15.
10. The PREPIC Study Group. Eight-year follow-up of patients with permanent vena cava filters in the prevention of pulmonary embolism: the PREPIC (Prevention du Risque d'Embolie Pulmonaire par Interruption Cave) randomized study. Circulation 2005;112:416–22.
11. Christie DB, Kang J, Ashley DW, et al. Accelerated migration and proliferation of smooth muscle cells cultured from neointima induced by a vena cava filter. Am Surg 2006;72:491–6.
12. Girard J, Philbrick J, Angle F, et al. Prophylactic vena cava filters for trauma patients: a systematic review of the literature. Thromb Res 2003;112:261–7.
13. Athanasoulis CA, Kaufman JA, Halpern EF, et al. Inferior vena cava filters: review of a 26-year single-center clinical experience. Radiology 2000; 216:54–66.
14. Karmy-Jones R, Jurkovich GJ, Velmahos GC, et al. Practice patterns and outcomes of retrievable vena cava filters in trauma patients: an AAST multicenter study. J Trauma 2007;62:17–24.
15. Piano G, Ketteler ER, Prachand V, et al. Safety, feasibility, and outcome of retrievable vena cava filters in high-risk surgical patients. J Vasc Surg 2007;45: 784–8.
16. Chung J, Owen RJT. Using inferior vena cava filters to prevent pulmonary embolism. Can Fam Physician 2008;54:49–55.
17. Stein PD, Dalen JE, Goldhaber SZ, et al. Opinions regarding the diagnosis and management of venous thromboembolic disease (Opinion statement II). Chest 1998;113:499–504.
18. Kirshner M. Eindurch die Trendelenburgs che Operation Grehefter fal von Embolie der art Pulmonalis. Arch Klin Chir 1924;133:312.
19. Stein PD, Alnas M, Beemath A, et al. Outcome of pulmonary embolectomy. Am J Cardiol 2007;99: 421–3.
20. Kasper W, Konstantinides S, Geibel A, et al. Management strategies and determinants of outcome in acute major pulmonary embolism: results of a multicenter registry. J Am Coll Cardiol 1997;30:1165–71.
21. Aklog L, Williams CS, Byrne JG, et al. Acute pulmonary embolectomy: a contemporary approach. Circulation 2002;105:1416.
22. Dauphine C, Omari B. Pulmonary embolectomy for acute massive pulmonary embolism. Ann Thorac Surg 2005;79:1240–4.
23. Ahmed P, Khan AA, Smith A, et al. Expedient pulmonary embolectomy for acute pulmonary embolism: improved outcomes. Interact Cardiovasc Thorac Surg 2008;7:591–4.
24. Verstraete M, Miller GA, Bounameaux H, et al. Intravenous and intrapulmonary recombinant tissue-type plasminogen activator in the treatment of acute massive pulmonary embolism. Circulation 1988;77: 353–60.
25. Kucher N. Catheter embolectomy for acute pulmonary embolism. Chest 2007;132:657–63.
26. Tapson VF, Gurbel PA, Stack RS. Pharmacomechanical thrombolysis of experimental pulmonary emboli: rapid low-dose intraembolic therapy. Chest 1994; 106:1558–62.
27. Eid-Lidt G, Gaspar J, Sandoval J, et al. Combined clot fragmentation and aspiration in patients with acute pulmonary embolism. Chest 2008;134: 54–60.
28. Torbicki A, Perrier A, Konstantinides S, et al. Guidelines on the diagnosis and management of acute pulmonary embolism. The task force for the diagnosis and management of acute pulmonary embolism of the European society of cardiology (ESC). Eur Heart J 2008;29:2276–315.

29. Greenfield LJ, Kimmell GO, McCurdy WC III. Transvenous removal of pulmonary emboli by vacuum-cup catheter technique. J Surg Res 1969;9:347–52.

30. Greenfield LJ, Proctor MC, Williams DM, et al. Long-term experience with transvenous catheter pulmonary embolectomy. J Vasc Surg 1993;18:450–7.

31. Brady AJ, Crake T, Oakley CM. Percutaneous catheter fragmentation and distal dispersion of proximal pulmonary embolus. Lancet 1991;338:1186–9.

32. Kucher N, Windecker S, Banz Y, et al. Percutaneous catheter thrombectomy device for acute pulmonary embolism: in vitro and in vivo testing. Radiology 2005;236:852–8.

33. Schmitz-Rode T, Janssens U, Schild HH, et al. Fragmentation of massive pulmonary embolism using a pigtail rotation catheter. Chest 1998;114:1427–36.

34. Schmitz-Rode T, Janssen U, Duda SH, et al. Massive pulmonary embolism: percutaneous emergency treatment by pigtail rotation catheter. J Am Coll Cardiol 2000;36:375–80.

35. Müller-Hülsbeck S, Brossmann J, Jahnke T, et al. Mechanical thrombectomy of major and massive pulmonary embolism with use of the Amplatz thrombectomy device. Invest Radiol 2001;36:317–22.

36. Erne P, Yamshidi P. Percutaneous aspiration of inferior vena cava thrombus. J Invasive Cardiol 2006;18:e149–51.

37. Fava M, Loyola S, Huete I. Massive pulmonary embolism: treatment with the hydrolyser thrombectomy catheter. J Vasc Interv Radiol 2000;11:1159–64.

38. Reekers JA, Baarslag HJ, Koolen MG, et al. Mechanical thrombectomy for early treatment of massive pulmonary embolism. Cardiovasc Intervent Radiol 2003;26:246–50.

39. Michalis LK, Tsetis DK, Rees MR. Case report: percutaneous removal of pulmonary artery thrombus in a patient with massive pulmonary embolism using the hydrolyser catheter; the first human experience. Clin Radiol 1997;52:158–61.

40. Siablis D, Karnabatidis D, Katsanos K, et al. AngioJet rheolytic thrombectomy versus local intrapulmonary thrombolysis in massive pulmonary embolism: a retrospective data analysis. J Endovasc Ther 2005;12:206–14.

41. Margheri M, Vittori G, Vecchio S, et al. Early and long-term clinical results of AngioJet rheolytic thrombectomy in patients with acute pulmonary embolism. Am J Cardiol 2008;101:252–8.

42. Angiojet Rheolytic Thrombectomy in Case of Massive Pulmonary Embolism. An ongoing clinical trial. Available at: http://clinicaltrials.gov/ct2/show/NCT00780767. Accessed January 7, 2010.

43. Fava M, Loyola S, Bertoni H, et al. Massive pulmonary embolism: percutaneous mechanical thrombectomy during cardiopulmonary resuscitation. J Vasc Interv Radiol 2005;16:119–23.

44. Vujic I, Young JWR, Gobien RP, et al. Massive pulmonary embolism treatment with full heparinization and topical low-dose streptokinase. Radiology 1983;148:671–5.

45. Gonzales-Juanatey JR, Valdes L, Amaro A, et al. Treatment of massive pulmonary thromboembolism with low intrapulmonary dosages of urokinase: short term angiographic and hemodynamic evolution. Chest 1992;102:341–6.

46. Molina HE, Hunter DW, Yedlick JW, et al. Thrombolytic therapy for post operative pulmonary embolism. Am J Surg 1992;163:375–81.

47. Kelly P, Carroll N, Grant C, et al. Successful treatment of massive pulmonary embolism with prolonged catheter-directed thrombolysis. Heart Vessels 2006;21:124–6.

48. Handa K, Sasaki Y, Kiyonaga A, et al. Acute pulmonary thromboembolism treated successfully by balloon angioplasty: a case report. Angiology 1988;8:775–8.

49. Schmitz-Rode T, Verma R, Pfeffer JG, et al. Temporary pulmonary stent placement as emergency treatment of pulmonary embolism: first experimental evaluation. J Am Coll Cardiol 2006;48:812–6.

50. Haskal ZJ, Soulen MC, Huetti EA, et al. Life-threatening pulmonary emboli and cor pulmonale: treatment with percutaneous pulmonary artery stent placement. Radiology 1994;191:473–5.

51. Koizumi J, Kusano S, Akima T, et al. Emergent Z stent placement for treatment of cor pulmonale due to pulmonary emboli after failed lytic treatment: technical considerations. Cardiovasc Intervent Radiol 1998;21:254–5.

52. Danetz JS, McLafferty RB, Ayerdi J, et al. Pancreatitis caused by rheolytic thrombolysis: an unexpected complication. J Vasc Interv Radiol 2004;15:857–60.

Upper Extremity Deep Vein Thrombosis

Peter S. Marshall, MD, MPH[a],*, Hilary Cain, MD[b]

KEYWORDS

- Upper extremity deep vein thrombosis
- Pulmonary embolus • Risk factors • Diagnosis
- Complications • Treatment

In the past, upper extremity deep vein thrombosis (UEDVT) was considered a rarely encountered, benign phenomenon. Thrombosis of the upper extremities has become more frequent since the 1970s because of the use of transvenous pacers and central venous catheters (CVCs).[1] Data published within the past 20 years suggests that UEDVT is associated with a significant prevalence of pulmonary embolus (PE).[2,3] Other complications include loss of vascular access, superior vena cava (SVC) syndrome, septic thrombophlebitis, and postthrombotic syndrome.[3]

UEDVT can be classified according to anatomic distribution or origin. Typically, UEDVT refers to thrombus in the axillary or subclavian veins.[4–6] The brachial vein also may be involved with thrombus.[7] The remaining vessels of interest are the central veins (brachiocephalic vein and SVC) and internal jugular vein.[8] The two etiologic groups of UEDVT are primary and secondary.[1] The primary category accounts for 20% of UEDVT and includes idiopathic and effort-related thrombosis (often referred to as Paget-Schroetter Syndrome).[9] Secondary causes account for 80% of UEDVT and include cancer, central venous pacers, CVCs, acquired thrombophilia, and inherited thrombophillia.[7,9,10]

EPIDEMIOLOGY

A recent study of 44,136 inpatients followed over 2 years found the prevalence of UEDVT to be 0.15% in patients of all ages and 0.19% in adults older than 20 years.[1] UEDVT constitutes 1% to 4% of all cases of DVT and 18% of deep vein thrombosis (DVT) among hospitalized patients.[1,9,11] At 3 months, the all-cause mortality of those with UEDVT is approximately 7% compared with 11% in those with lower extremity deep vein thrombosis (LEDVT).[12]

UEDVT often involves more than one vein, with the subclavian and axillary veins (74% and 38%, respectively) being most frequently affected.[1,13] The deep distal veins (brachial, ulnar, and radial) are affected only 14% of the time. SVC, brachiocephalic, and internal jugular vein thrombotic disease often accompanies axillosubclavian DVT but can also present in isolation. The main risk factors are similar (cancer, CVC, LEDVT, and anatomic abnormalities) to those identified for axillosubclavian DVT.[8,13]

Truly accurate estimates of the incidence and prevalence of UEDVT are difficult to obtain because studies do not always use contrast venography. When venography is used, the identification rate for UEDVT is higher than when either ultrasonography or impedance plethysmography are used.[14]

ETIOLOGY AND PATHOGENESIS
Risk Factors

The most common risk factors for UEDVT are cancer, CVCs, and thrombophilia. Cancer is found in as many as 63% of patients with UEDVT.[15] In non–CVC associated UEDVT, cancer diagnosed (within 6 months) or actively being treated (with chemotherapy or radiation) is a more significant

[a] Pulmonary & Critical Care Section, Department of Internal Medicine, Yale School of Medicine 333 Cedar Street, LCI 105B, PO Box 208057, New Haven, CT 06520-8057, USA
[b] CCU/MICU, Pulmonary and Critical Care Section, VA Connecticut Healthcare System – West Haven, Section of Pulmonary and Critical Care Medicine, 950 Campbell Avenue, West Haven, CT 06516, USA
* Corresponding author.
E-mail address: peter.marshall@yale.edu

Clin Chest Med 31 (2010) 783–797
doi:10.1016/j.ccm.2010.06.005
0272-5231/10/$ – see front matter. Published by Elsevier Inc.

risk factor for UEDVT than for LEDVT.[6] However, even in patients with cancer, spontaneous formation of an UEDVT is uncommon in the absence of a CVC, radiation therapy, or external compression of the vein from tumor.[16]

The presence of a CVC is the most powerful independent predictor of UEDVT (odds ratio [OR], 9.7; 95% CI, 7.8–12.2), and 55% of UEDVT occurs in patients who have a CVC or have had one within 30 days of the thrombosis diagnosis.[6] However, only an estimated 3% of patients with CVCs or pacemakers develop clinically evident UEDVT.[17] Some evidence shows that the type of catheter influences the rate of UEDVT. Central catheters have a 6-month DVT risk of 3% versus 9.3% for peripherally inserted catheters ($P = .007$). In one study of 422 patients, those who were not treated with prophylactic Coumadin had a 6-month risk of 4.9% versus 10.4% ($P = .002$).[18] The duration of catheter placement, type of fluid infused (chemotherapeutic agents, total parenteral nutrition, or crystalloid), number of lumens, and catheter-related infections all influence the risk of UEDVT when CVCs are used.[16] Patients with cancer with a CVC have a higher risk of UEDVT than those with a CVC and no cancer diagnosis ($P<.05$).[19]

UEDVT associated with implantable pacer devices has an estimated incidence of 5% or higher.[16] As with CVC-associated UEDVT, most instances are asymptomatic. In a prospective study, venography was obtained in 229 consecutive patients undergoing implantable pacemaker insertion 6 months after insertion. At 6 months, 13% had mild narrowing (up to 20% luminal narrowing), 30% had moderate narrowing (21%–69% narrowing), 15% had severe narrowing (70%–99% narrowing), and 6% had occlusive thrombi.[20] Similarly, other investigators have found the incidence of venous obstruction (severe narrowing or occlusion) at 6 months after pacer/implantable cardioversion device to be 13.9%.[21] Poor cardiac function (left ventricular ejection fraction <40%) and congestive heart failure likely contribute to the risk of UEDVT in these patients.[20]

Thrombophilic states are another major risk factor for UEDVT.[2,16] A five- to sixfold increase in the risk of UEDVT is noted when patients are deficient in protein C, protein S, or anti-thrombin III, or are heterozygotes for factor V Leiden and prothrombin G20210A.[22] Patients with inherited thrombophilia are also more likely to experience symptomatic recurrence of DVT.[22] The prevalence of inherited coagulation defects in patients with non–CVC-related UEDVT ranges from 10% to 62%.[23–25]

The presence of hyperhomocysteinemia is not a risk factor for the development of UEDVT, unlike LEDVT.[22] Pregnancy and oral contraceptive use may also be risk factors for UEDVT formation, but this is debated.[26,27] Oral contraceptives have an OR of 1.0 (95% CI, 0.5–2.0) for UEDVT alone, and 4.2 (95% CI, 1.4–12.6) for UEDVT and common inherited thrombophilia (factor V Leiden or prothrombin G20210A) alone.[22] The presence of a common inherited thrombophilia (factor V Leiden or prothrombin G20210A) together with oral contraceptive use results in a much greater risk of UEDVT (OR, 13.6; 95% CI, 2.7–67.3) than for either risk factor alone. A similar interaction has been documented for LEDVT; however, the use of oral contraceptives alone is a significant risk factor for LEDVT.[22]

Pathogenesis

UEDVT is less common than LEDVT for several reasons. The venous pathways of arms are less likely to form thromboses than those of legs because of a relatively high flow rate and less stasis from gravitational effects.[9] Even in bedridden patients, the upper limbs tend to be mobilized more than the lower limbs, resulting in less stasis.[16] In addition, arm veins have fewer valves that can serve as foci of thrombus formation. The veins in the upper extremity are shorter and therefore have lesser surface on which to form clot. Moreover, arm veins have been shown to generate higher levels of plasminogen activator and fibrinolytic activity.[11,28] To form UEDVTs, significant (or extreme) predisposing factors are necessary.[7]

Paget-Schroetter syndrome (thoracic outlet syndrome) is a rare condition typically seen in young men with overdeveloped anterior scalene muscles.[16] The channel between the skeletal and muscular components of the shoulder is narrow. During strenuous exercise the scalene muscles can compress the vein entering the thoracic cage. The combination of stasis (from the narrow thoracic outlet) and endothelial injury, caused by marked strenuous activity, results in UEDVT. Predisposing factors for effort-related upper extremity thrombosis include the presence of anatomic abnormalities contributing to thoracic outlet narrowing, such as a cervical rib or clavicular fracture. In combination with vigorous use of the dominant upper extremity or hyperabduction of the shoulder (eg, weightlifters, tennis players, wrestlers, rowers, painters, and baseball pitchers), thrombosis may occur.[9] A history of strenuous efforts, even in the absence of an anatomic abnormality, may result in thrombosis. Swelling of the upper extremity is a symptomatic manifestation of thoracic outlet syndrome and usually involves obstruction of the axillary or subclavian veins.[16]

Thrombi associated with CVCs may take several forms. The most frequently observed is the fibrin sleeve.[16] In an autopsy study of patients with subclavian catheters, circumferential sleeves were present in patients as early as 24 hours after insertion, and this observation has been documented in other studies.[29,30] A thin coating of fibrin forms on the outer surface of the catheter from its insertion point to the tip. The sleeves are asymptomatic, but can lead to formation of small thromboemboli that may lodge in the lungs.[14,16] Fibrin sleeves can also predispose the catheter to bacterial colonization.[30] Larger thrombi are classified as nonocclusive mural thrombi or occlusive thrombi, which cause complete occlusion of the vein. Mural thrombi are more likely to result in signs and symptoms of UEDVT than fibrin sleeves.[14,16]

In the absence of an obvious inciting event or anatomic abnormality (**Box 1**), the identification of UEDVT should prompt a search for acquired thrombophilia, inherited thrombophilia, or occult malignancy.

DIAGNOSIS
Clinical Presentation

Swelling of the upper extremity is the most prevalent sign of UEDVT; however, as many as 66% of patients with UEDVT are asymptomatic, and most of these occurrences are CVC-associated.[31] In one study in which all patients had arm swelling associated with UEDVT, pain was present in 40%, but only 6% had erythema of the affected area.[1] CVC-associated UEDVT is less likely to cause symptoms because clots develop more slowly and are less often occlusive.[14,16] For example, in non–CVC-associated UEDVT, limb pain is more frequent than CVC-associated UEDVT (17.1% vs 11.4%; $P = .02$).[6] Dyspnea is also less frequent in the CVC-associated UEDVT group (4.1% vs 18.5%; $P = .02$), implying lower frequency of pulmonary embolization of the clot.[6]

In CVC-associated UEDVT, the only apparent sign or symptom of thrombus may be an inability to draw blood from the catheter, increased dialysis pressures, or transient edema of the hand after dialysis.[14,16] Because of the subtleties of its presentation, clinicians must have a high index of suspicion of CVC-associated DVT or thrombosis can be missed, especially in patients with risk factors for thrombophilia or malignancy, and who practice strenuous upper extremity activity. A low threshold for confirmatory testing is advised in these patients.

> **Box 1**
> **Risk factors for UEDVT**
>
> *Inherited thrombophilia*
> Factor V Leiden
> Prothrombin (G20210A)
> Protein C
> Protein S
> Antithrombin III
> Fibrinogen
> *Acquired thrombophilia*
> Cancer
> Congestive heart failure
> Pregnancy
> Antiphospholipid syndrome
> Nephrotic syndrome
> Antineoplastic agents
> Liver disease
> Sepsis
> Vasculitic disorders
> Inflammatory bowel disease
> Oral contraceptives
> Heparin-induced thrombocytopenia
> Disseminated intravascular coagulation
> *Mechanical factors*
> Paget-Schroetter syndrome
> Central venous catheters
> Implanted pacemakers
> Trauma
> Previous DVT
> Clavicular fracture
> Cervical rib

Additional symptoms include neck swelling (implying that the central veins are involved), chest pain, cough, jaw pain, headache, arm warmth, arm paresthesias, and engorged superficial limb veins.[6,14] More serious presenting complications include SVC syndrome, venous gangrene, syncope, and PE.[16]

Objective Investigations

The clinical evaluation for UEDVT has not only poor sensitivity but also poor specificity, with only 50% of tests confirming DVT in patients with signs and symptoms of UEDVT.[2] Confirmation with testing is essential (**Table 1**).

Table 1
Imaging modalities in upper extremity deep vein thrombosis

Diagnostic Modality	Sensitivity	Specificity	Iodinated Contrast[c]	Image Central Veins	Comments
CV	Gold standard	Gold standard	Yes	Yes	Radiation exposure intravenous access
Ultrasound[a]	82%–97%	82%–96%	No	No	Portable No radiation Multiple techniques
CT venography[b]	NA	NA	Yes	Yes	No trials versus CV Pulmonary embolism diagnosis possible Radiation exposure
MR venography[d]	83%	NA	No	Yes	Expensive Chronic versus acute clot No trials versus CV Pulmonary embolism diagnosis possible

Abbreviations: CV, contrast venography; NA, not available.
[a] *Data from* Refs.[2,32]
[b] *Data from* Sabharwal R, Boshell D, Vladica P. Multidetector spiral CT venography in the diagnosis of upper extremity deep venous thrombosis. Australas Radiol 2007;51 Suppl:B253–56.
[c] Risk of severe allergy and nephrotoxicity with iodinated contrast.
[d] *Data from* Refs.[16,33,36]

Venography

Contrast venography is the test against which all other imaging techniques are measured.[2,32] Lack of filling of the brachial, axillary, or subclavian veins is most often encountered.[9] Contrast venography can also be used to image the central veins (SVC and innominate).[13] The technique is not without risk because it involves injection of iodinated contrast, which is potentially nephrotoxic and may precipitate severe allergic reactions. Between 6.4% and 12.9% of patients are unable to undergo contrast venography because of inaccessibility of arm veins, severe allergy, pregnancy, or renal insufficiency.[2,32] For safety and cost-containment reasons, contrast venography should only be used when other modalities have failed to diagnose or exclude UEDVT.

Ultrasound

Ultrasonography is frequently used as a diagnostic test for UEDVT. It is noninvasive and does not require the use of iodinated contrast or ionizing radiation. In most institutions it is widely available and may be performed at the bedside. Several modalities are used to diagnose UEDVT, including compression ultrasonography (CUS), color flow duplex/color duplex ultrasonography (CDUS), and Doppler ultrasonography.[2,33]

In 1997, a prospective comparison of these ultrasonographic techniques was completed in patients with suspected UEDVT.[2] Their performance was measured against contrast venography. The brachial, axillary, and subclavian veins were studied using ultrasound techniques. Compression ultrasonography had a sensitivity of 96.3% (95% CI, 81.0%–99.9%) and a specificity of 93.5% (95% CI, 78.6%–99.2%). Color flow Doppler imaging had a sensitivity of 100% (95% CI, 82.4%–100%) and specificity of 93.3% (95% CI, 68.0%–99.8%). Doppler ultrasonography had a sensitivity of 80.9% (95% CI, 58.1%–94.5%) and specificity of 76.9% (56.4%–91.0%). Compression ultrasonography and color flow Doppler imaging had greater accuracy than Doppler ultrasonography (94.6% and 97.1% vs 78.7%, respectively).

A more recent prospective trial evaluating the accuracy of color duplex ultrasonography (CDUS) using contrast venography as the gold standard imaged the basilic, cephalic, axillary, and subclavian veins.[32] DVT was diagnosed with duplex ultrasonography if noncompressibility of a venous segment, visible intraluminal thrombus, or abnormal flow pattern was present. The investigators found 82% (95% CI, 70%–93%) sensitivity and 82% (95% CI, 72%–92%) specificity for ultrasound.

CDUS and CUS are accurate tools for diagnosing UEDVT; however, these techniques cannot completely exclude the presence of an axillary, subclavian, SVC, or brachiocephalic clot. The presence of a central vein clot may be inferred from secondary signs such as absence of respiratory variation and absence of cardiac pulsatility.[34] In the presence of high clinical suspicion of UEDVT, an equivocal study, or suspicion of central vein clot (SVC/brachiocephalic), further testing may be necessary (**Fig. 1**).

CT venography

CT venography, like contrast venography, has the advantage of directly imaging central veins. It can diagnose other causes of venous obstruction caused by external compression by adjacent structures. It may also allow the simultaneous diagnosis of PE.[9] Spiral multidetector CT venography (with three-dimensional reconstructions) allows upper extremity venous anatomy to be mapped in reference to adjacent anatomy.[35] Unfortunately, it requires injection of iodinated contrast and exposure to radiation. Some patients will be excluded from this imaging technique because of lack of intravenous access, severe allergy to contrast, or renal insufficiency. Prospective comparisons with contrast venography and ultrasonography are required to determine its precise role in diagnosing UEDVT.

Magnetic resonance venography

Studies have shown magnetic resonance venography (MRV) to be an effective means of diagnosing UEDVT. In addition, MRV allows the central veins to be imaged. It has a sensitivity of almost 100% in assessing the SVC and internal jugular veins, but is less sensitive when assessing the shoulder region (83%).[16] In a prospective study of comparing MRI (using spin-echo sequences) with contrast venography in the imaging of patients with DVT (upper- and lower-limb), MRI had a sensitivity of 90% and specificity of 100%.[36] Other investigators have also noted good correlation between MRI and contrast venography.[9]

MRV can be performed without intravenous contrast, thereby making it available to patients with renal insufficiency and severe contrast allergy.[33] Many institutions perform MRV with and without gadolinium, and gadolinium may result in nephrogenic systemic fibrosis in patients with preexisting renal disease.[37] It does not require the use of ionizing radiation, making it safe for children and pregnant women.[33] Like CT venography, the anatomy of surrounding structures is visualized, and therefore causes of external

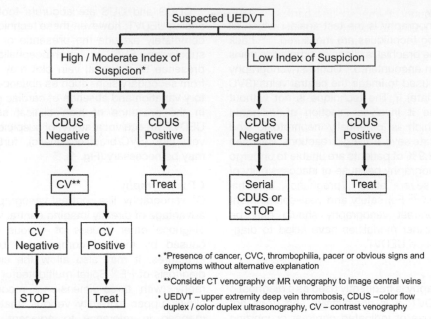

Fig. 1. Suspected upper extremity deep vein thrombosis.

compression may be determined. It is also capable of distinguishing chronic thrombus from acute thrombus.[33,36] Its use is limited, however, by cost and inconvenience. As with CT venography, a large prospective comparison of MRV versus contrast venography in patients suspected of UEDVT has not been completed.[33]

Other diagnostic techniques

Radionuclide venography also may be used for diagnosing UEDVT, and case reports have described its use.[38] Although few data are available on the use of D-dimer testing in the diagnosis of UEDVT, D-dimer assays, when combined with pretest probability and imaging modalities, may be useful as part of an algorithm for this diagnosis.

SEQUELAE AND COMPLICATIONS
Pulmonary Embolus

The reported prevalence of PE associated with UEDVT varies widely in the literature, from 2% to 35% of subjects with diagnosed thrombus.[9] It has long been observed that the incidence of PE is lower for UEDVT than it is for lower extremity clots. Recently published data from the ongoing Computerized Registry of Patients with Venous Thromboembolism (RIETE) of 11,564 cases of upper and lower extremity DVT or PE show that of 512 subjects with UEDVT, only 9% were associated with clinically apparent PE at clinical presentation, compared with a 29% incidence of PE

among those with LEDVT (OR, 0.24; 95% CI, 0.18–0.33).[12] The incidence if PE (formed after diagnosis of UEDVT) in untreated patients is difficult to estimate because retrospective studies report the rates of PE for treated and untreated patients as a group. No prospective studies exist that include an untreated arm.

Recurrent PE

The rate of recurrent PE after initial treatment for UEDVT is low. After 3 months of either low molecular weight heparin (LMWH) or vitamin K antagonist, the incidence of PE was 1.8% among the 512 subjects in the RIETE registry with UEDVT. Smaller studies have recorded even better success, with no reported PEs at 3 months among 46 outpatients treated with LMWH followed by 3 months of warfarin.[39] Similar success was reported for a high-risk cohort of 74 patients with cancer and UEDVT who required continued use of indwelling CVCs: no PEs were reported at 3 months after LWMH for a week or less followed by warfarin for 3 months.[40] Despite good early prevention of PE with anticoagulation strategies, longer follow-up intervals inevitably show increasing cumulative rates of PE over time. At 1 year, one PE was reported among 36 hospitalized patients (2.8%) treated for UEDVT with a similar anticoagulation strategy for up to an average of 5 months.[41] Another study reported cumulative PE rates of 2% at 1 year, 4.2% at 2 years, and 7.7% at 5 years after anticoagulation for a median of 3 months.[42]

The question of whether one particular site of UEDVT is more commonly associated with PE was studied in a cohort of 210 patients assembled over 5 years at a single institution.[8] DVT was identified with duplex ultrasound scanning in the subclavian–axillary veins (n = 126), internal jugular vein (n = 21), or both (n = 61). PE occurred in 4%, 0.5%, and 2.4% of subjects, respectively, but this did not constitute a statistically significant difference in incidence according to location of UEDVT.

Recurrent DVT

The rate of recurrent DVT after treatment of upper extremity thrombosis ranges from 2% to 13% over a 5-year follow-up. In the RIETE registry, the incidence of recurrent DVT was reported to be 2.8% for subjects without cancer over 3-month follow-up.[12] Longer follow-up intervals show an ongoing cumulative risk over time. In a cohort of 99 subjects with primary UEDVT followed for 5 years after treatment with anticoagulation for a mean duration of 6 months, the annual recurrence rate of UEDVT was 2.4%.[22] Similarly, a smaller study showed the cumulative incidence at sequential time points: 2% at 1 year, 4.2% at 2 years, and 7.7% at 5 years.[42]

Compared with the recurrence rate for clot in the lower extremity, the rate of recurrent thrombosis for unselected patients with UEDVT is lower, leading to the observation that UEDVT may be a more benign condition. For example, a 4% recurrence rate was reported in 50 patients with UEDVT followed for a mean of 59 months, compared with a 15% recurrence rate among 841 patients with LEDVT.[43]

Experts suggest that the choice of treatment (anticoagulation compared with thrombolysis/thrombectomy) may impact risk for rethrombosis of the affected vein. A recent review compiled data from 47 studies over 25 years (2557 patients with UEDVT) and reported a much higher overall recurrent clot rate of 13% among subjects treated with anticoagulation, and slightly better rates (9%) for those treated with thrombolysis or thrombectomy.[9] Although, both of these rethrombosis rates are higher than those reported in more recent studies, these results suggest a potential benefit from more aggressive initial therapy (thrombolysis or thrombectomy).

Patients with thrombophilias seem to have greater risk for recurrence of UEDVT than those with idiopathic or catheter-related UEDVT. Among patients with thrombophilia, the annual recurrence rate was 4.4% (95% CI, 1.2%–4.0%), compared with 1.6% (95% CI, 0.6%–3.2%) among those without thrombophilia.[22]

The recurrence rate was even higher among patients with cancer and UEDVT. Of 106 subjects with both cancer and UEDVT enrolled in the RIETE registry, a 6.1% recurrence rate of either PE or DVT was seen in a 3-month follow-up interval.[44]

Careful vigilance for rethrombosis is appropriate. More aggressive initial treatment of individuals at high risk for rethrombosis may be considered, but further studies are needed before formal recommendations can be made for treatment modification based on risk of recurrent UEDVT.

Postthrombotic Syndrome

Postthrombotic syndrome is characterized clinically by edema, pain, and skin hyperpigmentation of the affected limb. Symptoms may be as mild as an increase in arm girth. However, in more severe cases, venous stasis may be significant, leading to skin ulceration and a predisposition to superimposed infection. Even in the absence of serious sequelae, postthrombotic syndrome can significantly decrease quality of life in affected subjects, especially if the dominant arm is involved.

Because precise criteria for postthrombotic syndrome have not been established, most studies have used subjective symptoms to define the presence of postthrombotic syndrome. More formal scoring systems have been used in some studies, and these can be useful adjunctive tools to quantify the severity of postthrombotic syndrome and to follow signs and symptoms over time. The Villalta score, originally devised to quantify symptoms after lower extremity DVT, has been modified for use in the upper extremity.[45] A value from 0 (absent) to 3 (severe) is assigned to each of five symptoms (heaviness, pain, pruritis, cramps, and paresthesias) and five signs on examination (edema, induration, erythema, venous prominence, skin hyperpigmentation). A score of five or higher defines the presence of postthrombotic syndrome, and correlates well with validated scoring systems of upper extremity disability used for other causes.[46] The adoption of formal scoring of severity of postthrombotic syndrome would improve our ability to assess outcomes both clinically and in investigations.

The literature has described a prevalence of postthrombotic syndrome from 7% to 46%. This wide range in prevalence probably partly reflects the subjective definition of the condition. Postthrombotic syndrome may not develop until months or years after the initial UEDVT.[10] Therefore, a cumulative increase in the prevalence of postthrombotic syndrome occurs over time. Rates of postthrombotic syndrome after standard anti-coagulation have been reported as 21% at 6 months, 25% at 1 year, and 27% at 2 years with a subsequent stable rate.[42]

Even in the absence of clinically overt post-thrombotic syndrome, many patients treated for UEDVT with anticoagulant therapy have residual signs or symptoms, with 77% having at least mild persistent symptoms in one retrospective study.[47] In this study, 18 of 31 treated patients (58%) had an identifiable clot on ultrasound and 35% had abnormal obstruction to venous flow as measured with strain gauge plethysmography, although objective findings did not always corre-late well with symptoms.

Risk factors for the development of postthrom-botic syndrome include initial presence of clot in multiple vessels, delay in initiation of treatment, absence of clot resolution, elevated D-dimer and factor VII levels at diagnosis, and persistent eleva-tion after treatment.[48] Catheter-related DVTs seem to be associated with a lower incidence of postthrombotic syndrome compared with other DVTs.[10]

SVC Syndrome

SVC syndrome occurs when the SVC is ob-structed by extrinsic compression or intrinsic obstruction. Typically, SVC syndrome is caused by mediastinal malignancy, compressive lymph-adenopathy, or severe mediastinal fibrosis. It can occur in the setting of UEDVT if clot propagation into the SVC occurs, typically accompanied by bilateral subclavian or brachiocephalic stenosis.[49]

Phlegmasia Cerulea Dolens and Venous Gangrene

Phlegmasia cerulea dolens is rare in the upper extremity. It is more commonly seen in the lower extremity as a triad of profound edema, cyanosis, and severe pain from total or subtotal venous obstruction caused by thrombosis, stenosis, compression, or combinations of these events.[50,51] Untreated, the condition leads to distal venous gangrene (50%), digital amputation (50%), sepsis, and potentially hypovolemic shock from sequestration of a large volume of fluid in the limb.[48] Patients who develop the condition typically have the risk factors described for UEDVT, but also have significant comorbid disease and often advanced congestive heart failure.[50,51] Management hinges on prompt recog-nition and recanalization of the vein through anti-coagulation, thrombolytics, thrombectomy, or fasciotomy. Even in treated patients the mortality rate is reported to be between 25% and 40%.[47]

Infected Catheters and Blood Stream Infections

The association between CVC infection and clot formation has been established, although the precise causal relationship between the two events is less clear. Fibrinogen and fibronectin within clot have been shown to attract bacteria, especially Staphylococcus species, which adhere to the catheter, leading to the potential for clinical infection.[52] Children with UEDVT associated with long-term CVCs had an 18% bloodstream infec-tion rate, whereas those without clots had no infections.[53] Conversely, the relative risk of throm-bosis in the presence of CVC infection was 17.5 (95% CI, 4.1–74.1) compared with the absence of infection.[54] Thus, the association between clot and infection is apparent.

Mortality Associated With UEDVT

The mortality rate reported for UEDVT ranges widely depending on the underlying risk factors for clot formation. In the RIETE registry, the 3-month all-cause mortality for non–malignancy-associated UEDVT was 3.5%, compared with a 22% mortality at 3 months among 196 patients with both UEDVT and malignancy, most of whom were treated with low molecular weight heparin (LMWH).[12,44] Failure to document cause-specific mortality and variability in treatment strategy explains the wide range of mortality in the cohorts described.

The 3-month all-cause mortality for UEDVT is 11%, but the 3-month fatal PE rate is only 0.2%.[12] A similar pattern with respect to mortality for LEDVT exists, showing an overall mortality of 7% and a PE–specific mortality of 0.9% at 3 months.[12] Because rates of PE in UEDVT and mortality for catheter-related thrombosis in the absence of cancer are low (4.8%), it can be concluded that the high mortality rate reported in some case series of UEDVT cases is largely driven by comorbid disease.[7,12,55,56] UEDVT, much like LEDVT, usually seems to be a complication of underlying comorbid illness.

A study of internal jugular vein thrombosis (in the absence of cancer) noted increased mortality in elderly patients (>75 years of age), those with CVC, and those not anticoagulated.[8] The reported prevalence of PE was 4%, but because ventilation/perfusion (V/Q) scans were not performed in all patients, the true prevalence of PE was likely underestimated. Another investigation performing V/Q scans in all subjects, despite whether they were symptomatic, found the prevalence of PE to be 36%, supporting the notion that PE is often undiagnosed in UEDVT.[2]

The same cohort of 210 subjects with UEDVT confirmed on duplex ultrasound had an overall 1-year mortality of 40%.[8] No mortality difference was observed based on location of clot (subclavian–axillary or internal jugular vein). Although none of the patients died of clinically apparent PE, 43% of the cohort did not receive anticoagulation or thrombolytics.

Several conclusions can be made: (1) the prevalence of PE in UEDVT is underestimated in the current literature, and the contribution of PE in UEDVT deaths is uncertain, (2) deaths from PE in the setting of UEDVT are unlikely to occur in the absence of serious comorbid illness (such as cancer) but are possible, (3) deaths are more likely to occur in those who are not given long-term anticoagulation, and (4) the location of UEDVT does not influence mortality.

TREATMENT

Treatment options for UEDVT vary from conservative management with heat, rest, and arm elevation (advocated in the past) to anticoagulation, thrombolysis, thrombectomy, and surgical decompression. Adjunctive therapies such as ultrasound-enhanced lysis, percutaneous angioplasty, and stenting also may have roles in treatment algorithms. Each of these options is reviewed later.

In a recent meta-analysis, treatment algorithms described in the English language literature since the mid-1960s were complied and analyzed to determine overall efficacy and outcomes of the various treatment strategies.[4] The analysis included 41 studies of UEDVT and were categorized into one of four treatment algorithms: (1) rest, heat, and elevation, (2) anticoagulation alone, (3) surgical decompression, and (4) thrombolysis. The mean follow-up time was 2 to 8 years depending on algorithm.

Significant differences in presence and severity of residual upper extremity symptoms were found for each treatment algorithm. The greatest prevalence of symptoms was in the conservative option (after 8 years) of heat and elevation (74%). Symptom prevalence for subjects who had surgical treatment (after 6 years) was 60%, anticoagulation (after 6 years) resulted in a 44% symptom rate, and thrombolysis (after 3 years) resulted in persistent symptoms in 22% of patients. Similarly, the same analysis showed that incidence of PE was greatest among patients treated with heat and elevation (12%), intermediate in those in the anticoagulation-treated group (7%), and lowest for those undergoing thrombolysis (1%). Although prospective

head-to-head studies testing all of these treatments have not been performed, this analysis helps dispel the previously accepted notion that UEDVT may be treated successfully with conservative management using heat and elevation alone.

Anticoagulation

Anticoagulation is the primary preferred treatment for UEDVT. The initial treatment recommendations for anticoagulant for UEDVT are identical to options for LEDVT.[57] Patients with acute UEDVT should be initiated on LMWH, unfractionated heparin (UFH), or fondaparinux. If treatment is initiated with UFH, the recommendation is for an intravenous bolus of 80 U/kg or 5000 U, followed by a continuous infusion of 18 U/kg per hour or 1300 U/h, with dose adjustments to reach therapeutic activated partial thromboplastin times (aPTT) or prolongation that corresponds with plasma heparin levels of 0.3 to 0.7 IU/mL anti-Xa activity according to the amidolytic assay.[57] If treatment is initiated with LMWH, weight-adjusted doses may be delivered through subcutaneous injection once or twice daily without laboratory monitoring because of the more predictable pharmacokinetics and bioavailability of LWMH compared with UFH.

The use of weight-based LMWH regimens for significantly obese subjects is not well established. In the setting of renal failure or pregnancy, monitoring of anti-Xa activity may be useful. The American College of Chest Physicians (ACCP) 2008 guidelines recommend against using LMWH to treat DVTs in severe renal failure, suggesting that UFH and aPTT monitoring are the appropriate alternative in this population. Fondaparinux (a synthetic pentasaccharide) may be chosen for initial treatment of UEDVT based on noninferiority shown by the large Matisse trial, which compared fondaparinux with LMWH for treatment of DVT.[58] The ACCP 2008 guidelines give fondaparinux a grade 1A rating for noninferiority compared with LMWH. Initiation of a vitamin K antagonist along with UFH, LMWH, or fondaparinux is recommended once the diagnosis of UEDVT has been established. Treatment with UFH, LMWH, or fondaparinux should continue for at least 5 days and until the international normalized ratio (INR) of 2.0 or more has been maintained for 24 hours.[57]

Anticoagulation should then be maintained with a vitamin K antagonist or LMWH for at least 3 months. LMWH is considered superior to vitamin K antagonists in cancer patients because of the risk of rethrombosis and bleeding complications.

No studies have specifically investigated one particular regimen for UEDVT in cancer patients; however, LMWH has been shown to have a mortality benefit over UFH for treating venous thromboembolic disease in the setting of malignancy (OR, 0.53; 95% CI, 0.33–0.85).[59]

Many UEDVTs are associated with either long-term indwelling CVCs or central lines used in acute care settings. Therefore, the decision to leave the line in place or remove it is integral to the management of UEDVT. The ACCP guidelines recommend that if the line is needed and fully functional, it should be left in place as anticoagulation is undertaken. Nonessential lines may be removed; however, completion of 3 to 5 days of anticoagulation therapy is recommended before catheter removal.[57] Removal or maintenance of the central line should not affect the duration of full-dose anticoagulation therapy.

Considerations affecting the duration of treatment include the size of clot, ongoing risk of clot, individual patient characteristics, and comorbidities. Shorter courses of anticoagulation are not recommended but may be acceptable for very small clot burden. If a long-term indwelling catheter is still needed after the course of anticoagulation treatment is completed, no recommendations for anticoagulant prophylaxis exist for adults; however, low-dose anticoagulant therapy (vitamin K antagonist for goal INR 1.5–1.9 or LMWH for goal anti-Factor Xa range 0.1–0.3) is recommended for pediatric patients.[48,57,60]

The success of anticoagulation can be assessed through determining rates of recanalization or persistent thrombosis. The presence of thrombophilia was a predictor of incomplete recanalization and persistent clot (hazard ratio, 0.49; 95% CI, 0.38–0.63) in a cohort of patients with lower extremity clot but has not been adequately studied in UEDVT.[61]

Thrombolysis or Thrombectomy

Prospective investigations directly comparing thrombolysis or thrombectomy and subsequent anticoagulation with anticoagulation alone are lacking. Much of the literature consists of smaller case series and retrospective studies.[57] In one of the larger cohorts described in the literature, 118 cases of UEDVT were assembled retrospectively. Subjects were grouped according to treatment; urokinase for thrombolysis (n = 62) followed by anticoagulation was compared with anticoagulation alone (initial UFH or LMWH followed by a vitamin K antagonist for 6 months).[62] Subjects were assessed for venous patency on duplex sonography (Doppler ultrasonography), recurrent UEDVT,

postthrombotic syndrome, and major bleeding. In this cohort, thrombolysis was associated with better venous patency on ultrasound, but no significant difference was seen in incidence of recurrent DVT or postthrombotic syndrome at a median follow-up of 40 months. However, a significantly higher incidence of major bleeding was seen in the thrombolysis group compared with anticoagulation alone (0 of 62 vs 5 of 33 subjects; $P<.0001$).[62]

Compiled data from 41 studies (559 patients) were analyzed and found to suggest that thrombolysis followed by anticoagulation may have important benefits over anticoagulation alone in terms of persistence of symptoms (22% vs 44%) and risk of subsequent PE (1% vs 7%), However, the heterogeneity of the studies, their small size, and the absence of uniformly rigorous study design limit the conclusions that can be drawn.[4]

Catheter-directed thrombolysis (CDT) has been compared retrospectively with CDT with rheolytic percutaneous mechanical thrombectomy.[63] This study combined data for upper (n = 22) and lower (n = 45) extremity proximal DVTs treated with one of the two options. Among patients treated with catheter-directed urokinase alone, 29 of 40 limbs (73%) had complete clot resolution, compared with resolution in 22 of 27 limbs (82%) treated with CDT and rheolytic thrombectomy. Moreover, shorter urokinase infusion times and lower doses of lytics were used in the subjects treated with CDT and rheolytic thrombectomy.

Ultrasound-accelerated thrombolysis for DVT of upper or lower extremities has been advocated by some as a superior means of achieving lysis, with a reduction in average dose of thrombolytic and a shorter infusion time.[64] The technique uses a multilumen drug delivery catheter and matching ultrasound coaxial core wire through which ultrasound energy is delivered along the coaxial infusion zone. A case series of 53 patients described equivalent or better lysis compared with success rates reported in the recent literature and the National Venous Registry, with no intracranial or retroperitoneal bleeding.[64]

Overall, studies have not yet clearly shown the superiority of thrombolysis or thrombectomy followed by anticoagulation over anticoagulation alone for the treatment of most UEDVTs, although several studies have suggested potential benefit. The ACCP guidelines recommend against the use of systemic or catheter-directed thrombolytics for routine cases of UEDVT. For patients with severe symptoms, thrombolysis, either systemic or catheter-directed, may be considered if the patient is at low risk of bleeding. Similarly, the ACCP recommends against routine use of catheter extraction of clot or surgical thrombectomy for most UEDVTs. Experts have suggested, however, that Paget-Schroetter syndrome is best managed with primary thrombolysis, most often combined with surgical decompression of the thoracic outlet,[49,65,66] although even for these patients controversy exists, because some experts support conservative management.[67]

SVC Filters

SVC filters have a role in treating patients for whom anticoagulation therapy failed or who have contraindications to anticoagulation. Filters have been shown to be effective in preventing subsequent PE. The rate of secondary PE was 2.4% in a prospective cohort followed for a median of 3 months after placement of SVC filter, and one PE occurred among 41 subjects at 44 months after filter placement.[68] Similarly, no secondary PE or SVC syndrome was reported in a retrospective cohort of 72 patients who received SVC filters over a mean follow-up time of 7.8 months (range, 10 days to 78 months).[69] Longer-term follow-up is equally encouraging. In a retrospective cohort of 154 cases followed for up to 3750 days (mean 256 ± SD 576 days), no cases of symptomatic PE, SVC occlusion, or filter migration were seen.[70] Placement of an SVC filter does not preclude subsequent CVC or even pulmonary artery catheter placement, although reasonable caution should be used.[68] More serious complications such as pericardial tamponade from SVC perforation are reported, although rare.[70]

The ACCP recommends against the routine use of SVC filters in the management of UEDVT; however, studies have shown that filters are efficacious, and safe in selected populations.[57]

Venous Angioplasty, Stenting, and Bypass

Endovascular interventions such as angioplasty or stenting may be appropriate when anticoagulation or thrombolysis results in incomplete recanalization of the vein and persistent symptoms are present. If UEDVT is a result of thoracic outlet syndrome (as in Paget-Schroetter syndrome), venous angioplasty or stents rarely relieve symptoms adequately.[65] In these cases, surgical decompression with or without adjunctive venous stenting is typically necessary.[49] The ACCP recommends against routine use of transluminal angioplasty or stent placement, or the routine

use of these procedures after lytic therapy; however, the techniques can be successfully used in selected patients.[57] Long-term anticoagulation is typically still required and the durability of success in stenting procedures is still undetermined.

Venous bypass may be used when venous compression or thrombosis have resulted in vessel obliteration. Venous reconstruction or bypass may be the only options in these cases.[49]

Surgical Decompression

Surgical decompression of the thoracic outlet has been efficacious in the management of spontaneous or exertion-related UEDVT (Paget-Schroetter syndrome). Bone, muscles, and tendons may all contribute to the obstruction, and therefore surgical decompression procedures typically involve excision of the first rib, subclavius tendon, and the anterior scalene muscle insertion.[49]

The optimal timing of surgical decompression after initial thrombolysis and anticoagulation remains controversial, with some investigators advocating early decompression and others later intervention.[49] An individualized approach based on the degree of residual flow and venous emptying of the affected limb is the standard of care, with evidence of poor flow and emptying prompting early intervention.

Management of Postthrombotic Syndrome

Upper extremity postthrombotic syndrome is characterized by edema, pain, sensation of heaviness on exertion, skin hyperpigmentation, and, in extreme cases, skin ulceration from venous stasis. The therapeutic approach to postthrombotic syndrome focuses on symptom management. Simple approaches, such the use of elastic compression sleeves or elastic bandages similar to those used for management of lymphedema, can be beneficial.

PROPHYLAXIS FOR PATIENTS WITH CENTRAL LINES

Studies have repeatedly shown that the use of CVCs, both short- and long-term, predispose patients to UEDVT. Therefore, considerable interest has been shown in determining whether prophylactic anticoagulation should be used for certain subsets of patients. No firm consensus on benefit or harm from prophylactic anticoagulation for CVC use has been reached based on recent randomized, controlled trials in the literature.[71–73] No formal recommendation currently exists for routine prophylaxis against UEDVT in patients with CVCs. The incidence of CVC-related thrombosis in patients undergoing chemotherapy is reported to be between 10% and 18%, regardless of prophylactic anticoagulation.[73,74]

Additional factors have been identified to better characterize those at risk of UEDVT in the setting of malignancy, including (1) placement of catheter tip in an inappropriately high position within the SVC (sevenfold increased risk), (2) left-sided insertion of catheter, (3) chest radiotherapy, and (4) existence of distant metastasis.[75] It has been inferred from these studies that prophylactic anticoagulation may benefit certain high-risk subsets of patients with CVCs for chemotherapy.[76]

SUMMARY

UEDVT is clearly a significant clinical entity. Its presentation may be obvious or subtle. For individuals whose presentation is subtle, only a high index of suspicion and willingness to pursue the diagnosis beyond a negative ultrasound will result in accurate diagnosis. The main risk factors for development of UEDVT (cancer, CVC, thrombophilia, pacemaker insertion, and prior venous thromboembolism) are known, and patients with these risk factors should undergo a thorough evaluation if concern for UEDVT exists.

A community-based survey published in 2007 reported that only 56% of patients with UEDVT were discharged from the hospital on anticoagulation therapy.[77] This observation reflects the persistent notion that UEDVT does not necessitate prolonged anticoagulation. However, the current literature reflects a significant prevalence of serious sequelae of UEDVT. Accordingly, ACCP guidelines support at least 3 months of full anticoagulation for UEDVT and more aggressive therapies (thrombolysis, thrombectomy, or surgical decompression) for limited subsets of patients.[4,57] Treatment of UEDVT (anticoagulation, surgical decompression, thrombolysis, and SVC filters) followed by long-term anticoagulation improves outcomes.

REFERENCES

1. Mustafa S, Stein P, Patel K, et al. Upper extremity deep venous thrombosis. Chest 2003;123(6): 1953–6.
2. Prandoni P, Polistena P, Bernardi E, et al. Upper-extremity deep vein thrombosis. Risk factors, diagnosis, and complications. Arch Intern Med 1997;157(1):57–62.
3. Becker D, Philbrick J, Walker FT. Axillary and subclavian venous thrombosis. Prognosis and treatment. Arch Intern Med 1991;151(10):1934–43.
4. Thomas I, Zierler B. An integrative review of outcomes in patients with acute primary upper extremity deep venous thrombosis following no treatment or treatment with anticoagulation, thrombolysis, or surgical algorithms. Vasc Endovascular Surg 2005;39(2):163–74.
5. Joffe H, Goldhaber S. Upper-extremity deep vein thrombosis. Circulation 2002;106(14):1874–80.
6. Joffe H, Kucher N, Tapson V, et al. Upper-extremity deep vein thrombosis: a prospective registry of 592 patients. Circulation 2004;110(12):1605–11.
7. Hingorani A, Ascher E, Marks N, et al. Morbidity and mortality associated with brachial vein thrombosis. Ann Vasc Surg 2006;20(3):297–300.
8. Ascher E, Salles-Cunha S, Hingorani A. Morbidity and mortality associated with internal jugular vein thromboses. Vasc Endovascular Surg 2005;39(4): 335–9.
9. Sajid M, Ahmed N, Desai M, et al. Upper limb deep vein thrombosis: a literature review to streamline the protocol for management. Acta Haematol 2007;118(1):10–8.
10. Elman E, Kahn S. The post-thrombotic syndrome after upper extremity deep venous thrombosis in adults: a systematic review. Thromb Res 2006; 117(6):609–14.
11. Hill S, Berry R. Subclavian vein thrombosis: a continuing challenge. Surgery 1990;108(1):1–9.
12. Muñoz F, Mismetti P, Poggio R, et al. Clinical outcome of patients with upper-extremity deep vein thrombosis: results from the RIETE Registry. Chest 2008;133(1):143–8.
13. Otten T, Stein P, Patel K, et al. Thromboembolic disease involving the superior vena cava and brachiocephalic veins. Chest 2003;123(3):809–12.
14. Monreal M, Davant E. Thrombotic complications of central venous catheters in cancer patients. Acta Haematol 2001;106(1-2):69–72.
15. Lindblad B, Tengborn L, Bergqvist D. Deep vein thrombosis of the axillary-subclavian veins: epidemiologic data, effects of different types of treatment and late sequelae. Eur J Vasc Surg 1988;2(3): 161–5.
16. Kommareddy A, Zaroukian M, Hassouna H. Upper extremity deep venous thrombosis. Semin Thromb Hemost 2002;28(1):89–99.
17. Malhotra S, Punia V. Upper extremity deep vein thrombosis. J Assoc Physicians India 2004;52: 237–41.
18. Kuriakose P, Colon-Otero G, Paz-Fumagalli R. Risk of deep venous thrombosis associated with chest versus arm central venous subcutaneous port

catheters: a 5-year single-institution retrospective study. J Vasc Interv Radiol 2002;13(2 Pt 1):179–84.

19. Whigham C, Greenbaum M, Fisher R, et al. Incidence and management of catheter occlusion in implantable arm ports: results in 391 patients. J Vasc Interv Radiol 1999;10(6):767–74.

20. Da Costa S, Scalabrini Neto A, Costa R, et al. Incidence and risk factors of upper extremity deep vein lesions after permanent transvenous pacemaker implant: a 6-month follow-up prospective study. Pacing Clin Electrophysiol 2002;25(9):1301–6.

21. Korkeila P, Nyman K, Ylitalo A, et al. Venous obstruction after pacemaker implantation. Pacing Clin Electrophysiol 2007;30(2):199–206.

22. Martinelli I, Battaglioli T, Bucciarelli P, et al. Risk factors and recurrence rate of primary deep vein thrombosis of the upper extremities. Circulation 2004;110(5):566–70.

23. Prandoni P, Bernardi E. Upper extremity deep vein thrombosis. Curr Opin Pulm Med 1999;5(4):222–6.

24. Hendler M, Meschengieser S, Blanco A, et al. Primary upper-extremity deep vein thrombosis: high prevalence of thrombophilic defects. Am J Hematol 2004;76(4):330–7.

25. Héron E, Lozinguez O, Alhenc-Gelas M, et al. Hypercoagulable states in primary upper-extremity deep vein thrombosis. Arch Intern Med 2000;160(3):382–6.

26. Rozmus G, Daubert J, Huang D, et al. Venous thrombosis and stenosis after implantation of pacemakers and defibrillators. J Interv Card Electrophysiol 2005;13(1):9–19.

27. Vayá A, Mira Y, Mateo J, et al. Prothrombin G20210A mutation and oral contraceptive use increase upper-extremity deep vein thrombotic risk. Thromb Haemost 2003;89(3):452–7.

28. Pandolfi M, Robertson B, Isacson S, et al. Fibrinolytic activity of human veins in arms and legs. Thromb Diath Haemorrh 1968;20(1):247–56.

29. Starkhammar H, Bengtsson M, Morales O. Fibrin sleeve formation after long term brachial catheterisation with an implantable port device. A prospective venographic study. Eur J Surg 1992;158(9):481–4.

30. Raad I, Luna M, Khalil S, et al. The relationship between the thrombotic and infectious complications of central venous catheters. JAMA 1994;271(13):1014–6.

31. Chastre J, Cornud F, Bouchama A, et al. Thrombosis as a complication of pulmonary-artery catheterization via the internal jugular vein: prospective evaluation by phlebography. N Engl J Med 1982;306(5):278–81.

32. Baarslag H, van Beek E, Koopman M, et al. Prospective study of color duplex ultrasonography compared with contrast venography in patients suspected of having deep venous thrombosis of the upper extremities. Ann Intern Med 2002;136(12):865–72.

33. Baarslag H, Koopman M, Reekers J, et al. Diagnosis and management of deep vein thrombosis of the upper extremity: a review. Eur Radiol 2004;14(7):1263–74.

34. Katz D, Hon M. Current DVT imaging. Tech Vasc Interv Radiol 2004;7(2):55–62.

35. Sabharwal R, Boshell D, Vladica P. Multidetector spiral CT venography in the diagnosis of upper extremity deep venous thrombosis. Australas Radiol 2007;51(Suppl):B253–6.

36. Erdman W, Jayson H, Redman H, et al. Deep venous thrombosis of extremities: role of MR imaging in the diagnosis. Radiology 1990;174(2):425–31.

37. Chrysochou C, Power A, Shurrab A, et al. Low risk for nephrogenic systemic fibrosis in nondialysis patients who have chronic kidney disease and are investigated with gadolinium-enhanced magnetic resonance imaging. Clin J Am Soc Nephrol 2010;5(3):484–9.

38. Silverstein A, Turbiner E. Technetium-99m red blood cell venography in upper extremity deep venous thrombosis. Clin Nucl Med 1987;12(6):421–3.

39. Savage K, Wells P, Schulz V, et al. Outpatient use of low molecular weight heparin (Dalteparin) for the treatment of deep vein thrombosis of the upper extremity. Thromb Haemost 1999;82(3):1008–10.

40. Kovacs M, Kahn S, Rodger M, et al. A pilot study of central venous catheter survival in cancer patients using low-molecular-weight heparin (dalteparin) and warfarin without catheter removal for the treatment of upper extremity deep vein thrombosis (The Catheter Study). J Thromb Haemost 2007;5(8):1650–3.

41. Karabay O, Yetkin U, Onol H. Upper extremity deep vein thrombosis: clinical and treatment characteristics. J Int Med Res 2004;32(4):429–35.

42. Prandoni P, Bernardi E, Marchiori A, et al. The long term clinical course of acute deep vein thrombosis of the arm: prospective cohort study. BMJ 2004;329(7464):484–5.

43. Lechner D, Wiener C, Weltermann A, et al. Comparison between idiopathic deep vein thrombosis of the upper and lower extremity regarding risk factors and recurrence. J Thromb Haemost 2008;6(8):1269–74.

44. Monreal M, Munoz F, Rosa V, et al. Upper extremity DVT in oncological patients: analysis of risk factors. Data from the RIETE registry. Exp Oncol 2006;28(3):245–7.

45. Villalta S, Prandoni P, Cogo A, et al. The utility of noninvasive tests for detection of previous proximal-vein thrombosis. Thromb Haemost 1995;73(4):592–6.

46. Arnhjort T, Persson L, Rosfors S, et al. Primary deep vein thrombosis in the upper limb: A retrospective

study with emphasis on pathogenesis and late sequelae. Eur J Intern Med 2007;18(4):304–8.

47. Persson L, Arnhjort T, Lärfars G, et al. Hemodynamic and morphologic evaluation of sequelae of primary upper extremity deep venous thromboses treated with anticoagulation. J Vasc Surg 2006;43(6): 1230–5 [discussion: 1235].

48. Baskin J, Pui C, Reiss U, et al. Management of occlusion and thrombosis associated with long-term indwelling central venous catheters. Lancet 2009;374(9684):159–69.

49. Sharafuddin M, Sun S, Hoballah J. Endovascular management of venous thrombotic diseases of the upper torso and extremities. J Vasc Interv Radiol 2002;13(10):975–90.

50. Bolitho D, Elwood E, Roberts F. Phlegmasia cerulea dolens of the upper extremity. Ann Plast Surg 2000; 45(6):644–6.

51. Kammen B, Soulen M. Phlegmasia cerulea dolens of the upper extremity. J Vasc Interv Radiol 1995;6(2): 283–6.

52. Mehall J, Saltzman D, Jackson R, et al. Fibrin sheath enhances central venous catheter infection. Crit Care Med 2002;30(4):908–12.

53. Barzaghi A, Dell'Orto M, Rovelli A, et al. Central venous catheter clots: incidence, clinical significance and catheter care in patients with hematologic malignancies. Pediatr Hematol Oncol 1995;12 (3):243–50.

54. van Rooden C, Schippers E, Barge R, et al. Infectious complications of central venous catheters increase the risk of catheter-related thrombosis in hematology patients: a prospective study. J Clin Oncol 2005;23(12):2655–60.

55. Hingorani A, Ascher E, Lorenson E, et al. Upper extremity deep venous thrombosis and its impact on morbidity and mortality rates in a hospital-based population. J Vasc Surg 1997;26(5): 853–60.

56. Hingorani A, Ascher E, Hanson J, et al. Upper extremity versus lower extremity deep venous thrombosis. Am J Surg 1997;174(2):214–7.

57. Kearon C, Kahn S, Agnelli G, et al. Antithrombotic therapy for venous thromboembolic disease: American College of Chest Physicians Evidence-Based Clinical Practice Guidelines (8th edition). Chest 2008;133(Suppl 6):454S–545S.

58. Büller H, Agnelli G, Hull R, et al. Antithrombotic therapy for venous thromboembolic disease: the Seventh ACCP Conference on Antithrombotic and Thrombolytic Therapy. Chest 2004;126(Suppl 3): 401S–28S.

59. van Dongen C, van den Belt A, Prins M, et al. Fixed dose subcutaneous low molecular weight heparins versus adjusted dose unfractionated heparin for venous thromboembolism. Cochrane Database Syst Rev 2004;4:CD001100.

60. Monagle P, Chalmers E, Chan A, et al. Antithrombotic therapy in neonates and children: American College of Chest Physicians Evidence-Based Clinical Practice Guidelines (8th edition). Chest 2008; 133(Suppl 6):887S–968S.

61. Spiezia L, Tormene D, Pesavento R, et al. Thrombophilia as a predictor of persistent residual vein thrombosis. Haematologica 2008; 93(3):479–80.

62. Sabeti S, Schillinger M, Mlekusch W, et al. Treatment of subclavian-axillary vein thrombosis: long-term outcome of anticoagulation versus systemic thrombolysis. Thromb Res 2002;108(5–6): 279–85.

63. Kim H, Patra A, Paxton B, et al. Catheter-directed thrombolysis with percutaneous rheolytic thrombectomy versus thrombolysis alone in upper and lower extremity deep vein thrombosis. Cardiovasc Intervent Radiol 2006;29(6):1003–7.

64. Parikh S, Motarjeme A, McNamara T, et al. Ultrasound-accelerated thrombolysis for the treatment of deep vein thrombosis: initial clinical experience. J Vasc Interv Radiol 2008;19(4):521–8.

65. Urschel HJ, Patel A. Paget-Schroetter syndrome therapy: failure of intravenous stents. Ann Thorac Surg 2003;75(6):1693–6 [discussion: 1696].

66. Urschel HJ, Razzuk M. Paget-Schroetter syndrome: what is the best management? Ann Thorac Surg 2000;69(6):1663–8 [discussion: 1668–9].

67. Lee J, Karwowski J, Harris E, et al. Long-term thrombotic recurrence after nonoperative management of Paget-Schroetter syndrome. J Vasc Surg 2006;43(6):1236–43.

68. Spence L, Gironta M, Malde H, et al. Acute upper extremity deep venous thrombosis: safety and effectiveness of superior vena caval filters. Radiology 1999;210(1):53–8.

69. Ascher E, Hingorani A, Tsemekhin B, et al. Lessons learned from a 6-year clinical experience with superior vena cava Greenfield filters. J Vasc Surg 2000; 32(5):881–7.

70. Usoh F, Hingorani A, Ascher E, et al. Long-term follow-up for superior vena cava filter placement. Ann Vasc Surg 2009;23(3):350–4.

71. Couban S, Goodyear M, Burnell M, et al. Randomized placebo-controlled study of low-dose warfarin for the prevention of central venous catheter-associated thrombosis in patients with cancer. J Clin Oncol 2005;23(18):4063–9.

72. Karthaus M, Kretzschmar A, Kröning H, et al. Dalteparin for prevention of catheter-related complications in cancer patients with central venous catheters: final results of a double-blind, placebo-controlled phase III trial. Ann Oncol 2006; 17(2):289–96.

73. Verso M, Agnelli G, Bertoglio S, et al. Enoxaparin for the prevention of venous thromboembolism

associated with central vein catheter: a double-blind, placebo-controlled, randomized study in cancer patients. J Clin Oncol 2005;23(18):4057–62.

74. Ong B, Gibbs H, Catchpole I, et al. Peripherally inserted central catheters and upper extremity deep vein thrombosis. Australas Radiol 2006;50(5): 451–4.

75. Verso M, Agnelli G, Kamphuisen P, et al. Risk factors for upper limb deep vein thrombosis associated with the use of central vein catheter in cancer patients. Intern Emerg Med 2008;3(2):117–22.

76. Prandoni P. Should cancer patients receive thromboprophylaxis to prevent catheter-related upper limb deep vein thrombosis? Intern Emerg Med 2008;3(2):85–6.

77. Spencer F, Emery C, Lessard D, et al. Upper extremity deep vein thrombosis: a community-based perspective. Am J Med 2007;120(8):678–84.

Index

Note: Page numbers of article titles are in **boldface** type.

Clin Chest Med 31 (2010) 799–804
doi:10.1016/S0272-5231(10)00117-6

United States Postal Service

Statement of Ownership, Management, and Circulation
(All Periodicals Publications Except Requestor Publications)

1. Publication Title: Clinics in Chest Medicine

2. Publication Number: 0 0 0 - 7 0 6

3. Filing Date: 9/15/10

4. Issue Frequency: Mar, Jun, Sep, Dec

5. Number of Issues Published Annually: 4

6. Annual Subscription Price: $274.00

7. Complete Mailing Address of Known Office of Publication (Not printer) (Street, city, county, state and ZIP+4®):
Elsevier Inc.
360 Park Avenue South
New York, NY 10010-1710

Contact Person: Stephen Bushing
Telephone (Include area code): 215-239-3688

8. Complete Mailing Address of Headquarters or General Business Office of Publisher (Not printer):
Elsevier Inc., 360 Park Avenue South, New York, NY 10010-1710

9. Full Names and Complete Mailing Addresses of Publisher, Editor, and Managing Editor (Do not leave blank)

Publisher (Name and complete mailing address):
Kim Murphy, Elsevier, Inc., 1600 John F. Kennedy Blvd. Suite 1800, Philadelphia, PA 19103-2899

Editor (Name and complete mailing address):
Sarah Barth, Elsevier, Inc., 1600 John F. Kennedy Blvd. Suite 1800, Philadelphia, PA 19103-2899

Managing Editor (Name and complete mailing address):
Catherine Bewick, Elsevier, Inc., 1600 John F. Kennedy Blvd. Suite 1800, Philadelphia, PA 19103-2899

10. Owner (Do not leave blank. If the publication is owned by a corporation, give the name and address of the corporation immediately followed by the names and addresses of all stockholders owning or holding 1 percent or more of the total amount of stock. If not owned by a corporation, give the names and addresses of the individual owners. If owned by a partnership or other unincorporated firm, give its name and address as well as those of each individual owner. If the publication is published by a nonprofit organization, give its name and address.)

Full Name	Complete Mailing Address
Wholly owned subsidiary of	4520 East-West Highway
Reed/Elsevier, US holdings	Bethesda, MD 20814

11. Known Bondholders, Mortgagees, and Other Security Holders Owning or Holding 1 Percent or More of Total Amount of Bonds, Mortgages, or Other Securities. If none, check box ☐ None

Full Name	Complete Mailing Address
N/A	

12. Tax Status (For completion by nonprofit organizations authorized to mail at nonprofit rates) (Check one)
The purpose, function, and nonprofit status of this organization and the exempt status for federal income tax purposes:
☐ Has Not Changed During Preceding 12 Months
☐ Has Changed During Preceding 12 Months (Publisher must submit explanation of change with this statement)

PS Form 3526, September 2007 (Page 1 of 3 (Instructions Page 3)) PSN 7530-01-000-9931 PRIVACY NOTICE: See our Privacy policy in www.usps.com

---

13. Publication Title: Clinics in Chest Medicine

14. Issue Date for Circulation Data Below: September 2010

15. Extent and Nature of Circulation

		Average No. Copies Each Issue During Preceding 12 Months	No. Copies of Single Issue Published Nearest to Filing Date
a. Total Number of Copies (Net press run)		2471	2365
b. Paid Circulation (By Mail and Outside the Mail)	(1) Mailed Outside-County Paid Subscriptions Stated on PS Form 3541. (Include paid distribution above nominal rate, advertiser's proof copies, and exchange copies)	1231	1121
	(2) Mailed In-County Paid Subscriptions Stated on PS Form 3541 (Include paid distribution above nominal rate, advertiser's proof copies, and exchange copies)		
	(3) Paid Distribution Outside the Mails Including Sales Through Dealers and Carriers, Street Vendors, Counter Sales, and Other Paid Distribution Outside USPS®	560	541
	(4) Paid Distribution by Other Classes Mailed Through the USPS (e.g. First-Class Mail®)		
c. Total Paid Distribution (Sum of 15b (1), (2), (3), and (4))		1791	1662
d. Free or Nominal Rate Distribution (By Mail and Outside the Mail)	(1) Free or Nominal Rate Outside-County Copies Included on PS Form 3541	89	77
	(2) Free or Nominal Rate In-County Copies Included on PS Form 3541		
	(3) Free or Nominal Rate Copies Mailed at Other Classes Through the USPS (e.g. First-Class Mail)		
	(4) Free or Nominal Rate Distribution Outside the Mail (Carriers or other means)		
e. Total Free or Nominal Rate Distribution (Sum of 15d (1), (2), (3) and (4))		89	77
f. Total Distribution (Sum of 15c and 15e)		1880	1739
g. Copies not Distributed (See instructions to publishers #4 (page #3))		591	626
h. Total (Sum of 15f and g)		2471	2365
i. Percent Paid (15c divided by 15f times 100)		95.27%	95.57%

16. Publication of Statement of Ownership
If the publication is a general publication, publication of this statement is required. Will be printed in the December 2010 issue of this publication. ☐ Publication not required

17. Signature and Title of Editor, Publisher, Business Manager, or Owner

Stephen R. Bushing
Stephen R. Bushing – Fulfillment/Inventory Specialist

Date: September 15, 2010

I certify that all information furnished on this form is true and complete. I understand that anyone who furnishes false or misleading information on this form or who omits material or information requested on the form may be subject to criminal sanctions (including fines and imprisonment) and/or civil sanctions (including civil penalties).

PS Form 3526, September 2007 (Page 2 of 3)

Moving?

Make sure your subscription moves with you!

To notify us of your new address, find your **Clinics Account Number** (located on your mailing label above your name), and contact customer service at:

Email: journalscustomerservice-usa@elsevier.com

800-654-2452 (subscribers in the U.S. & Canada)
314-447-8871 (subscribers outside of the U.S. & Canada)

Fax number: 314-447-8029

Elsevier Health Sciences Division
Subscription Customer Service
3251 Riverport Lane
Maryland Heights, MO 63043

*To ensure uninterrupted delivery of your subscription, please notify us at least 4 weeks in advance of move.

Printed and bound by CPI Group (UK) Ltd, Croydon, CR0 4YY

03/10/2024

01040354-0018